Bioinformatics of the Brain

The brain consisting of billions of neurons is probably the most complex and mysterious organ of the body. Understanding the functioning of the brain in its health and disease states has baffled the researchers working in this area for many years. The diversity of brain diseases and disorders makes the analysis of brain functions an even more challenging area of research. *In vitro* and *in vivo* studies regarding the brain may be laborious, however, *bioinformatics* using *in silico approaches* may take the burden off the experimental studies and give us a clearer perspective on disease and healthy states of the brain, its functions, and disease mechanisms.

Recent advancements in neuroimaging technologies, the development of high-performance computers and the development of software, algorithms and methods to analyze data obtained from various neuroimaging processes have opened new frontiers in neuroscience enabling unprecedented finer analysis of the brain functions. This relatively new approach of brain analysis which may be termed *Bioinformatics of the Brain* is the main subject of this volume aiming to provide a thorough review of various bioinformatics approaches for analyzing the functioning of the brain and understanding brain diseases such as neurodegenerative diseases, brain tumors, and neuropsychiatric disorders. Authors from various disciplines in this volume each focus on a different aspect aiming to expand our understanding of this area of research. Topics included are:

Brain diseases and disorders
Stem cell therapy of neurodegenerative diseases
Tissue engineering applications of gliomas
Brain tumor detection and modeling
Brain tumor growth simulation
Brain-computer interface
Bioinformatics of brain diseases
Graph-theoretical analysis of complex brain networks
Brain proteomics

This book is intended to aid scientists, researchers, and graduate students in carrying out interdisciplinary research in the areas of bioinformatics, bioengineering, computer engineering, software engineering, mathematics, molecular biology, genetics, and biotechnology.

Bioinformatics of the Brain

Edited by
Kayhan Erciyes and Tuba Sevimoglu

CRC Press
Taylor & Francis Group
Boca Raton London New York

CRC Press is an imprint of the
Taylor & Francis Group, an **informa** business

Designed cover image: © Liu zishan/Shutterstock

First edition published 2025
by CRC Press
2385 NW Executive Center Drive, Suite 320, Boca Raton FL 33431

and by CRC Press
4 Park Square, Milton Park, Abingdon, Oxon, OX14 4RN

CRC Press is an imprint of Taylor & Francis Group, LLC

Library of Congress Cataloging-in-Publication Data
Names: Erciyes, Kayhan, editor. | Sevimoğlu, Tuba, editor.
Title: Bioinformatics of the brain / edited by Kayhan Erciyes and Tuba Sevimoğlu.
Description: First edition. | Boca Raton : CRC Press, 2025. | Includes bibliographical references and index.
Identifiers: LCCN 2024014430 (print) | LCCN 2024014431 (ebook) | ISBN 9781032610726 (hbk) | ISBN 9781032610733 (pbk) | ISBN 9781003461906 (ebk)
Subjects: LCSH: Brain--Diseases--Diagnosis--Data processing. | Brain--Data processing. | Bioinformatics.
Classification: LCC RC386.2 .B565 2025 (print) | LCC RC386.2 (ebook) | DDC 616.800285--dc23/eng/20240613
LC record available at https://lccn.loc.gov/2024014430
LC ebook record available at https://lccn.loc.gov/2024014431

ISBN: 978-1-032-61072-6 (hbk)
ISBN: 978-1-032-61073-3 (pbk)
ISBN: 978-1-003-46190-6 (ebk)

DOI: 10.1201/9781003461906

Typeset in Latin Modern font
by KnowledgeWorks Global Ltd.

For Humanity
and Peace...

Contents

Preface

Bioinformatics uses computational methods and tools to analyze and produce meaningful information from biological data. This discipline mainly comprises studies in biology, computer science, and statistics. Bioinformatics of the brain is the employment of computational methods to analyze and understand the functioning of the brain with emphasis on its health and disease states. Recent advancements in neuroimaging technologies and developments of high-performance computers along with computer algorithms and tools provided unprecedented finer analysis of brain functions to understand the operation of cognitive processes and neurological disorders such as Alzheimer's Disease, Parkinson's Disease, and schizophrenia.

Our aim in bringing researchers in this field together to have this volume is to review the contemporary research in this new and exciting field of bioinformatics of the brain to aid research studies in computational analysis of the brain. To this end, we provide a thorough review of brain functions using computational processes stressing the analysis of the brain during various diseases and disorders. The detailed contents of each chapter are as follows.

The first chapter delves into the intricate workings, structure, and diverse neurological conditions that can affect an individual's brain. It looks at various neurological conditions under three headings. The first category includes neurological diseases, such as multiple sclerosis, Alzheimer's, Parkinson's, and Huntington's. These illnesses produce excruciating symptoms and pose significant challenges to patient care. Second, brain tumors—primary and metastatic—often require radiation, chemotherapy, and surgery and pose challenging diagnostic and therapeutic issues. Meningeal tumors, brain lymphomas, and gliomas represent a representative subset of the diverse spectrum of brain cancers, and each one has unique therapeutic challenges. Third, the intricate interplay between neurological and psychological phenomena is highlighted by neuropsychiatric disorders. These illnesses include major depressive disorders, autism spectrum disorder, attention deficit hyperactivity disorder, schizophrenia, and bipolar disorder. Neuropsychological rehabilitation is crucial to the treatment of different disorders because it highlights the complex connection between the brain and behavior.

In reference to the neurodegenerative conditions covered in Chapter 1, stem cell treatment is discussed in Chapter 2. Many advances in the biological sciences have been accelerated by stem cells, which have been the subject of constant attention in recent years. Stem cells are excellent cellular resources for research on molecular mechanisms, regenerative medicine, tissue engineering, biological modeling, and drug screening. As more and more people are enduring the symptoms of neurodegenerative disorders every day, stem cells seem to hold promise for treating these conditions.

Brain tumor tissue engineering applications are covered in Chapter 3. Glioblastoma (GBM) in particular is the deadliest of these tumors because of its aggressiveness, ability to invade, and late diagnosis, all of which necessitate the use of modern biotechnologies. The range of GBM diagnosis and treatment modalities now employed in clinics calls for the enhancement of current care. Tissue engineering can be a very useful tool for researchers and doctors to better understand the biology of the tumor and increase patient's life.

The focus of Chapter 4 is imaging-based brain tumor detection. Early brain tumor identification is essential for an early diagnosis and a well-thought-out treatment plan. Over the past few years, MRI scanning has played an increasingly important role in medical research. Digital image processing plays a major role in medical image analysis. Image segmentation is a crucial step in image processing since it makes data extraction from complex medical images easier. Dividing of aberrant brain tissue (a tumor) from healthy brain tissue is known as brain tumor segmentation. Brain tumor segmentation algorithms have shown promise in the analysis and detection of tumors in clinical images. Since the beginning locations of metastatic gliomas are unpredictable, Chapter 5 focuses on spatiotemporal simulation of initial glioma growth. Several reaction diffusion equation techniques have been used to simulate the growth of gliomas in both the reaction and diffusion phases. The spatiotemporal state of glioma growth has been simulated using three response equations and five distinct diffusion techniques. The life expectancy of a patient, the future effects of brain damage on perception and attitude, and the efficacy of present treatments can all be predicted with the use of brain tumor development simulator modeling.

In Chapter 6, fractional operators are discussed in the mathematical modeling of brain tumors. Partial differential equations and ordinary differential equations are examples of mathematical models, as are mathematical structures. Although there are several ways to solve the problem, information about fractional operators in glioma modeling is provided in this chapter. The impact of fractional calculus on the formation of brain tumors is also investigated.

Applications of the Brain-Computer Interface (BCI) are the main topic of Chapter 7. The development of BCI systems has the potential to significantly improve our knowledge of, and ability to treat neuropsychiatric disorders such as Parkinson's disease, Alzheimer's disease, and other mood and mental disorders. The first section of the chapter explains the basic ideas behind electroencephalography (EEG) and why it is useful for recording brain activity in real time. It then explores the complex field of neurodegenerative diseases and neuropsychiatric disorders, highlighting how EEG-based BCIs can improve diagnostic, therapeutic, and rehabilitative approaches.

The research on brain bioinformatics utilizing RNA-seq and Microarray techniques is the main topic of Chapter 8. We have discussed the high throughput approaches for evaluating brain transcriptomics, the repositories used to store the information collected through them, and the data processing and visualization tools. Each technique's benefits and drawbacks have been presented. Additionally, examples of current RNA-seq and microarray research on the neurological conditions covered in this book are provided. Several proposals have been pointed out that could assist researchers in comprehending the data now accessible on brain diseases and disorders, such as combining different methodologies (such as imaging techniques, transcriptomics data, and artificial intelligence approaches).

An analysis of brain health and disease states using graph theory forms the basis topics of Chapter 9, which first describes the main graph analysis parameters and complex network models. Then, three main topics in brain studies using graph theory which are module detection, brain network motif search and network alignment are reviewed. The final part of this chapter outlines the brain network alterations due to various neurological disorders such as Alzheimer's disease and Parkinson's disease.

Our final chapter covers brain proteomics, or more precisely, the use of mass spectrometry (MS) for extensive analysis of the brain proteome. Shotgun proteomics is widely used in MS-based proteomics. This technique provides a comprehensive protein profile of a tissue or cell and is made possible by high-resolution equipment. Additionally, rapid technological developments in bioinformatics have greatly improved the field's ability to conduct high-throughput studies that involve the analysis of massive volumes of data. Proteome analysis using high-throughput technology holds enormous potential for advancing our understanding of neurodegenerative disorders such as Alzheimer's disease (AD), Parkinson's disease, and schizophrenia.

We express our gratitude to each and every one of our contributors for their valuable work on this book.

Kayhan Erciyes
Yaşar University
Tuba Sevimoglu
University of Health Sciences

List of Figures

List of Tables

Editors

Kayhan Erciyes holds a B.Sc. (Hons.) in Electrical Engineering and Electronics from the University of Manchester Institute of Science and Technology, England, an M.Sc. degree in Electronic Control Engineering from the University of Salford, England and a Ph.D. degree in Computer Engineering from Ege University, Turkiye with part of the Ph.D. study realized at Edinburgh University, Scotland. He has worked as a professor in a number of institutions including Ege University, Yasar University, Uskudar University, Izmir Institute of Technology , UC Davis, Oregon State University, and California State University San Marcos. He is currently working at Yaşar University and has published several books including Distributed and Sequential Algorithms for Bioinformatics by Springer Computational Biology Series. His research interests are broadly in graph theory and its applications in bioinformatics and brain networks, and parallel and distributed algorithms.

Tuba Sevimoglu holds a B.Sc. in Chemical Engineering from Yildiz Technical University, Türkiye, an M.Sc. degree in Industrial Engineering from Florida International University, USA, and a Ph.D. degree in Bioengineering from Marmara University, Türkiye. She is currently a professor of Bioengineering at University of Health Sciences in Istanbul, Türkiye. Her research interests include bioinformatics approaches to analyzing big data, gene expression, biological networks and the bioinformatics of genetic, neurodegenerative, and autoimmune diseases.

Contributors

Tugba Bal
Üsküdar University
İstanbul, Türkiye

Kristin Surpuhi Benli
Üsküdar University
İstanbul, Türkiye

Zihni Onur Çalışkaner
Biruni University
İstanbul, Türkiye

Ihab Elaff
Üsküdar University
İstanbul, Türkiye

Kayhan Erciyes
Yaşar University
İzmir, Türkiye

Arife Aysun Karaaslan
Üsküdar University
İstanbul, Türkiye

Çağla Özdemir
University of Health Sciences
İstanbul, Türkiye

Tuba Sevimoglu
University of Health Sciences
İstanbul, Türkiye

Mustafa Gani Sürmen
University of Health Sciences
İstanbul, Türkiye

Saime Sürmen
University of Health Sciences
İstanbul, Türkiye

Emine Elif Tülay
Muğla Sıtkı Koçman University
Muğla, Türkiye

1

Brain Diseases and Disorders

Tuba Sevimoglu, Tugba Bal, Çağla Özdemir

University of Health Sciences, İstanbul, Türkiye
Üsküdar University, İstanbul, Türkiye

The brain coordinates critical physiological and mental processes by sending signals throughout the central nervous system (CNS). Comprehending the anatomy and physiology of the brain is essential to appreciating its intricate growth and mastery over both voluntary and involuntary movements, sensory perception, and emotional reactions. This chapter explores the complex functioning, architecture, and wide range of neurological illnesses that can impact the human brain. The degeneration of nerve cells and synaptic connections is a hallmark of neurodegenerative illnesses, which include Alzheimer's disease (AD), Parkinson's disease (PD), Huntington's disease (HD), Amyotrophic Lateral Sclerosis (ALS), and Multiple Sclerosis (MS). These diseases cause severe symptoms and present substantial obstacles to patient care. Analogously, brain tumors—both primary and metastatic—present difficult diagnostic and treatment challenges and frequently call for radiotherapy, chemotherapy, and surgery. The wide range of brain cancers is typified by meningeal tumors, brain lymphomas, and gliomas, each of which presents particular therapeutic difficulties. Furthermore, neuropsychiatric conditions emphasize the complex interaction between neurological and psychological events. Examples of these conditions include schizophrenia (SCZ), bipolar disorder (BD), attention deficit hyperactivity disorder (ADHD), major depressive disorder (MDD), and autism spectrum disorder (ASD). Neuropsychological rehabilitation emphasizes the intricate relationship between the brain and behavior and is essential in the management of these disorders. This review offers significant insights into the complex mechanisms of the brain and the wide range of neurological conditions that affect the health and quality of life of humans.

DOI: 10.1201/9781003461906-1

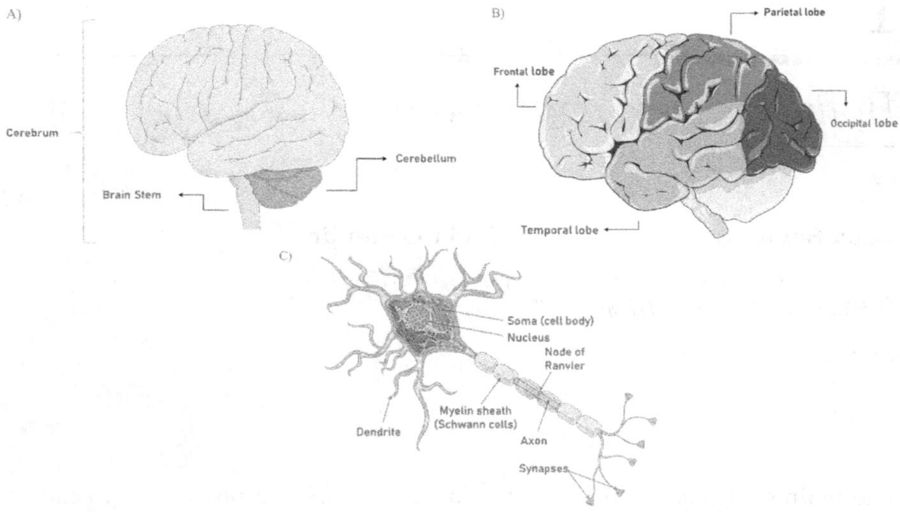

FIGURE 1.1
A. Main parts of the brain **B.** Lobes of the brain **C.** A neuron and its parts. The figure was partly generated using Servier Medical Art, provided by Servier, licensed under a Creative Commons Attribution 4.0 unported license.

1.1 Introduction

The most intricate organ in the body, the brain, is essential for maintaining and regulating bodily functions. There are three main parts of the brain: cerebrum, cerebellum, and brain stem (Figure 1.1A). It has a volume of about 1370 ml, is approximately 1400–1500 grams, made up of more than 100 billion nerves, and can accommodate around 2.5 million gigabytes of memory [1].

The brain is responsible for mental functions such as thinking, producing, and learning, as well as the harmonious functioning of all vital functions such as walking, breathing, and sweating. As a part of the CNS, it transmits signals through nerve cells to the spinal cord and throughout the body. Additionally, the control of all voluntary and involuntary movements, reactions and thoughts are shaped in the brain. The biological elements that are decisive in this control process are directly related to the physical structure of the brain stemming from its chemistry. Therefore, parts of the brain, their structure, and functions need to be well understood to comprehend brain function and development [1, 2].

1.2 Brain: The Command Center of the Body

The brain performs a multitude of vital tasks. It is the reason we are capable of evaluating and interpreting the events that are transpiring around us. All five of our senses—sight, smell, hearing, touch, and taste—can all be used to simultaneously transmit instructions to the brain. The brain is responsible for many bodily functions, including thinking, memory, speech, and movement of the limbs. The brain's body control determines how a person responds to stress (such as exam excitement, losing a job, illness) by changing respiration and heart rates.

The brain is organized, and each part is divided into certain functions [2]. Considering the anatomy of the brain, it is clear that the cerebrum also known as the telencephalon is the largest and main part of the brain, and, together with the diencephalon, they assemble into the forebrain. The cerebrum consists of right and left hemispheres connected to each other by the corpus callosum and fornix which provides signal transmission of nerve cells and consists of axon fibers. Each hemisphere of the brain is divided into 4 different lobes: Frontal lobe, occipital lobe, temporal lobe, and parietal lobe forming the front, posterior, lower, and upper parts of the brain, respectively (Figure 1.1B) [3]. The frontal lobe directs purposeful actions such as creativity, problem solving, decision making, and planning [4]. The occipital lobe in the upper posterior region carries out processes involving vision. The temporal lobe (right and left) is located around and above the ears. This region is mainly responsible for hearing, memory, emotion, smell, and comprehension of language. In contrast, the parietal lobe is crucial for perception and visual processing [5]. The diencephalon region consists of the hippocampus, thalamus, hypothalamus, and amygdala. Also known as the limbic system, this section of the brain is required for the production of emotions, sleep, attention, body functioning, hormones, sex, smell, and many of the brain chemicals [6].

The outermost part of the cerebrum (cerebral cortex, gray matter) contains neurons which are unmyelinated and have slower conduction. This cortex is the region where the most important perceptual functions such as memory, attention, perceptual awareness, thought, language, and consciousness are created. Therefore, this region is significant for the body and is of interest for routine functions. The walnut-shaped brain shell contains folds called gyrus, while the slits between the folds are called sulcus [7]. One of the most interesting facts about the cerebrum is that it contains tens of billions of neurons, forming nerve fibers, and these nerve fibers produce behaviors that "we think we are doing consciously" by constantly evaluating the data coming from the environment [8].

The diencephalon is the region between the cerebrum and the brain stem. This structure consists of the thalamus, hypothalamus, and epithalamus. Another nucleus known as the subthalamic nucleus often has been under debate whether it should be a part of the ventral thalamus or the hypothalamus [9]. As the largest part of the diencephalon, thalamus is reported to relay information for motor, sensory, limbic, cognitive, and high-order functions [10–12]. The hypothalamus is the hormonal output regulatory center, located at the base of the brain. It is the main mediator for the activity of the pituitary gland on the target organs. In this axis, the pituitary gland secretes adrenocorticotropic hormone, thyroid-stimulating hormone, growth hormone, prolactin, and the gonadotrophs to manipulate the cellular activity throughout the body [13]. Located dorsal to the thalamus, epithalamus-based outputs are essential for motor control, biological clock, and stress responses [14]. The brain stem forms the connection between cerebrum to spinal cord and cerebellum and, consists of the medulla, the pons, and the midbrain [15].

The path of all nerve fibers that transmit signals between the cortex and spinal cord passes through the brain stem. Therefore, it receives information from all areas of the CNS and processes this information by integrating it. Its main functions are control of circulation and respiration, control of sleep and attention, gastrointestinal activity, and other neurological activities [16]. Additionally, the medulla plays a crucial role in breathing, blood pressure, blood rhythm, coughing, sneezing, and swallowing reflexes [17]. As a result, the prominent role of the brain stem and its part is significant to sustain life. Another subunit, pons, (meaning "bridge" in Latin) acts as a bridge to the brain. It receives and distributes signals from and to the brain [18]. It also has many important tasks such as biological clock, control of swallowing, hearing, tasting, and posture. Finally, the midbrain, rostral to the pons and caudal to the thalamus and the basal ganglia carry out the tasks of motor movements, visual and auditory senses, balance, sleep/wake cycles, alertness, arousal and control and regulation of eye movements [19]. The cerebellum as the largest section of the brain is assembled with two hemispheres and midline vermis. It is suggested that this brain section is involved in cognitive function and movements [20]. Although the cerebellum occupies around 10% of the entire brain mass, it accounts for nearly 80% of cerebral neurons [21].

1.3 Body Under Control of Brain

The brain is a perfect composition of fine structural and functional units composed of groups of neurons arranged together as a clear anatomical model. These neurons pass signals to each other and to other types of cells such as glia to communicate. Neurons consist of three parts: Cell body, axon, and dendrites (Figure 1.1C). The greater the number of network patterns formed by neurons, the stronger the information processing process occurs. Each neuron has many short extensions called dendrites and one long extension called axon surrounded by a myelin sheath. Neurons communicate with each other through junctions called synapses which are located between axon terminals, dendrite, or cell body [22]. All activities and memory in the nervous system are related to the electrical current arising in and traveling between neurons [23].

The corpus callosum network, which consists of a dense neural network, acts as a bridge between the right and left lobes of the brain, which ensures the continuous exchange of information. When the corpus callosum is cut, the communication between these two parts is interrupted and therefore, information exchange between them is not possible in any direction. Accordingly, every learning experience means the formation of new synaptic connections. Here, learning is observed as a biochemical change. Hebb, who systematized this theory, also known as the "brain-based learning theory", argues that the nature of learning cannot be understood without knowing how the circuits in the brain work. Within the framework of the findings of the neurophysiology theory put forward by Hebb, the two hemispheres of the brain process different information [24]. It has been proven that no hemisphere is superior to the other and that both are needed. In most people, the left hemisphere is responsible for speech and the right hemisphere is responsible for spatial and perceptual functions [25].

Expanding upon research on individual mental activity and applying it to the field of education, Herman developed the theory of brain dominance, which holds that certain brain regions are used more frequently by different persons. For instance, it's suggested that people who learn best with their left hemispheres of the brains typically learn by reading, whereas people with their right hemispheres actively learn through seeing and doing [26].

As the studies on the brain hemispheres deepened, it became necessary to examine the brain by dividing it into quarters. Kolb developed the four-quarter brain concept in depth. In this model, the brain is divided into four quadrants: upper-left (A), lower-left (B), lower-right (C), and upper-right (D). According to this, while logical, factual, critical, technical, quantitative, and discriminative features are mainly listed as the characteristics of the quadrant A, the structural, sequential, planned, organized, detailed, and preserving features constitute the structure of the quadrant B. Relational, emotional, spiritual, and tactile aspects are revealed in quadrant C, while the dominant brain's quadrant D emphasizes visual, intuitive, inventive, imaginative, logical, and traditional aspects (Figure 1.2) [27]. Information that is verbal, mathematical, or logical is better processed by the left hemisphere of the brain whereas information that is perceptual, startling, spatial, holistic, or creative is better processed by the right hemisphere. Even if it is easy to distinguish between the two hemispheres of the brain's functioning as mentioned, this distinction cannot be made in day-to-day situations since a person's thought process on a given topic is typically linked to the functions of both hemispheres [25]. Despite having distinct centers for diverse functions, both hemispheres work together to accomplish these goals. For instance, by employing color graphs and diagrams, we can improve the efficiency of the right hemisphere function when evaluating data with left hemisphere functions. We cannot develop our

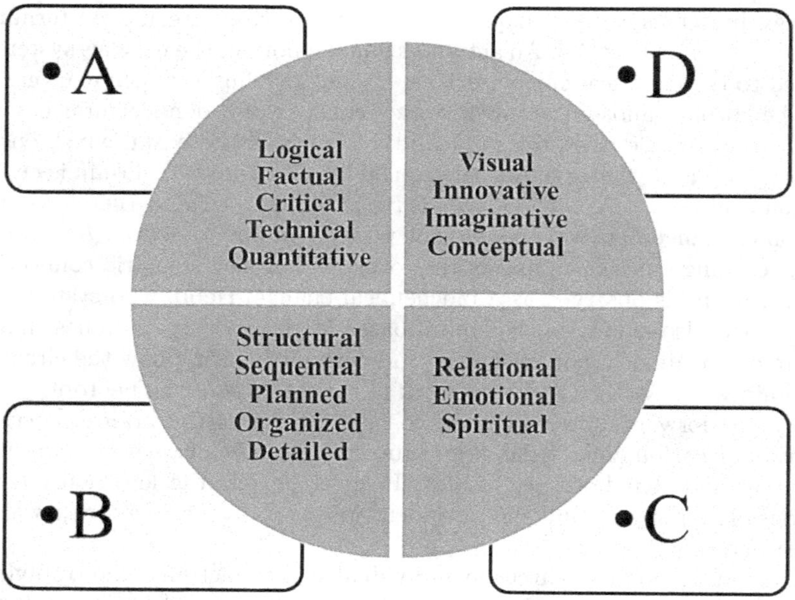

FIGURE 1.2
A four-quarter brain model.

logic by neglecting our creativity and creativity without using our logic. Logic and creativity are complementary ways of thinking. That is, creative thinking generates the idea, while logical thinking tests and develops the idea. For learning to be effective and create a lasting memory, learning activities need to engage with both halves of the brain [28].

1.4 Tools to Diagnose Brain Conditions

Other than physical exams, brain conditions can be diagnosed through biopsies, tests such as electroencephalogram (EEG), imaging tests such as magnetic resonance imaging (MRI), computed tomography (CT) and positron emission tomography (PET) scans, and laboratory tests with samples from blood, urine or spinal fluid. There are also new genetic/bioinformatics tools to understand these conditions such as microarrays that work with predefined transcripts and RNA-sequencing that allows the sequencing of the whole transcriptome [29]. Brain research has focused on the identification, modeling, categorization, imaging, and analysis of various brain diseases to gain a better understanding of the structure and function of the brain as well as to develop

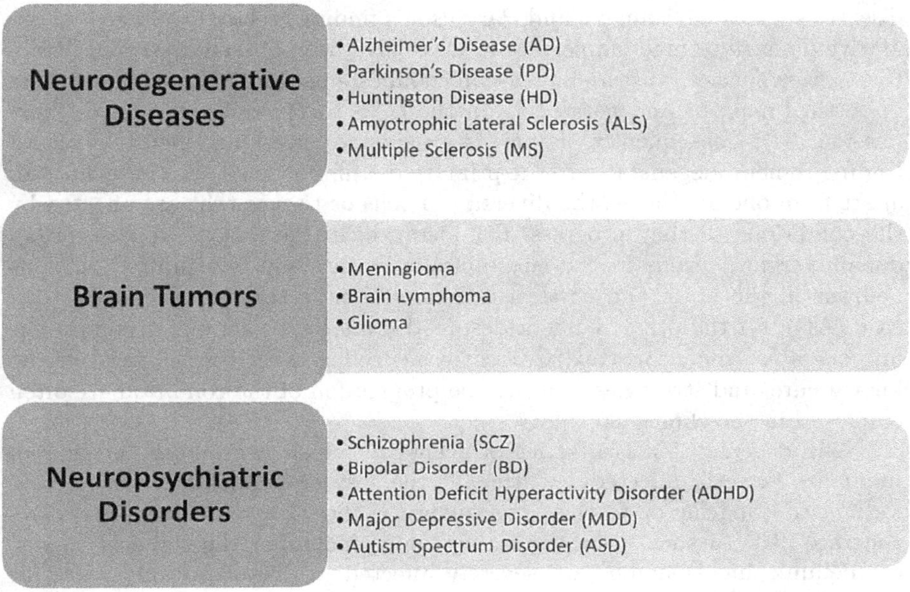

Neurodegenerative Diseases
• Alzheimer's Disease (AD)
• Parkinson's Disease (PD)
• Huntington Disease (HD)
• Amyotrophic Lateral Sclerosis (ALS)
• Multiple Sclerosis (MS)
Brain Tumors
• Meningioma
• Brain Lymphoma
• Glioma
Neuropsychiatric Disorders
• Schizophrenia (SCZ)
• Bipolar Disorder (BD)
• Attention Deficit Hyperactivity Disorder (ADHD)
• Major Depressive Disorder (MDD)
• Autism Spectrum Disorder (ASD)

FIGURE 1.3
Brain diseases and disorders included in this chapter.

improved diagnostic and therapeutic approaches. The aim of this book is to shed light on what is being done in these areas and offer some future work [29].

1.5 Diversity of Brain Disease and Disorders

There are a wide range of conditions that affect the normal activities of the brain. These include but are not limited to neurodegenerative, mental diseases and tumors (Figure 1.3). It should be acknowledged that the complexity of the brain limits treatment strategies and diagnosis of associated diseases. Especially the nature of the blood-brain barrier is an obstacle to drug delivery to CNS [30].

1.6 Neurodegenerative Diseases

Neurodegenerative diseases are multifactorial diseases that negatively affect patient life quality and progress rapidly and are characterized by structural and functional degeneration and/or death of nerve cells. In neurodegenerative diseases such as Alzheimer's and Parkinson's findings related to increased oxidative damage to macromolecules in CNS have been observed [31, 32]. Reactive oxygen species cause an increase in cholinesterase and tyrosinase activities in cortical neurons and nerve cells in the CNS to prevent cholinergic transmission [33]. Consequently, it increases oxidative stress and neuronal death leading to neurodegeneration. The primary distinction that sets these illnesses apart from one another is the diversity of cells or tissues that are affected by the conditions as they progress. For instance, in Parkinson's disease (PD), dopaminergic neurons in the substantia nigra are severely injured whereas neurons in the brain and cortical region are unaffected. In Alzheimer's disease (AD), on the other hand, widespread damage to neurons occurs in the hippocampus and neocortex. Currently, neurodegenerative diseases have no known cure, and strategies to delay the progression of the condition are often employed in the clinics [30].

Neurodegeneration is a series of events in which neurons in the human brain are directly affected resulting in the loss of neural function. A major contributing factor to this consequence is the inability of neurons to regenerate [34]. In such diseases, brain regions including the cerebral cortex, cerebellum, and thalamus are severely affected in disease-specific patterns. Neurodegenerative diseases arise from the contribution of diverse factors of environmental (diet, age and exercise), metabolic stress, neuroinflammation, neurovascular coupling and genetics (GWAS sex-linked inheritance) leading to loss of neurons and synapses, and alteration of the key pathways [35, 36]. These alterations manifest as physical symptoms such as exhaustion, contractions, amnesia, and issues with movement [34].

1.6.1 Alzheimer's Disease (AD)

Alzheimer's disease (AD) is a progressive neurodegenerative disease marked by diminished cognitive abilities, difficulties in self-care, and a variety of behavioral and neuropsychiatric abnormalities. It is caused by the loss of neurons and synapses in the different regions of the CNS [37].

There are two types of diagnostic criteria for AD: The Diagnostic and Statistical Manual (DSM) criterion and the one created by the National Institute of Neurological and Communication Diseases and the Stroke-Alzheimer Disease and Associated Diseases Association (NINCDSADRDA) [38]. These criteria can be used to evaluate and confirm the diagnosis of AD. Evaluations include determining whether the patient has learning and memory disorders, aphasia, apraxia, agnosia, impairment in executive functions (e.g., planning, organizing, sequencing, abstraction), and whether there is any other CNS-related pathology [39]. A variety of imaging modalities, including positron emission tomography (PET), single photon emission tomography (SPECT), magnetic resonance imaging (MRI imaging), and computed tomography (CT) are utilized to rule out other potential causes and differentiate AD from other brain disorders [40].

Memory impairment is the primary clinical indication of AD in its early stages. As the disease progresses, dysfunctions related to other cognitive areas such as attention and executive functions, thought and behavior, language, apraxia and visuospatial functions also manifest themselves [40]. Owing to the disease's progressive nature, patients experience worsening motor abilities, decreased social functioning, and increased memory loss as the stages advance. Patients in the latter stages need assistance with everyday tasks [41]. In most patients with AD, cognitive decline coexists with noticeable behavioral abnormalities and psychiatric symptoms. Depression, anxiety, apathy, phobia of being alone, aimless wanderings, agitation, aggression, hallucinations, delusions, and sleep disorders are among these behavioral changes and psychiatric symptoms. Extrapyramidal symptoms such as bradykinesia and rigidity are observed in the majority of patients, while myoclonus and seizures occur in a few of them [37].

Pharmacological treatments are applied to slow down the disease and reduce the symptoms [42]. Tacrine is a centrally and peripherally acting reversible cholinesterase inhibitor with a duration of action of 4–6 hours, but its effect is nonspecific. It inhibits acetylcholinesterase, yet high doses are moderately effective in AD. Further, its hepatotoxicity and gastrointestinal side effects limit its use. Therefore, liver function tests should be performed weekly for the first 16 weeks of treatment. In cases where enzymes are elevated, the drug should be discontinued. However, it positively affects behavioral problems in AD patients [42]. Another drug called methyl folate, is an organophosphorus with partial selectivity to inhibit choline esterase and it passes easily into the brain. It improves behavioral issues and has less negative effects in addition to cognitive difficulties [43]. Rivastigmine is also an acetylcholinesterase inhibitor and it binds to the esoteric site of the target enzyme and dissociates very slowly causing false reversible inhibition. As it rapidly travels into the CNS, rivastigmine inhibits acetylcholinesterase in cortical and hippocampal areas more than in other areas of the brain. The consequence of this activity leads to specific treatment of memory disorders without causing respiratory and extrapyramidal system side effects [44].

In recent years, there has been a growing interest in general workouts designed for those suffering from dementia or cognitive impairments since exercise promotes the creation of new neurons and provides neuroplasticity [45]. An exercise regimen can help patients in a variety of ways, regardless of their stage. The Finnish Alzheimer's Disease Exercise (FINALEX) study suggests that exercise regimens carried out twice a week for a year, under the guidance of a physiotherapist, improve patients' physical functioning in cases of mild dementia and reduce their risk of falls in cases of advanced dementia [46].

1.6.2 Parkinson's Disease (PD)

Parkinson's disease (PD) occurs as a progressive and degenerative disorder with the deficiency of dopaminergic neurons in the nigro-striatal system [47].

PD typically affects 5–6 persons out of every 1000 [48, 49]. About 1–2% of persons over 65 and 4% of adults over 80 are affected [50]. In PD, α-synuclein proteins accumulate as Lewy bodies in the nervous system. Lewy bodies destroy relevant nerve cells and connections and, stop the exchange of neurotransmitters [51]. As a result, signals can no longer be sent over these lines, and issues arise with activities such as mobility and attention management. Tremor, bradykinesia, and postural instability thus arise as the distinctive indicators of this disease [50].

Many different underlying mechanisms have been proposed in the pathophysiology of PD such as genetic causes, congenital causes, toxic agent exposure, mitochondrial dysfunction, trauma, inflammation, and oxidative stress, [52]. Outcome of PD is defined by the loss of dopaminergic neurons in the substantia nigra as well as localization of the Lewy bodies in the midbrain leading to the gradual loss of movement capacity [53].

Observation of the response to dopamine drugs (dopamine agonists and L-dopa) is the most widely used diagnostic method, but imaging techniques such as MRI and tomography fail to diagnose PD [54]. The diagnosis of PD typically relies on clinical findings and patient history [55]. Laboratory tests may be sought to exclude other forms of parkinsonism. However, there are no specific biological markers for antemortem diagnosis of PD. Particularly in the early stages of the disease, diagnoses made immediately after the onset of symptoms can change in approximately one-third of patients within the first five years [56]. The diagnostic accuracy of patients treated for PD based on clinical assessment is found to be 76% in postmortem studies [57]. However, under the supervision of a specialist experienced in movement disorders, the diagnostic specificity of the presence of resting tremor, asymmetric bradykinesia, rigidity, and a good response to L-Dopa is 98%, with a sensitivity of 91%. Final confirmation of the diagnosis based on current clinical features is often possible through neuropathological examination.

Distinguishing PD from atypical parkinsonisms and other parkinsonian syndromes is crucial not only for determining treatment response and prognosis but also for selecting appropriate patients for clinical trials, especially those related to potential neuroprotective therapies. Although various criteria have been proposed for the diagnosis of PD [58], the most used criteria today are the Clinical Diagnostic Criteria of the United Kingdom Parkinson's Disease Society Brain Bank, published in the late 1980s. According to these criteria, bradykinesia is essential for diagnosis, and the presence of at least one additional symptom such as rigidity, resting tremor, or postural instability is required [59]. There are four main symptoms in PD acronymized as TRAP: Tremor at rest, rigidity, akinesia, and postural instability [55].

Clinical findings in PD are usually asymmetrical, and not all of them may be found together. Secondary motor symptoms are hypoxemia, dysarthria, dysphagia, sialorrhea, micrographia, shuffling, festination, freezing, slowing of activities of daily living, blepharospasm, and dystonia. The first symptoms are resting tremors in one extremity, clumsiness of the hand especially in fine movements, slowing down or slowing down of all movements, especially walking, bending the body forward. These symptoms start insidiously and progress slowly. A decrease in the sense of smell or shoulder pain may be one of the first symptoms that go unnoticed. Over time, rigidity and bradykinesia become evident and postural changes begin to occur. The patient's mobility gradually decreases as a result of decreased trunk rotation, arm swing during walking, disappearance of spontaneous facial expressions, and increasing difficulty initiating movement [60]. Another symptom is a form of freezing akinesia known as a motor block, which is characterized by an abrupt, transient (less than 10 seconds) immobility, primarily affecting the legs when walking. This causes anxiety when the patient first starts to walk and makes it difficult to move quickly when turning, crossing, or getting through tight spaces, which can lead to falls.

Bradykinesia is the most common sign of the diseases affecting the basal ganglia. It is characterized by trouble with movement-based activities including coordination, purposeful movement initiation, direction changes, halting, switching between movements, and simultaneous performance of two movements. Activities and reaction times generally slow down, particularly in the case of handling the sophisticated technologies. The clinical signs of bradykinesia includes spontaneous cessation of movement, dribbling from the mouth due to difficulties in swallowing, monotone and hypokinetic dysarthria, loss of facial expression, decreased blinking, and decreased arm swing while walking. It can be easily detected by rapid, repetitive, and alternating movements of the extremities in neurological examination. The degree of bradykinesia is linked to a shortfall in dopamine and is considered to be the consequence of a reduction in the dopaminergic activity leading to a decrease in activation of the motor cortex, premotor cortex, and supplementary motor cortex [61].

The term "rigidity" describes the rise in muscular tone due to simultaneous antagonist and agonist muscle contractions. The voluntary movement of the opposing limb, commonly referred to as the "froment maneuver," enhances rigidity; this strengthening effect is crucial for exposing moderate rigidity [62]. Postural instability is a condition that develops after other PD signs and symptoms. It is the weakening or loss of postural reflexes, which ordinarily automatically maintain the body position taken while standing or sitting in healthy individuals. In contrast, patients struggle to get up from their sitting positions without assistance due to postural instability. PD patients frequently experience balance issues, falls, and especially backward falls. Postural instability is also closely linked to other parkinsonian symptoms, orthostatic hypotension, age-related sensory alterations, and kinesthetic impairments in the control of vestibular, proprioceptive, and visual stimulations. The flexion posture, bradykinesia, tremor, and stiffness associated with PD impede the development of balance techniques and increases reaction times [63].

As PD symptoms are based on the lack of dopamine, for almost 40 years, the best treatment for PD has been levodopa combined with peripheral decarboxylase inhibitors (carbidopa, benserazide) to prevent levodopa from being converted to dopamine. Bradykinesia and stiffness can be effectively reduced with levodopa treatment, yet early onset of the disease, prolonged illness, and prolonged levodopa administration are risk factors for the development of dyskinesia [64, 65]. PD patients may experience variations in their motor function and a progressive reduction in the duration of a single levodopa dosage (wearing-off phenomena) following years of stability with the medication. In more severe situations, episodes of immobility occur for whatever length of time that levodopa is taken. PD patients are also treated with dopamine receptor agonists, which stimulate postsynaptic dopamine receptors to enhance dopaminergic transmission [65].

While senior individuals are more vulnerable to the neuropsychiatric side effects of other anti-Parkinsonian medications, they are also less likely to experience motor issues from levodopa. For this reason, it is more advisable to start levodopa usage early in the older population. Levodopa can be used for both standard and controlled releases when initiating treatment [66]. Contrary to expectations, however, there was no evidence to back up the theory that the controlled release type can stop the onset of motor problems. The absorption of the controlled-release formulations is irregular, and their effectiveness is roughly two-thirds to three-quarters that of a typical tablet. This is because levodopa is only absorbed from the small intestine, and even then, only a portion of the levodopa in the slow-release pill is released into the large intestine. It's common practice to take slow-releasing levodopa right before bed. As a result, mobility is offered for an extended amount of time while you sleep [67]. The basis of pharmacokinetic problems is that levodopa is a neutral amino acid. Therefore, it competes with other amino acids both during intestinal absorption and during blood-brain barrier passage. If it is taken with protein-rich food, the amount transferred to the brain decreases and therefore the clinical efficacy is weakened. The best efficacy for levodopa is achieved when taken on an empty stomach [64]. In the postrema region, where the blood-brain barrier is absent, peripheral dopamine induces both nausea and vomiting. It also causes peripheral dopaminergic side effects which affect the cardiovascular system resulting the abnormalities such as orthostatic hypotension and arrhythmia.

Dopamine receptor agonists are medications to stimulate postsynaptic dopamine receptors to lower symptoms; they accomplish this without metabolizing dopamine and are therefore not affected by the neurodegenerative process. Dopamine agonists are preferred over levodopa due to their effectiveness to treat PD symptoms and lowered risk of the development of motor impairments. While monotherapy with dopamine agonists is successful, the percentage of patients who actively use it decreases over time and drops below 20% after a few years of treatment [68, 69]. For this reason, most individuals are given additional treatments—typically levodopa—after receiving medication for a few years. Neuralgia, vomiting, and orthostatic hypotension are examples of peripheral dopaminergic adverse effects that typically manifest early in treatment and improve with time. However, at first, the medication must be gradually increased, and domperidone (a peripheral dopamine antagonist) may need to be used. Agonists also experience more central side effects than levodopa, including mental and cognitive side effects. Serious issues might arise in the form of hallucinations and psychotic symptoms [70]. To improve the effectiveness of levodopa or dopamine agonists various strategies such as adding another dopamine agonist, dividing the dose of levodopa into smaller but more frequent doses, or adding a catechol-O-methyltransferase inhibitor or monoaminoxidase (MAO) inhibitors are frequently applied [54, 55].

Amantadine is synthetic tricyclic amine manufactured as salt, as immediate or extended-release oral formulations and as intravenous (IV) infusion [71]. Although it has been suggested for PD, this drug is not as potent as any other dopaminergic medication. It is hypothesized that it works by enhancing dopamine release from vesicles, blocking dopamine absorption from the synaptic cleft, and having an anticholinergic effect. Livedo reticularis, or red, mottled skin around the knees, ankle edema, visual hallucinations, and confusion are common adverse effects of amantadine [72]. Anticholinergic medications are expected to work by reversing the imbalance caused by lower dopamine levels between acetylcholine and striatal dopamine activity. They have a minor impact on PD symptoms, and there is currently inadequate evidence to support its specific effect on the tremors [73]. Due to their modest anticholinergic and hypnotic properties, antihistamines like diphenhydramine can also be utilized, particularly in elderly individuals for whom anticholinergics are contraindicated [73]. Dry mouth, constipation, urine retention, tachycardia, and hazy vision from trouble adapting are examples of peripheral adverse effects of anticholinergics [74].

1.6.3 Huntington's Disease (HD)

The neurodegenerative condition known as Huntington's disease (HD) is an autosomal dominant condition that manifests as physical, cognitive, and mental symptoms emerging in middle age [75]. Chorea—unusual, uncontrollable movement—is the most definitive sign of HD. A substantial portion of the body is involved in these uncontrollable moving jumps that occur continuously [76]. HD is marked by abnormal facial expressions, expression disorder, and difficulty swallowing and chewing due to physical instability and weakening of muscle function. Dysphagia and related weight loss are also present. Moreover, irregularities in sleep cycles, insomnia, and fast eye movements during sleep are noted [77]. Given that the condition is inherited autosomal dominantly, inheriting the mutant gene from one parent who has been diagnosed with HD carries a 50% risk. This danger is alarmingly high given the progressive nature and the lack of a conclusive cure for the disease at present [78].

The neuropathology of HD shows that different areas of the brain are affected by the disease to diverse degrees [79]. Patients with HD have impaired glucose metabolism, especially in the striatum, according to PET imaging results. This is the earliest pathological change in HD. This defect in cell metabolism causes cell death in the striatum and a decrease in metabolic enzymes for energy production in the brain [80]. The HD gene is located on the short arm of chromosome 4 [81]. The mutation in exon 1 of this gene causes an increase in the repeats of CAG trinucleotides. While there are less than 35 CAG repeats in healthy individuals, this number increases to 37 and above in individuals with HD. Increased CAG trinucleotide repeats result in the addition of abnormally long polyglutamine sequences to the mutant huntingtin (HTT) protein [82]. This is an indication that the gene defect does not eliminate an essential gene, rather the enzyme activity decreases or completely disappears due to repeat copy number changes in HD [82].

In HD, cognitive symptoms occur due to the weakening of selective cognitive abilities. Accordingly, executive functions (planning, cognitive flexibility), psychomotor functions (slowing down in intellectual processes related to muscle control), perceptual and environmental abilities, choosing the right method in remembering information and choosing new disorders in learning skills show parallelism with the pathology in the individual [83]. In addition to various physical and cognitive symptoms, the disease also includes psychiatric symptoms such as depression, anxiety, decreased emotional expression (emotional limitation), and compulsive behaviors. Performance at work or in daily life also declines in patients suffering from HD, and they must continue taking medicine to maintain their quality of life [84]. In 80% of patients, psychiatric symptoms rather than cognitive symptoms occur within the first 10–15 years of the disease. The risk of suicide in HD patients is higher than in the general population [85]. Furthermore, aggression and irritability have been reported to be higher among Huntingtin gene carriers compared to the general population. In contrast, obsessive-compulsive disorder (OCD), schizophrenia, and delusional disorders can be observed less frequently in Huntington's patients [86].

There is currently no treatment option to reverse or stop the degenerative process in HD, but the treatment of HD is based on the symptoms [87]. Dopamine receptor blockers, benzodiazepines, drugs that empty dopamine stores, and valproate can be used for the treatment of chorea. Drugs that reduce dopaminergic neurotransmission should be used with extreme caution, as they may increase parkinsonism in advanced stages of the disease and in juvenile-onset patients. Serotonin reuptake inhibitors can be used for depressive symptoms [88]. While genetic testing is the gold standard for making the final diagnosis of HD, neuroimaging tests can also provide valuable guidance. Although striatal volume loss and increased volume in the frontal horn of the lateral ventricles are findings supporting HD in structural brain imaging studies, it should be underlined that these findings may not be detected in the early stages of the disease. However, with functional neuroimaging techniques, brain dysfunctions in, for example, lateral prefrontal and cingulate regions can be demonstrated before the symptoms begin [89].

Even though the clinical diagnosis of HD is based on the presence of the aforementioned motor symptoms, cognitive dysfunctions and psychiatric symptoms constitute the major reasons for the burden on families and are considered the most important predictors of a decrease in daily functions and placement in care institutions and hospitalizations [90]. To properly address genetic testing counseling, a multidisciplinary team effort with a psychiatrist or psychologist is required, considering all hereditary factors and risks [91]. Sufficient genetic and clinical information should be given to the at-risk individual. The consultant should adopt a neutral stance, neither endorsing nor opposing the prognostic test. A decision to get tested must take into account factors such as depression, hopelessness, anxiety, suicidal thoughts, and the existence of social support [92].

1.6.4 Amyotrophic Lateral Sclerosis (ALS)

Amyotrophic lateral sclerosis (ALS) is a progressive disease characterized by degeneration of upper and lower motor neurons of the brain and spinal cord. The disease is usually inherited as an autosomal dominant (OD) [93] and clinical findings usually begin between the ages of 50 and 60 [94]. In familial cases, the age of onset of the disease is earlier. This disease occurs due to the loss of motor nerve cells in the CNS. Various combinations of findings resulting from upper and lower motor neuron involvement determine the clinical picture. Sleep-related respiratory disorders are quite common in ALS patients. It rises with phrenic denervation and diaphragm weakness, develops in proportion to the severity of respiratory and upper airway muscle weakness, and increases significantly during rapid eye movement (REM) sleep, when postural muscular inhibition takes place [95].

Familial ALS cases account for approximately 10% of all ALS cases and, are phenotypically and genetically heterogeneous. It has been suggested that genetic causes, glutamate excitotoxicity, viral infections, autoimmune reactions, and heavy metal intoxications such as lead, mercury and aluminum play a role in the onset of the disease [96]. In 20% of familial cases and 1–5% of sporadic cases, there is a mutation on the gene encoding the Cu/Zn-superoxide dismutase 1 (SOD1) enzyme localized on chromosome 21. While only 2% of the disease was predicted to be genetically transmitted in the 1990s, with the increase in scientific studies on the subjects over the recent years, this rate has increased to approximately 23% today [93].

The etiology of ALS is not fully known. Due to its complex pathophysiology, which involves multiple pathways including oxidative stress, mitochondrial failure, endoplasmic reticulum stress, and axonal transport problem, the disease is challenging to detect. The precursors of ALS are usually not specific to this disease and may mimic other neuromuscular diseases. These diseases are often called mimic syndromes. Errors in early diagnosis could postpone the identification of ALS [97]. After clinical diagnosis, ALS symptoms gradually worsen over time [98]. Factors leading to a delay in diagnosis include familial form of the disease, place of initial involvement, and gender [99]. Current diagnostic criteria are based on clinical examination and electrophysiological measurements. Early diagnosis is important for potential treatments to be more effective. One possible way to enable early detection is to use ALS-specific biomarkers [100]. These biomarkers (such as NfL, Tregs, miRNAs, CK, hs-cTnT) have also gained importance in ALS patients to determine the stage and to follow the progression of the disease. Studies on cerebrospinal fluid (CSF) have been shown that the protein level detected by the ELISA method increases during the progression of the disease [101].

ALS usually presents with weakness in the extremities, i.e., with spinal onset, or with difficulty in speaking and swallowing. Respiratory failure and the problems that result from it typically cause death. Patients with progressed muscle weakness to the point where they are unable to speak, swallow, move their hands, or walk have significant difficulty in daily interactions [102]. Muscle cramps are one of the most common symptoms of patients with ALS and often occur several months before the onset of symptoms. Although muscle cramps occur in healthy individuals and most commonly in the calf muscles, ALS can occur in unusual muscles such as the thighs, abdomen, back, or tongue [103].

Symptoms of muscle weakness vary depending on the motor dysfunction. For instance, patients may find it difficult to turn keys, fasten buttons, open bottle lids, or turn doorknobs as they start to lose strength in their hands and fingers [104]. Patients may suffer low foot or instability as a result of the weakening in the legs [105]. In bulbar muscle involvement, progressive deterioration in bulbar functions such as babbling, hoarseness, and inability to whistle or shout is observed. Fasciculations are often not the initial manifestation of ALS but develop in almost all patients soon after onset. The absence of fasciculations is a condition that requires a review of the diagnosis. In some patients, fasciculation waves sometimes appear to spread towards the chest or back [106].

Dysphagia and aspiration are troubling and dangerous complications and are especially important in bulbar ALS. Muscle weakness, weight loss, and malnutrition is accelerated with a decrease in oral intake. It should be questioned whether the patient is coughing or choking while swallowing [104]. High-calorie food supplementation should be used, and the form, as well as structure of the meals, should be altered to prevent dysphagia and aspiration [103]. In a prospective study on cognition in ALS, one-third of the patients were found to have cognitive disabilities, and most patients diagnosed with ALS have late-onset progressive personality, behavioral, and language impairment without signs of motor neuron disease. ALS patients lose physical abilities such as speaking, manual dexterity, using a pencil and pressing a button over time due to progressive muscle weakness [107]. ALS has made a name for itself with the advances made in its treatment in recent years. Riluzole is the first approved drug used in the treatment of ALS and acts as a glutamatergic transmission modulator [108]. In addition, Edaravone is a powerful antioxidant and has been used in Japan in the treatment of ischemic stroke since 2001 and in the treatment of ALS since 2015. The oxidative stress pathway is affected by the edaravone molecule, which is used to treat ALS patients. This results in a 33% decline in the ALS functional assessment scale, which measures motor and bulbar functions, when compared to placebo [109].

1.6.5 Multiple Sclerosis (MS)

Multiple sclerosis (MS) is an autoimmune, multifocal, and neurodegenerative disease that affects the brain, spinal cord, and optic nerves. In MS, demyelination, axonal loss, and a glial scar (sclerosis) develop in the white matter of the CNS, and neurological dysfunctions are present in the related systems [110]. Viral infections, environmental factors such as the immune system and climate play a role in the etiology of the disease [111]. It is a chronic disease that can affect the patient's life in physical, economic, psychological, and social aspects, and often leads to disability. Due to the presence of various symptoms and their unpredictable nature, patients are faced with uncertainty about their future [112]. Since there is no definitive treatment, it can create a financial burden on the patient and their families [113].

In MS, diagnosis is made using the clinical features of the cases, the course of the disease, and auxiliary laboratory methods [114]. Although the diagnosis is based on clinical findings, para-clinical tests, especially MRI examination, are very helpful in making the diagnosis. To conclude the diagnosis, the neurologist must examine clinical parameters, and results of evaluations such as MRI, CSF, and evoked potential studies [115]. The disease can be seen in three different clinical types: symptoms that worsen from the beginning (primary progressive), progressive course after recurrent-remission attacks (secondary progressive) or recurrent-progressive (relapsing-progressive) attacks [116].

Somatosensory findings, motor findings, fatigue, vision loss, brain stem findings, cerebellar findings, cognitive problems, bladder, bowel, and sexual disorders are the most prevalent symptoms of multiple sclerosis [117]. Somatosensory symptoms constitute the majority of the initial manifestations of MS [118]. Stress is an important factor affecting the onset and course of MS [119, 120]. Negative perspective, ineffective coping, depression, and insufficient social support together with stress affect the trigger of MS attacks, and the importance of effective coping with stress in adaptation to illness is emphasized [121].

Treatments in MS include treatment of attacks, disease-modifying treatments, and management of various symptoms and complications. The aim of relapse treatment is to shorten the recovery time in the acute period, to reduce the severity of the attack, and to control, reduce, or cope with the symptoms that occur in the attack [122, 123]. Early diagnosis is very important in controlling the disability and its negative effects on quality of life. Planning interventions for individuals diagnosed with MS from a holistic perspective requires understanding the coping strategies used by these patients as well as defining the psychological symptoms that have been identified [124].

1.7 Brain Tumors

A mass created by uncontrollably multiplying and growing brain cells is called a brain tumor [125]. Not only brain tumors are difficult to diagnose and cure, but they are also ranked among the most serious and potentially fatal illnesses [126].

Brain tumors can be seen as primary, metastatic (secondary), benign or malignant [127]. Primary brain tumors (PBT) are tumors originating from cells and structures in the brain [128]. Secondary brain tumors or metastatic brain tumors start anywhere in the body and spread to the brain [129]. A benign brain tumor grows within the limited skull, and pressurizes the surrounding tissues, disrupts venous and arterial circulation, causing local symptoms [130]. A malignant brain tumor grows rapidly and spreads to the tissues of the brain and spinal cord. However, spread outside the CNS is rare [131]. Neoplastic structures consist of heterogeneous cells. These cells differ in their immunogenicity, growth rate, and tissue invasive potential, and are generally very aggressive. Generally, the tumor cell uses a hematogenous route to spread. It passes through the tissues adjacent to the vascular bed and through the lymph. When they reach the lymph node, they are subjected to a mechanical barrier and filter, from where they drain into the venous system. Since there is no lymphatic system in the brain, all metastases must come through the internal carotid artery, vertebral artery or blood [132].

1.7.1 Meningeal Tumors (Meningiomas)

Meningiomas usually arise from arachnoid cells in the meninges [133]. Meningioma are benign, highly vascular tumors that do not infiltrate the brain tissue and can be easily removed by surgery [134]. Treatment of meningioma includes surgery, chemotherapy, and radiotherapy. In its treatment, partial resection is sometimes performed in order to preserve functions, and radiotherapy is used in slowly growing tumors. In addition, stereotactic surgery is used in regions such as sphenoid, parasagittal, orbital, tentorial, or clivus [129].

1.7.2 Brain Lymphomas

Lymphomas are primary tumors of the lymphoreticular system and are divided into two as Hodgkin lymphoma and non-Hodgkin lymphoma. Hodgkin lymphoma usually presents as lymph node involvement, and extranodal involvement is more common in non-Hodgkin lymphomas [135]. CNS lymphomas are divided into two groups as primary and secondary. While lymphomas originating from the brain, medulla spinalis, and meninges are called primary brain lymphomas, lymphomas caused by a systemic lymphoma involving the CNS are called secondary brain lymphomas. In order for a lymphoma to be called primary brain lymphoma, there must be no involvement other than CNS at the time of diagnosis [136].

While brain lymphomas are usually seen as leptomeningeal involvement, brain parenchymal infiltration is rare and usually seen in advanced stages. Primary brain lymphomas are the second most common extranodal lymphomas that can develop as a result of immunodeficiency in organ transplantation and autoimmune diseases, use of immunosuppressant drugs, AIDS (acquired immunodeficiency syndrome) and other causes such as congenital immunodeficiencies and Hodgkin lymphoma treatment. Brain metastases can be seen in approximately 1/3 of systemic cancer patients [137].

1.7.3 Glioma

Gliomas are tumors originating from neuroglia and are grouped into four stages. Stages I and II are low-grade tumors, and III and IV are high-stage tumors [138]:

- *Stage I:* Tumors that grow slowly and show the most distant feature from the natural structure.
- *Stage II:* Tumors that grow slowly, are adherent to adjacent tissue, have the ability to invade, and can recur with higher grades of malignancy.
- *Stage III:* Tumors in which abnormal cells actively proliferate and can infiltrate into healthy tissue.
- *Stage IV:* Tumors that spread quickly and immediately invade nearby tissues. As a result of the tumors' rapid growth, new blood vessels are formed, and the center region exhibits necrosis. This type is the most malignant.

These neuroepithelial tumors also have different sub-titles such as Ependymoma, Glioblastoma, Medulloblastoma, and Oligodendroglioma [138].

Ependymomas are gliomas that originate from ependymal cells in the wall of the ventricles, grow inside the ventricle, and adhere to the brain tissue [133]. 70% of ependymomas occur in the fourth ventricle and cause deterioration in balance, walking, muscle coordination, and especially fine motor skills. Shunt intervention is useful in the treatment of hydrocephalus, which develops when the tumor obstructs the CSF circulation pathways. When ependymoma occurs anatomically in the brain stem or upper spinal cord, it causes neck pain in patients [133].

Glioblastoma multiforme (GBM) is the most common and aggressive malignant primary CNS tumor in adults [139]. GBM accounts for approximately 70% of all adult brain tumors [140]. Standard treatment includes surgical resection with radiation therapy and temozolomide chemotherapy, which does not improve overall patient survival [141]. Despite maximum treatment, in the majority of cases, cancer relapses. High resistance to established treatments, and the blood brain-barrier resistance to the diverse types of medicine are some of the factors contributing to the difficulty of the treatment [142, 143]. At the population level, primary GBM develops more frequently in males, while secondary GBM occurs more frequently in females. Primary and secondary GBM constitute different disease subtypes. People are affected at different ages and occur through different genetic pathways [144]. There are clinical and cytogenetic differences between primary and secondary GBM tissues. On a genetic basis, TP53 mutation is frequently encountered and can be detected at an early stage [145]. Primary and secondary GBM cannot be distinguished morphologically, and both have a poor prognosis regardless of the patient's age. As in all cancers, tumor cells belonging to GBM tissue show an increase in the activation of life signals, angiogenesis, uncontrolled proliferation, tissue invasion, and resistance to apoptosis [146].

Oligodendroglioma develops from neoplastic oligodendrocytes responsible for myelin production [147]. Oligodendroglioma is low stage, anaplastic, and about half is associated with astrocytoma and is defined as a mixed type. About one-third of oligodendrogliomas show malignant degeneration, which is then called oligodendroblastoma, but rarely becomes GBM [133]. Most of these tumors occur deep in the white matter of the frontal and temporal lobes, but also in the cerebrum, third ventricle, brain stem, cerebellum, and spinal cord. These tumors grow slowly, but at the time of clinical manifestation of symptoms, they are quite large, well-defined and can be diagnosed by X-ray. Partial removal of the tumor and radiotherapy are used together in the treatment of oligodendroglioma [148].

1.8 Neuropsychiatric Disorders

Neuropsychology is the branch of science that deals with how psychological phenomena correspond to the systems in the brain. As a sub-branch, clinical/applied neuropsychology deals with how neurological disorders in the brain affect the psychological functionality and how this functionality can be corrected through neuropsychological rehabilitation [149]. The brain-behavior relationship is quite complex [150]. No psychiatric disease has a specific localization, but loops involving certain neuroanatomical regions can be mentioned. It is possible to see relatively similar psychiatric and behavioral "symptoms" in diseases involving certain regions of the brain [151].

Cognitive, emotional, and behavioral functioning of the individual should all be considered while discussing neuropsychological functionality. For instance, a person with any kind of damage to the prefrontal cortex, which is part of the brain's frontal lobe, will have issues with both cognitive and psychosocial functioning [152]. While patients with frontal lobe damage can perform close to healthy individuals in traditional neuropsychological tests, they may have difficulties in daily life activities. The fact that one's intelligence and knowledge are preserved and cannot be used to regulate their thoughts and behaviors is called the "frontal lobe paradox" [153]. In addition to the classical tests in neuropsychological evaluation, it is important to measure the skills of the person in daily life activities that require cognitive ability, in creating a more accurate neuropsychological evaluation profile. Unfortunately, there are no psychotropics specially developed for the treatment of psychiatric diseases. Although the symptom profiles of the diseases differ from the primary psychiatric disorders, there is still an obligation to treat the indications with drugs that are the primary psychiatric diseases [151].

1.8.1 Schizophrenia (SCZ)

Schizophrenia (SCZ) is a mental disorder characterized by symptoms such as delusions, hallucinations, behavioral and speech disorders, and lack of emotion, distorting one's thoughts, actions, expression of emotions, and perception of reality [154]. It is a heterogeneous disorder associated with metabolic changes, hormonal regulation, and immune status [155]. Subtypes of SCZ, which were included in the psychiatric diagnosis classifications in the past, are not included in the new classifications due to their limited diagnostic stability, low reliability and weak validity, and are currently considered as a single disease [156]. Although there are several risk factors for SCZ, the exact cause has not yet been determined. There is strong evidence of genetic causes. It is common to think that stressful events play a role in the emergence of the disease. Although certain schizophrenic brains show structural abnormalities, particularly in the temporal lobes, this is insufficient to explain the illness [157]. Initial studies investigating the genetic etiology of SCZ focused on family, twin, and adoption studies. With these studies, the role of heredity in the etiology of SCZ has been confirmed as a risk factor. According to research results, while genetics has a major role in the etiology of SCZ with a heritability rate of 81%, it has been stated that the environmental effect is around 11% [158].

Since SCZ is a chronic disease that affects every aspect of a patient's life, the goal of treatment is to reduce or eliminate symptoms, increase the quality of patient life and improve social adaptation, and reduce the devastating effects of the disease [159]. Today, with an appropriate treatment method, approximately 25% of SCZ patients show great improvement and continue their social lives, and 50% show moderate and good improvement and continue their social lives relatively independently or with support [160]. First-episode SCZ patients are typically hospitalized. Despite regular antipsychotic treatment after being treated and discharged, the probability of having a second attack within the first year is approximately 35%–40% [161]. Apart from the explanation provided for the symptoms, factors such as age, personality traits, education level, socioeconomic status, disease severity and type, family and social environment structure, and the quality of available health services are crucial when assessing psychotic symptoms and seeking assistance [162]. The role of psychosocial treatment in the treatment of SCZ patients is increasing. Psychosocial treatments are beneficial for social recovery, whereas antipsychotics reduce the symptoms of the illness, hospitalizations, and the chance of recurrence, as well as the abilities the patient loses [162, 163].

1.8.2 Bipolar Disorder (BD)

Bipolar Disorder (BD) is a chronic disease that requires serious and continuous treatment, and lasts a lifetime. Since it is far more common than anticipated and has a high fatality rate due to high morbidity and suicide risk, it is a significant public health concern. It negatively affects the lives of both patients and those around them, and, causes significant disability [164]. The prevalence of bipolar disorder in men is 9–15/100,000 and in women it is 7.4–30/100,000 [165, 166]. 69% of these patients cannot be diagnosed at the time of their first visit to a psychiatrist [167]. The high number of comorbid conditions is one of the most important factors that makes diagnosis difficult. On average, it takes approximately 10 years from the onset of symptoms to a diagnosis. Similar to SCZ, whose etiology is still unknown, BD is also attributed to the same biological components that are to blame for SCZ [168]. The person with BD often experiences mood swings that range from highs to lows to highs, often with periods of normal mood in between [169, 170]. SCZ and BD affect more than 2% of the world's population. These two diseases greatly affect the quality of life of people, and both disorders are characterized by similar symptoms such as thought, mood, perception, and behavior disorders [163].

One of the steps in the treatment of the disease, which is at least as important as the acute period treatment, is preventive treatment. Preventing relapses, eliminating subthreshold symptoms, and maintaining patients' premorbid levels of functionality are the main goals of preventive treatment. For this purpose, lithium and some antiepileptics (valproic acid, carbamazepine, lamotrigine) are used as mood stabilizers. Recently, atypical antipsychotics have begun to be preferred by clinicians in preventive treatment [171].

1.8.3 Attention Deficit Hyperactivity Disorder (ADHD)

Attention deficit hyperactivity disorder (ADHD) is a neuropsychiatric disorder that begins before the age of seven and presents with inattention, hyperactivity and impulsivity. In the past, ADHD was considered a specific disorder, limited to childhood, resolving in adolescence, and having a developmental delay in behavioral controls [172]. ADHD diagnosis is now widely accepted for both children and adults. Whether in childhood or adulthood, ADHD affects not only patients but also their environment, families, and parents. In the presence of ADHD, smoking, and substance abuse, legal problems, poor peer relations, loss of self-confidence, low school and work success, and psychiatric comorbidity are observed in adolescents and young adults who are under threat in terms of risky health behaviors. In these people, risky behaviors such as accidents, suicide attempts, and violence are determined and evaluated [173]. People with ADHD have cognitive impairments similar to people with traumatic frontal lobe damage, but they do not exhibit obvious pathology. As a result of poor executive functions, frontal lobe disinhibition occurs, and individuals with ADHD remain risk-taking adolescents rather than adults [174].

Neuropsychological testing of patients with ADHD shows problems with response inhibition. The capacity to suppress the expected physical or mental response has the effect of keeping impulsive responses in check. The neuropsychological impairment in adults with ADHD increases as cognitive needs increase or as tasks become more complex. This explains why adult patients seek treatment when challenging changes occur in their lives [175]. Dopamine and noradrenaline are involved in related cognitive functions that require adequate arousal and focus, such as motivation, interest, and learning [173]. Prefrontal noradrenergic pathways mediate energy, fatigue, motivation, and interest processes, as well as their role in maintaining and focusing attention. Mesocortical dopamine projection is important for verbal fluency, sequential learning, alertness for executive functions, maintaining and focusing attention, prioritizing behaviors, and adjusting behaviors according to social behavior patterns. Arousal is usually associated with an increase in dopamine and noradrenaline, and inattention reflects the inadequacy of the neurotransmitters mentioned in these pathways [82].

1.8.4 Major Depressive Disorders (MDD)

Major depressive disorders (MDD) are syndromes that include mood disorders, symptoms, and symptom clusters. These diseases can last weeks to months, drastically alter a person's ordinary functioning, and have a tendency to reoccur on a regular or cyclical basis [176]. MDD is one of the most studied depressive disorders [177]. One of the syndromes that determines the clinical appearance of mood disorders is depression. The word depression is an emotional experience that includes the feelings of grief used in meanings such as collapse, feeling sad, and decrease in functional and vital activity [178]. Every similar emotional state that arises should not be considered as depression. Depression imposes a heavy burden on society in terms of treatment costs, and these are due to expenditures such as treatment process, insufficiency in functionality and suicide [179]. Depression is typified by depressive and hopeless feelings, as well as psychomotor slowdown, which is a lack of energy in both the mental and physical domains and is usually expressed as an inability to enjoy routine activities and once-pleasurable situations as well as a loss of interest in them. It shows itself as a reduction in mental content, a noticeable slowdown in cognitive performance, and diminished functionality [178]. MDD (unipolar depression) is the most common mood disorder. Although the course of acute episodes is good in most patients, relapses persist throughout life in 1 of 3 patients with MDD, and residual symptoms of varying degrees are observed in the period between seizures [178]. MDD can be seen at any age, but it is more common in the middle ages, especially between the ages of 40–50. However, in many studies, the mean age of onset was found to be in the late 20s [180]. The age at which MDD manifests itself is significant due to its association with worsening social and occupational functioning, a decline in quality of life, an increase in depressive episodes, and the severity of symptoms, as well as a rise in suicide attempts and comorbid psychotic and physical illnesses. The risk of MDD is higher in singles, separated, widowed and divorced than married people [180, 181].

Changes in neuronal and glial cell density and size have been reported in many different frontolimbic brain regions such as the prefrontal cortex, orbitofrontal cortex, anterior cingulate cortex, amygdala, and hippocampus in depression [182]. Ventricular enlargement has been observed in patients with depression by CT and MRI studies, but these findings were not considered specific [183]. It is suggested that SPECT and PET findings obtained from depression patients can provide information about depression subtypes or can be used in the differential diagnosis of treatment-resistant and complicated cases [184].

The analysis of the hereditary component of MDD in individuals has revealed that, in comparison to the general population, there is a greater likelihood of a patient's first-generation relatives receiving a diagnosis of depression [185]. Various therapies and medications are used today in the treatment of depression. Electroconvulsive therapy is a technique utilized to treat depression. A single type of therapy method will not be sufficient to alleviate the symptoms of the disorder, as the causes of depression are not observed in the same way in every individual, and individuals respond differently to the treatment methods applied [186].

1.8.5 Autism Spectrum Disorder (ASD)

Autism spectrum disorder (ASD) is a neurodevelopmental condition that manifests in early childhood. The term "autism" was first used by Swiss psychiatrist Eugen Bleur in 1911. The term "autistic", which Bleur defines as "adult schizophrenia", comes from the Greek word "otos" and means "self". Bleur used this term to describe the negative behavior of individuals who completely isolate themselves from the outside world and are not interested in what is happening there [187]. ASD symptoms vary depending on developmental level and chronological age. A newborn with autism is different from other babies and is described as a well-behaved baby. He acts as if he does not need his mother, and is indifferent to her closeness, distance, presence, absence, and strangers [188]. Children diagnosed with ASD have deficiencies in eye-to-eye communication, understanding social stimuli, using body language, and facial expressions. They exhibit problematic behaviors due to these deficiencies [189]. Delay in speech is often the first symptom that attracts attention in the families of children with ASD [190]. Although the same diagnostic criteria were applied, the initial estimate of the frequency of autism was roughly 4/10,000 in the 1940s. However, throughout the past few decades, there have been significant increases in the prevalence of autism [191]. In large-scale studies, the frequency of autism has been reported to be 1–2% [192]. This increase in autism cases appears to be more closely associated with factors like improved autism awareness and recognition, easy access to health services, geographic differences, the inclusion of mild cases without intellectual disability in the diagnosis, and earlier diagnosis ages, even though the role of risk factors in the increase of incidence of autism cannot be excluded [192]. In clinical studies, ASD was found to be 4–6 times more common in boys than girls, and in community samples, it was 2–3 times more common in boys [191]. Early diagnosis of ASD is of great importance in terms of the path to be followed in the treatment process of the disease. When children are correctly guided through early diagnosis, they benefit more from the treatment and education process than other autistic individuals due to their tendency [193].

Common treatments used in ASD include behavioral training programs, floor play therapy, pharmacological treatments, and alternative treatments (such as allergy, diet, occupational and emotional integration therapy). The symptoms of individuals with ASD are controlled through lifelong education programs and they are no different from their peers when they reach adolescence. However, for these treatment methods to play an effective role with early diagnosis, awareness-raising activities about autism are a must. In recent years, studies and research on early diagnosis of autism have gained momentum, and attention has been drawn to various factors that reduce the age of diagnosis. The fact that the mysterious nature of the disease has rapidly attracted experts interested in this subject, the increasing number of studies conducted, the importance society attaches to quality communication, and the technological requirements of the information age are just some of the reasons that enable early diagnosis [194].

Many genetic diseases such as Fragile X Syndrome, Tuberous Sclerosis, Phenyl Ketonuria, Williams Syndrome, Cornelia de Lange Syndrome, Cohen Syndrome, and WAGR Syndrome are also observed in individuals with ASD. 44% of children with Tuberous Sclerosis and 12–21% of children with Fragile X Syndrome (FXS) have autistic symptoms [195]. Medical disorders such as Fragile X Syndrome and Rett Syndrome are also called "secondary autism", and 5–10% of cases of ASD are accompanied by secondary autism [187]. The occurrence of ASD together with genetic disorders suggests that two separate genes that lead to two separate disorders are closely related to each other [196]. Although the genetic effects are pronounced in the etiology of ASD, it does not seem possible to talk about a genetically based treatment method at present.

Autism is a lifelong disease that has no cure. However, alternative therapies and treatments may be used to reduce some problems that occur in individuals with ASD. Among these treatments are acupuncture, cleansing therapy, gluten and casein-free diet, animal therapy, hyperbaric oxygen therapy, medication, meditation, neurofeedback, art therapy, and vitamin and mineral support [196] There are no medications yet developed to reduce or eliminate the core symptoms of ASD. However, there are psychotropic medications used for conditions such as inattention, impulsivity/hyperactivity, sleep problems, anxiety, agitation, aggression, and repetitive and self-harming behaviors seen in individuals with ASD [197].

1.9 Concluding Remarks

Since the brain is the center of the body, the nervous system is in charge of all bodily functions, and even the smallest neural error can result in a variety of diseases at different intensities. This chapter explains the structure of the brain, various brain disorders and cancer kinds, how these diseases are diagnosed, and available treatment options. It's crucial to give the best possible care, starting with an early diagnosis and focusing on psychological well-being before moving on to medical interventions.

Bibliography

[1] S. Herculano-Houzel, "The human brain in numbers: A linearly scaled-up primate brain," *Frontiers in Human Neuroscience*, vol. 3, 2009.

[2] A. Beretta, "The language-learning brain," 2009.

[3] N. P. Friedman and T. W. Robbins, "The role of prefrontal cortex in cognitive control and executive function," *Neuropsychopharmacology*, vol. 47, pp. 72–89, 2021.

[4] L. C. de Souza, H. C. Guimarães, A. L. Teixeira, *et al.*, "Frontal lobe neurology and the creative mind," *Frontiers in Psychology*, vol. 5, 2014.

[5] J. Moini, J. Koenitzer, and A. LoGalbo, *Global Emergency of Mental Disorders.* 2021.

[6] R. Wlodkowski and M.Ginsberg, *Enhancing adult motivation to learn: A comprehensive guide for teaching all adults.* 2019.

[7] S. Shipp, "Structure and function of the cerebral cortex," *Current Biology*, vol. 17, pp. R443–R449, 2007.

[8] C. R. Brewin, J. D. Gregory, M. G. Lipton, *et al.*, "Intrusive images in psychological disorders," *Psychological Review*, vol. 117, pp. 210–232, 2010.

[9] A. Imam, A. Bhagwandin, M. S. Ajao, *et al.*, "The brain of the tree pangolin (manis tricuspis). v. the diencephalon and hypothalamus," *Journal of Comparative Neurology*, vol. 527, pp. 2413–2439, 2019.

[10] S. Younis, A. Hougaard, R. Noseda, *et al.*, "Current understanding of thalamic structure and function in migraine," *Cephalalgia*, vol. 39, pp. 1675–1682, 2018.

[11] V. J. Kumar, C. F. Beckmann, K. Scheffler, *et al.*, "Relay and higher-order thalamic nuclei show an intertwined functional association with cortical-networks," *Communications Biology*, vol. 5, 2022.

[12] F. Capone, S. Collorone, R. Cortese, *et al.*, "Fatigue in multiple sclerosis: The role of thalamus," *Multiple Sclerosis Journal*, vol. 26, pp. 16–26, 2019.

[13] U. Feldt-Rasmussen, G. Effraimidis, and M. Klose, "The hypothalamus-pituitary-thyroid (hpt)-axis and its role in physiology and pathophysiology of other hypothalamus-pituitary functions," *Molecular and Cellular Endocrinology*, vol. 525, 2021.

[14] B. Liu, K. Zhou, X. Wu, *et al.*, "Foxg1 deletion impairs the development of the epithalamus," *Molecular Brain*, vol. 11, 2018.

[15] M. A. Fernández-Gil, R. Palacios-Bote, M. Leo-Barahona, *et al.*, "Anatomy of the brainstem: a gaze into the stem of life.," *Seminars in ultrasound, CT, and MR*, vol. 31 3, pp. 196–219, 2010.

[16] S. J. Yong, "Persistent brainstem dysfunction in long-covid: A hypothesis," *ACS Chemical Neuroscience*, vol. 12, pp. 573–580, 2021.

[17] R. Ambalavanar, Y. Tanaka, W. S. Selbie, *et al.*, "Neuronal activation in the medulla oblongata during selective elicitation of the laryngeal adductor response.," *Journal of neurophysiology*, vol. 92 5, pp. 2920–2932, 2004.

[18] D.-D. Rosmus, C. A. Lange, F. Ludwig, *et al.*, "The role of osteopontin in microglia biology: Current concepts and future perspectives," *Biomedicines*, vol. 10, 2022.

[19] S. Benghanem, A. Mazeraud, E. Azabou, *et al.*, "Brainstem dysfunction in critically ill patients," *Critical Care*, vol. 24, 2020.

[20] M. King, C. R. Hernandez-Castillo, R. A. Poldrack, *et al.*, "Functional boundaries in the human cerebellum revealed by a multi-domain task battery," *Nature Neuroscience*, vol. 22, pp. 1371–1378, 2019.

[21] F. A. C. Azevedo, L. R. Carvalho, L. T. Grinberg, *et al.*, "Equal numbers of neuronal and nonneuronal cells make the human brain an isometrically scaled-up primate brain," *Journal of Comparative Neurology*, vol. 513, 2009.

[22] P. Wolfe, "Brain matters: Translating research into classroom practice, 2nd edition," 2001.

[23] F. Uğur, "Evaluation of activities in secondary school level turkish workbooks according to types of memory and revised bloom's taxonomy," *International Education Studies*, 2019.

[24] D. O. Hebb, "The role of neurological ideas in psychology," *Journal of personality*, vol. 20 1, pp. 39–55, 1951.

[25] P. W. Burgess and J. S. Simons, "Theories of frontal lobe executive function: Clinical applications," 2012.

[26] S. Dehaene, "Reading in the brain: The science and evolution of a human invention," 2009.

[27] B. E. Kolb, R. L. Gibb, and T. E. Robinson, "Brain plasticity and behavior," *Current Directions in Psychological Science*, vol. 12, pp. 1–5, 2003.

[28] R. L. Buckner and L. M. DiNicola, "The brain's default network: updated anatomy, physiology and evolving insights," *Nature Reviews Neuroscience*, vol. 20, pp. 593–608, 2019.

[29] R. Hitzemann, P. Darakjian, N. A. R. Walter, *et al.*, "Introduction to sequencing the brain transcriptome.," *International review of neurobiology*, vol. 116, pp. 1–19, 2014.

[30] R. Daneman and A. Prat, "The blood-brain barrier," *Cold Spring Harbor perspectives in biology*, vol. 7 1, p. a020412, 2015.

[31] M. I. Teixeira, C. M. Lopes, M. H. Amaral, *et al.*, "Current insights on lipid nanocarrier-assisted drug delivery in the treatment of neurodegenerative diseases.," *European journal of pharmaceutics and biopharmaceutics: official journal of Arbeitsgemeinschaft fur Pharmazeutische Verfahrenstechnik e. V*, 2020.

[32] H. Scheiblich, M. I. Trombly, A. Ramírez, *et al.*, "Neuroimmune connections in aging and neurodegenerative diseases," *Trends in immunology*, 2020.

[33] T. Cassano, R. Villani, L. Pace, *et al.*, "From cannabis sativa to cannabidiol: Promising therapeutic candidate for the treatment of neurodegenerative diseases," *Frontiers in Pharmacology*, vol. 11, 2020.

[34] S. Guerreiro, A. Privat, L. Bressac, *et al.*, "Cd38 in neurodegeneration and neuroinflammation," *Cells*, vol. 9, 2020.

[35] L. Gan, M. R. Cookson, L. Petrucelli, *et al.*, "Converging pathways in neurodegeneration, from genetics to mechanisms," *Nature Neuroscience*, vol. 21, pp. 1300–1309, 2018.

[36] L. K. Wareham, S. A. Liddelow, S. Temple, *et al.*, "Solving neurodegeneration: common mechanisms and strategies for new treatments," *Molecular Neurodegeneration*, vol. 17, 2022.

[37] S. Gilman and D. Pushkar, "Subject–volume 11 - number 1-6, january - december 1996," *American Journal of Alzheimer's Disease and Other Dementias*, vol. 12, pp. 45–47, 1997.

[38] M. T. Koyun, S. Şirin, S. A. Erdem, *et al.*, "Pyocyanin isolated from pseudomonas aeruginosa: Characterization, biological activity and its role in cancer and neurodegenerative diseases," *Brazilian Archives of Biology and Technology*, 2022.

[39] B. J. Kelley and R. C. Petersen, "Alzheimer's disease and mild cognitive impairment," 2009.

[40] M. K. Samanta, B. Wilson, K. Santhi, *et al.*, "Alzheimer disease and its management: A review," *American Journal of Therapeutics*, vol. 13, pp. 516–526, 2006.

[41] F. Aragón, M. A. Zea-Sevilla, J. Montero, *et al.*, "Oral health in alzheimer's disease: a multicenter case-control study," *Clinical Oral Investigations*, vol. 22, pp. 3061–3070, 2018.

[42] N. B. Mutlu, Z. Değim, S. Yılmaz, *et al.*, "New perspective for the treatment of alzheimer diseases: Liposomal rivastigmine formulations," *Drug Development and Industrial Pharmacy*, vol. 37, pp. 775–789, 2011.

[43] M. Racchi, M. Mazzucchelli, E. Porrello, *et al.*, "Acetylcholinesterase inhibitors: novel activities of old molecules," *Pharmacological research*, vol. 50 4, pp. 441–451, 2004.

[44] P. M. Arabi, V. Deepa, D. Susheel, *et al.*, "Early detection and characterization of alzheimer's using medical image analysis," 2018.

[45] S. P. Cass, "Alzheimer's disease and exercise: A literature review," *Current Sports Medicine Reports*, vol. 16, p. 19–22, 2017.

[46] H. Öhman, N. Savikko, T. E. Strandberg, *et al.*, "Effects of exercise on functional performance and fall rate in subjects with mild or advanced alzheimer's disease: Secondary analyses of a randomized controlled study," *Dementia and Geriatric Cognitive Disorders*, vol. 41, pp. 233–241, 2016.

[47] A. U. Khan, M. Akram, M. Daniyal, *et al.*, "Awareness and current knowledge of parkinson's disease: a neurodegenerative disorder," *International Journal of Neuroscience*, vol. 129, pp. 55–93, 2018.

[48] M. Rodríguez-Violante, A. Cervantes-Arriaga, S. Fahn, *et al.*, "Two-hundred years later: Is parkinson's disease a single defined entity?," *Revista de investigacion clinica; organo del Hospital de Enfermedades de la Nutricion*, vol. 69 6, pp. 308–313, 2017.

[49] L. de Lau, P. C. Giesbergen, M. C. de Rijk, *et al.*, "Incidence of parkinsonism and parkinson disease in a general population," *Neurology*, vol. 63, pp. 1240–1244, 2004.

[50] E. R. Dorsey, R. Constantinescu, R. Constantinescu, *et al.*, "Projected number of people with parkinson disease in the most populous nations, 2005 through 2030," *Neurology*, vol. 68, pp. 384–386, 2007.

[51] C. W. Olanow, J. H. Kordower, A. E. Lang, *et al.*, "Dopaminergic transplantation for parkinson's disease: Current status and future prospects," *Annals of Neurology*, vol. 66, 2009.

[52] J. Tran, H. Anastacio, and C. Bardy, "Genetic predispositions of parkinson's disease revealed in patient-derived brain cells," *NPJ Parkinson's Disease*, vol. 6, 2020.

[53] C. Blauwendraat, M. A. Nalls, and A. B. Singleton, "The genetic architecture of parkinson's disease," *The Lancet Neurology*, vol. 19, pp. 170–178, 2020.

[54] L. V. Kalia, S. K. Kalia, and A. E. Lang, "Disease-modifying strategies for parkinson's disease," *Movement Disorders*, vol. 30, 2015.

[55] J. Jankovic, "Parkinson's disease: Clinical features and diagnosis," *J Neurol Neurosurg Psychiatry*, vol. 79, pp. 368–376, 2008.

[56] J. M. Miyasaki, W. R. W. Martin, O. Suchowersky, *et al.*, "Practice parameter: Initiation of treatment for parkinson's disease: An evidence-based review," *Neurology*, vol. 58, pp. 11–17, 2002.

[57] E. Tolosa, A. Garrido, S. W. Scholz, *et al.*, "Challenges in the diagnosis of parkinson's disease," *The Lancet Neurology*, vol. 20, pp. 385–397, 2021.

[58] N. R. McFarland, "Diagnostic approach to atypical parkinsonian syndromes," *CONTINUUM: Lifelong Learning in Neurology*, vol. 22, p. 1117–1142, 2016.

[59] C. Váradi, "Clinical features of parkinson's disease: The evolution of critical symptoms," *Biology*, vol. 9, 2020.

[60] J. Jankovic and A. S. Kapadia, "Functional decline in parkinson disease.," *Archives of neurology*, vol. 58 10, pp. 1611–5, 2001.

[61] C. Raza, R. Anjum, and N. U. A. Shakeel, "Parkinson's disease: Mechanisms, translational models and management strategies," *Life Sciences*, vol. 226, p. 77–90, 2019.

[62] T. Endo, N. Yoshikawa, H. Fujimura, *et al.*, "Parkinsonian rigidity depends on the velocity of passive joint movement," *Parkinson's Disease*, vol. 2015, 2015.

[63] F. Bloch, J. L. Houeto, S. T. du Montcel, *et al.*, "Parkinson's disease with camptocormia," *Journal of Neurology, Neurosurgery & Psychiatry*, vol. 77, pp. 1223–1228, 2006.

[64] D. K. Kwon, M. Kwatra, J. Wang, *et al.*, "Levodopa-induced dyskinesia in parkinson's disease: Pathogenesis and emerging treatment strategies," *Cells*, vol. 11, 2022.

[65] M. W. I. M. Horstink, E. Tolosa, U. Bonuccelli, *et al.*, "Review of the therapeutic management of parkinson's disease. report of a joint task force of the european federation of neurological societies (efns) and the movement disorder society-european section (mds-es). part ii: late (complicated) parkinson's disease," *European Journal of Neurology*, vol. 13, 2006.

[66] N. Tambasco, M. Romoli, and P. Calabresi, "Levodopa in parkinson's disease: Current status and future developments," *Current Neuropharmacology*, vol. 16, pp. 1239–1252, 2017.

[67] D. Nyholm and H. Lennernäs, "Irregular gastrointestinal drug absorption in parkinson's disease," *Expert Opinion on Drug Metabolism & Toxicology*, vol. 4, pp. 193–203, 2008.

[68] C. Zhuo, X. Zhu, R.-H. Jiang, *et al.*, "Comparison for efficacy and tolerability among ten drugs for treatment of parkinson's disease: A network meta-analysis," *Scientific Reports*, vol. 7, 2017.

[69] P. Huot, T. H. Johnston, J. B. Koprich, *et al.*, "The pharmacology of l-dopa-induced dyskinesia in parkinson's disease," *Pharmacological Reviews*, vol. 65, pp. 171–222, 2013.

[70] G. A. Demaagd and A. Philip, "Parkinson's disease and its management: Part 1: Disease entity, risk factors, pathophysiology, clinical presentation, and diagnosis," *P & T: a peer-reviewed journal for formulary management*, vol. 40 8, pp. 504–32, 2015.

[71] O. Rascol, M. Fabbri, and W. Poewe, "Amantadine in the treatment of parkinson's disease and other movement disorders," *The Lancet Neurology*, vol. 20, pp. 1048–1056, 2021.

[72] J. J. Ferreira, R. Katzenschlager, B. R. Bloem, *et al.*, "Summary of the recommendations of the efns/mds-es review on therapeutic management of parkinson's disease," *European Journal of Neurology*, vol. 20, 2013.

[73] P. Maiti, J. Manna, and G. L. Dunbar, "Current understanding of the molecular mechanisms in parkinson's disease: Targets for potential treatments," *Translational Neurodegeneration*, vol. 6, 2017.

[74] R. Katzenschlager, C. Sampaio, J. Costa, *et al.*, "Anticholinergics for symptomatic management of parkinson's disease," *The Cochrane database of systematic reviews*, vol. 2, p. CD003735, 2002.

[75] L. M. Fox, K. Kim, C. W. Johnson, *et al.*, "Huntington's disease pathogenesis is modified in vivo by alfy/wdfy3 and selective macroautophagy," *Neuron*, vol. 105, pp. 813–821.e6, 2019.

[76] M. D. Thompson, W. M. Burnham, and D. E. C. Cole, "The g protein-coupled receptors: Pharmacogenetics and disease," *Critical Reviews in Clinical Laboratory Sciences*, vol. 42, pp. 311–389, 2005.

[77] F. Zhang, L. Niu, X. Liu, *et al.*, "Rapid eye movement sleep behavior disorder and neurodegenerative diseases: An update," *Aging and Disease*, vol. 11, pp. 315–326, 2020.

[78] A. Semaka, S. Creighton, S. C. Warby, *et al.*, "Predictive testing for huntington disease: interpretation and significance of intermediate alleles," *Clinical Genetics*, vol. 70, 2006.

[79] M. D. Lezak, D. Howieson, D. W. Loring, *et al.*, "Neuropsychological assessment, 4th ed.," 2004.

[80] M. P. Mattson and T. V. Arumugam, "Hallmarks of brain aging: Adaptive and pathological modification by metabolic states," *Cell metabolism*, vol. 276, pp. 1176–1199, 2018.

[81] P. McColgan and S. J. Tabrizi, "Huntington's disease: a clinical review," *European Journal of Neurology*, vol. 25, 2018.

[82] F. Saudou and S. Humbert, "The biology of huntingtin," *Neuron*, vol. 89, pp. 910–926, 2016.

[83] S. A. Johnson, J. C. Stout, A. C. Solomon, *et al.*, "Beyond disgust: impaired recognition of negative emotions prior to diagnosis in huntington's disease," *Brain: a journal of neurology*, vol. 130 Pt 7, pp. 1732–44, 2007.

[84] J. Y. Li, N. Popovic, and P. Brundin, "The use of the r6 transgenic mouse models of huntington's disease in attempts to develop novel therapeutic strategies," *NeuroRX*, vol. 2, pp. 447–464, 2005.

[85] J. G. Fiedorowicz, J. A. Mills, A. Ruggle, *et al.*, "Suicidal behavior in prodromal huntington disease," *Neurodegenerative Diseases*, vol. 8, pp. 483–490, 2011.

[86] B. J. Sadock and V. A. Sadock, "Kaplan and sadock's comprehensive textbook of psychiatry," 2017.

[87] K. E. Anderson, E. van Duijn, D. Craufurd, *et al.*, "Clinical management of neuropsychiatric symptoms of huntington disease: Expert-based consensus guidelines on agitation, anxiety, apathy, psychosis and sleep disorders," *Journal of Huntington's Disease*, vol. 7, pp. 355–366, 2018.

[88] A. J. Hughes, S. E. Daniel, Y. Ben-Shlomo, *et al.*, "The accuracy of diagnosis of parkinsonian syndromes in a specialist movement disorder service," *Brain: a journal of neurology*, vol. 125 Pt 4, pp. 861–70, 2002.

[89] J. S. Paulsen, "Functional imaging in huntington's disease," *Experimental Neurology*, vol. 216, pp. 272–277, 2009.

[90] L. S. Ishihara, D. Oliveri, and E. J. Wild, "Neuropsychiatric comorbidities in huntington's and parkinson's disease: A united states claims database analysis," *Annals of Clinical and Translational Neurology*, vol. 8, pp. 126–137, 2020.

[91] M. Groves, "The highly anxious individual presenting for huntington disease-predictive genetic testing: the psychiatrist's role in assessment and counseling," *Handbook of clinical neurology*, vol. 144, pp. 99–105, 2017.

[92] T.-B. R. Wahlin, "To know or not to know: a review of behaviour and suicidal ideation in preclinical huntington's disease," *Patient education and counseling*, vol. 65 3, pp. 279–87, 2007.

[93] O. Goldstein, O. Nayshool, B. Nefussy, *et al.*, "Optn 691_692insag is a founder mutation causing recessive als and increased risk in heterozygotes," *Neurology*, vol. 86, pp. 446–453, 2016.

[94] M. H. Hastings and M. Goedert, "Circadian clocks and neurodegenerative diseases: time to aggregate?," *Current Opinion in Neurobiology*, vol. 23, pp. 880–887, 2013.

[95] R. M. Ahmed, R. E. A. Newcombe, A. J. Piper, *et al.*, "Sleep disorders and respiratory function in amyotrophic lateral sclerosis," *Sleep medicine reviews*, vol. 26, pp. 33–42, 2016.

[96] S. Byrne, C. Walsh, C. Lynch, *et al.*, "Rate of familial amyotrophic lateral sclerosis: a systematic review and meta-analysis," *Journal of Neurology, Neurosurgery & Psychiatry*, vol. 82, pp. 623–627, 2010.

[97] M. Agrawal and A. Biswas, "Molecular diagnostics of neurodegenerative disorders," *Frontiers in Molecular Biosciences*, vol. 2, 2015.

[98] P. Masrori and P. van Damme, "Amyotrophic lateral sclerosis: a clinical review," *European Journal of Neurology*, vol. 27, pp. 1918–1929, 2020.

[99] I. Kacem, I. Sghaier, S. Bougatef, *et al.*, "Epidemiological and clinical features of amyotrophic lateral sclerosis in a tunisian cohort," *Amyotrophic Lateral Sclerosis and Frontotemporal Degeneration*, vol. 21, pp. 131–139, 2019.

[100] M. E. Cudkowicz, S. Titus, M. Kearney, *et al.*, "Safety and efficacy of ceftriaxone for amyotrophic lateral sclerosis: a multi-stage, randomised, double-blind, placebo-controlled trial," *The Lancet Neurology*, vol. 13, pp. 1083–1091, 2014.

[101] Z. Xu, R. D. Henderson, M. David, *et al.*, "Neurofilaments as biomarkers for amyotrophic lateral sclerosis: A systematic review and meta-analysis," *PLoS ONE*, vol. 11, 2016.

[102] D. Hartzfeld, N. Siddique, D. E. Victorson, *et al.*, "Reproductive decision-making among individuals at risk for familial amyotrophic lateral sclerosis," *Amyotrophic Lateral Sclerosis and Frontotemporal Degeneration*, vol. 16, pp. 114–119, 2015.

[103] M. R. O'brien, "Management of patients with motor neurone disease," 2011.

[104] L. C. Wijesekera and P. N. Leigh, "Amyotrophic lateral sclerosis," *Orphanet Journal of Rare Diseases*, vol. 4, pp. 3–3, 2009.

[105] A. Radunović, H. Mitsumoto, and N. P. Leigh, "Clinical care of patients with amyotrophic lateral sclerosis," *The Lancet Neurology*, vol. 6, pp. 913–925, 2007.

[106] J. D. Michael Swash, "Motor neuron disease: Classification and nomenclature," *Amyotrophic Lateral Sclerosis and Other Motor Neuron Disorders*, vol. 1, pp. 105–112, 2000.

[107] A. Al-Chalabi, O. Hardiman, M. C. Kiernan, *et al.*, "Amyotrophic lateral sclerosis: moving towards a new classification system," *The Lancet Neurology*, vol. 15, pp. 1182–1194, 2016.

[108] R.G. Miller, J.D., Mitchell, M. Lyon, D.H. Moore, Riluzole for amyotrophic lateral sclerosis (ALS)/motor neuron disease (MND). *Cochrane Database Syst Rev.* 2002;(2):CD001447. doi: 10.1002/14651858.CD001447.

[109] J.-M. Park, S.-Y. Kim, D. Park, and J.-S. Park, "Effect of edaravone therapy in Korean amyotrophic lateral sclerosis (als) patients," *Neurological Sciences*, vol. 41, pp. 119–123, 2019.

[110] H. Lassmann, "Multiple sclerosis pathology," *Cold Spring Harbor perspectives in medicine*, vol. 8 3, 2018.

[111] Şeyda Figül Gökçe, B. Çiğdem, S. N. Karaca, *et al.*, "Prevalence of multiple sclerosis in an urban population of sivas province in Turkey," *Turkish Journal of Medical Sciences*, vol. 49, pp. 288–294, 2019.

[112] M. Ahmadi, M. Gheibizadeh, M. Rassouli, *et al.*, "Experience of uncertainty in patients with thalassemia major: A qualitative study," *International Journal of Hematology-Oncology and Stem Cell Research*, vol. 14, pp. 237–247, 2020.

[113] H. Naci, R. L. Fleurence, J. A. Birt, *et al.*, "Economic burden of multiple sclerosis," *PharmacoEconomics*, vol. 28, pp. 363–379, 2012.

[114] I. I. Kehayov, B. D. Kitov, C. B. Zhelyazkov, *et al.*, "Neurocognitive impairments in brain tumor patients," in *Folia Medica*, 2012.

[115] N. Oudrer, A. Aidi, A. Bahmani, *et al.*, "The clinical course of multiple sclerosis patients in oran," *Multiple Sclerosis and Related Disorders*, 2023.

[116] M. B. Brodkey, A. B. Ben-Zacharia, and J. D. Reardon, "Living well with multiple sclerosis," *AJN, American Journal of Nursing*, vol. 111, pp. 40–48, 2011.

[117] N. Ghasemi, S. Razavi, and E. Nikzad, "Multiple sclerosis: Pathogenesis, symptoms, diagnoses and cell-based therapy," *Cell Journal (Yakhteh)*, vol. 19, pp. 1–10, 2016.

[118] J. Halper, K. Costello, and C. Harris, "Nursing practice in multiple sclerosis: A core curriculum," 2003.

[119] A. K. Artemiadis, M. C. Anagnostouli, and E. C. Alexopoulos, "Stress as a risk factor for multiple sclerosis onset or relapse: A systematic review," *Neuroepidemiology*, vol. 36, pp. 109–120, 2011.

[120] R. F. Brown, C. Tennant, M. J. Sharrock, *et al.*, "Relationship between stress and relapse in multiple sclerosis: part i. important features," *Multiple Sclerosis*, vol. 12, pp. 453–464, 2006.

[121] C. Heesen, D. C. Mohr, I. Huitinga, *et al.*, "Stress regulation in multiple sclerosis – current issues and concepts," *Multiple Sclerosis Journal*, vol. 13, pp. 143–148, 2007.

[122] N. A. A. Corso, A. P. S. Gondim, P. C. R. Dalmeida, *et al.*, "Nursing care systematization for outpatient treatment care of patients with multiple sclerosis," *Revista da Escola de Enfermagem da U S P*, vol. 47 3, pp. 750–755, 2013.

[123] S. Onat, S. Ü. Delialioğlu, Z. Özişler, *et al.*, "Demographic and clinical features of hospitalized multiple sclerosis patients undergoing a rehabilitation program at our clinic," vol. 61, 2015.

[124] E. Faraclas, "Interventions to improve quality of life in multiple sclerosis: New opportunities and key talking points," *Degenerative Neurological and Neuromuscular Disease*, vol. 13, pp. 55–68, 2023.

[125] R. Azzarelli, B. D. Simons, and A. Philpott, "The developmental origin of brain tumours: a cellular and molecular framework," *Development (Cambridge, England)*, vol. 145, 2018.

[126] R. Grant, T. Dowswell, E. Tomlinson, *et al.*, "Interventions to reduce the time to diagnosis of brain tumours," *The Cochrane database of systematic reviews*, vol. 9, p. CD013564, 2020.

[127] T. S. Armstrong, M. Z. Cohen, L. Eriksen, *et al.*, "Symptom clusters in oncology patients and implications for symptom research in people with primary brain tumors," *Journal of nursing scholarship: an official publication of Sigma Theta Tau International Honor Society of Nursing*, vol. 36 3, pp. 197–206, 2004.

[128] T. S. Armstrong and M. R. Gilbert, "Metastatic brain tumors: diagnosis, treatment, and nursing interventions," *Clinical journal of oncology nursing*, vol. 4 5, pp. 217–25, 2000.

[129] A. E. Elia, H. A. Shih, and J. S. Loeffler, "Stereotactic radiation treatment for benign meningiomas," *Neurosurgical focus*, vol. 23 4, p. E5, 2007.

[130] D. Camp-Sorrell, "Brain tumors: Facing trouble head-on," *Nursing made Incredibly Easy*, vol. 4, pp. 20–28, 2006.

[131] R. Srinivasan, M. Kalyani, K. Jyothi, *et al.*, "Review of brain and brain cancer treatment," *International journal of pharma and bio sciences*, 2011.

[132] L. E. Tobar, R. H. Farnsworth, and S. A. Stacker, "Brain vascular microenvironments in cancer metastasis," *Biomolecules*, vol. 12, 2022.

[133] C. T. Ogasawara, B. D. Philbrick, and D. C. Adamson, "Meningioma: A review of epidemiology, pathology, diagnosis, treatment, and future directions," *Biomedicines*, vol. 9, 2021.

[134] M. M. Vargo, "Brain tumor rehabilitation," *American Journal of Physical Medicine & Rehabilitation*, vol. 90, pp. S50–S62, 2011.

[135] N. Zhou, X. Xu, Y. ming Liu, *et al.*, "A proposed protocol of intravitreal injection of methotrexate for treatment of primary vitreoretinal lymphoma," *Eye*, vol. 36, pp. 1448–1455, 2021.

[136] D. Ricard, A. Idbaih, F. Ducray, *et al.*, "Primary brain tumours in adults," *The Lancet*, vol. 379, pp. 1984–1996, 2003.

[137] L. E. Abrey, T. T. Batchelor, A. J. M. Ferreri, *et al.*, "Report of an international workshop to standardize baseline evaluation and response criteria for primary cns lymphoma.," *Journal of clinical oncology : official journal of the American Society of Clinical Oncology*, vol. 23 22, pp. 5034–43, 2005.

[138] S. Chandana, S. Movva, M. L. Arora, *et al.*, "Primary brain tumors in adults.," *American family physician*, vol. 77 10, pp. 1423–30, 2008.

[139] F. Hanif, K. Muzaffar, K. Perveen, *et al.*, "Glioblastoma multiforme: A review of its epidemiology and pathogenesis through clinical presentation and treatment," *Asian Pacific Journal of Cancer Prevention: APJCP*, vol. 18, pp. 3–9, 2017.

[140] T. C. Hirst, H. M. Vesterinen, E. S. Sena, *et al.*, "Systematic review and meta-analysis of temozolomide in animal models of glioma: was clinical efficacy predicted?," *British Journal of Cancer*, vol. 108, pp. 64–71, 2013.

[141] N. Fathi and N. Rezaei, "Lymphopenia in covid-19: Therapeutic opportunities," *Cell Biology International*, vol. 44, pp. 1792–1797, 2020.

[142] R. Stupp, W. P. Mason, M. J. van den Bent, *et al.*, "Radiotherapy plus concomitant and adjuvant temozolomide for glioblastoma," *The New England journal of medicine*, vol. 352 10, pp. 987–996, 2005.

[143] F. Bernard-Arnoux, M. P. Lamure, F. Ducray, *et al.*, "The cost-effectiveness of tumor-treating fields therapy in patients with newly diagnosed glioblastoma," *Neuro-oncology*, vol. 18 8, pp. 1129–1136, 2016.

[144] H. Ohgaki and P. Kleihues, "Genetic pathways to primary and secondary glioblastoma," *The American journal of pathology*, vol. 170 5, pp. 1445–53, 2007.

[145] H. Ohgaki and P. Kleihues, "Genetic alterations and signaling pathways in the evolution of gliomas," *Cancer Science*, vol. 100, 2009.

[146] C. Krakstad and M. Chekenya, "Survival signalling and apoptosis resistance in glioblastomas: opportunities for targeted therapeutics," *Molecular Cancer*, vol. 9, pp. 135–135, 2010.

[147] S. E.-S. Amin and M. Z. A. Megeed, "Brain tumor diagnosis systems based on artificial neural networks and segmentation using mri," *2012 8th International Conference on Informatics and Systems (INFOS)*, pp. MM–119–MM–124, 2012.

[148] M. R. Wrensch, Y. A. Minn, T. Chew, *et al.*, "Epidemiology of primary brain tumors: current concepts and review of the literature.," *Neuro-oncology*, vol. 4 4, pp. 278–99, 2002.

[149] J. Li, Y. Zhong, Z. Ma, *et al.*, "Emotion reactivity-related brain network analysis in generalized anxiety disorder: a task fmri study," *BMC Psychiatry*, vol. 20, 2020.

[150] S. A. Langenecker, H. J. Lee, and L. A. Bieliauskas, "Neuropsychology of depression and related mood disorders," In I. Grant & K. M. Adams (Eds.), Neuropsychological assessment of neuropsychiatric and neuromedical disorders, *Oxford University Press*, 3rd ed., pp. 523–559, 2009.

[151] J. L. Levenson, "The american psychiatric publishing textbook of psychosomatic medicine: psychiatric care of the medically ill," American Psychiatric Publishing, 2005.

[152] D. Badre and D. E. Nee, "Frontal cortex and the hierarchical control of behavior," *Trends in Cognitive Sciences*, vol. 22, pp. 170–188, 2018.

[153] E. Lugaresi and P. L. Parmeggiani, "Somatic and autonomic regulation in sleep : physiological and clinical aspects," Springer, 1997.

[154] J. P. Pandarakalam, "Where scizophrenia and consciousness intersect: Disorders of consciousness in schizophrenia," *Neuroquantology*, vol. 17, pp. 121–139, 2019.

[155] J. Tomasik, E. Schwarz, P. C. Guest, *et al.*, "Blood test for schizophrenia," *European Archives of Psychiatry and Clinical Neuroscience*, vol. 262, pp. 79–83, 2012.

[156] W. T. Carpenter and R. Tandon, "Psychotic disorders in dsm-5: summary of changes," *Asian journal of psychiatry*, vol. 6 3, pp. 266–8, 2013.

[157] K. H. Karlsgodt, D. Sun, and T. D. Cannon, "Structural and functional brain abnormalities in schizophrenia," *Current Directions in Psychological Science*, vol. 19, pp. 226–231, 2010.

[158] P. V. Gejman, A. R. Sanders, and J. Duan, "The role of genetics in the etiology of schizophrenia," *The Psychiatric clinics of North America*, vol. 33 1, pp. 35–66, 2010.

[159] M. I. Herz, J. S. Lamberti, J. Mintz, *et al.*, "A program for relapse prevention in schizophrenia: a controlled study," *Archives of general psychiatry*, vol. 57 3, pp. 277–283, 2000.

[160] K. R. Patel, J. Cherian, K. Gohil, *et al.*, "Schizophrenia: overview and treatment options," *P & T: a peer-reviewed journal for formulary management*, vol. 39 9, pp. 638–645, 2014.

[161] M. Carbon and C. U. Correll, "Clinical predictors of therapeutic response to antipsychotics in schizophrenia," *Dialogues in Clinical Neuroscience*, vol. 16, pp. 505–524, 2014.

[162] A. P. Behere, P. Basnet, and P. A. Campbell, "Effects of family structure on mental health of children: A preliminary study," *Indian Journal of Psychological Medicine*, vol. 39, pp. 457–463, 2017.

[163] C. U. Correll, J. B. Penzner, A. M. Frederickson, *et al.*, "Differentiation in the preonset phases of schizophrenia and mood disorders: evidence in support of a bipolar mania prodrome," *Schizophrenia bulletin*, vol. 33 3, pp. 703–714, 2007.

[164] J. Angst and R. Sellaro, "Historical perspectives and natural history of bipolar disorder," *Biological Psychiatry*, vol. 48, pp. 445–457, 2000.

[165] H. S. Akiskal, M. L. Bourgeois, J. Angst, *et al.*, "Re-evaluating the prevalence of and diagnostic composition within the broad clinical spectrum of bipolar disorders," *Journal of affective disorders*, vol. 59 Suppl 1, pp. S5–S30, 2000.

[166] R. C. Kessler, D. R. Rubinow, C. Holmes, *et al.*, "The epidemiology of dsm-iii-r bipolar i disorder in a general population survey," *Psychological Medicine*, vol. 27, pp. 1079–1089, 1997.

[167] H. S. Akiskal, "Classification, diagnosis and boundaries of bipolar disorders," *Wiley*, 2002.

[168] S. Bahn and E. Schwarz, "[serum-based biomarkers for psychiatric disorders]," *Der Nervenarzt*, vol. 82 11, pp. 1395–6, 1398, 1400 passim, 2011.

[169] S. M. Strakowski, "Diagnostic boundaries between bipolar disorder and schizophrenia: Implications for pharmacologic intervention," *Advanced Studies in Medicine*, vol. 3, 2003.

[170] E. Yang, D. Tadin, D. M. Glasser, *et al.*, "Visual context processing in bipolar disorder: a comparison with schizophrenia," *Frontiers in Psychology*, vol. 4, 2013.

[171] D. J. Muzina, O. Elhaj, P. Gajwani, *et al.*, "Lamotrigine and antiepileptic drugs as mood stabilizers in bipolar disorder," *Acta Psychiatrica Scandinavica*, vol. 111, 2005.

[172] R. C. Kessler, "The prevalence and correlates of adult adhd in the united states: results from the national comorbidity survey replication," *The American journal of psychiatry*, vol. 163 4, pp. 716–23, 2006.

[173] R. Cools, M. I. Froböse, E. Aarts, *et al.*, "Dopamine and the motivation of cognitive control.," *Handbook of clinical neurology*, vol. 163, pp. 123–143, 2019.

[174] B. B. Doyle, "Understanding and treating adults with attention deficit hyperactivity disorder," *American Psychiatric Publishing*; 1st ed., 2006.

[175] N. N. J. Rommelse, M. E. Altink, L. M. J. Sonneville, *et al.*, "Are motor inhibition and cognitive flexibility dead ends in adhd?," *Journal of Abnormal Child Psychology*, vol. 35, pp. 957–967, 2007.

[176] S. H. Kennedy, "Core symptoms of major depressive disorder: relevance to diagnosis and treatment," *Dialogues in Clinical Neuroscience*, vol. 10, pp. 271–277, 2008.

[177] P. Chen, Y. Feng, X. Li, *et al.*, "Systematic reviews and meta-analyses on major depressive disorder: a bibliometric perspective," *Frontiers in Psychiatry*, vol. 14, 2023.

[178] T. Martinek, M. N. Jarczok, E. Rottler, *et al.*, "Typical disease courses of patients with unipolar depressive disorder after in-patient treatments–results of a cluster analysis of the inddep project," *Frontiers in Psychiatry*, vol. 14, 2023.

[179] N. Olchanski, M. M. Myers, M. Halseth, *et al.*, "The economic burden of treatment-resistant depression," *Clinical therapeutics*, vol. 35 4, pp. 512–22, 2013.

[180] E. Mcintosh, D. Gillanders, and S. Rodgers, "Rumination, goal linking, daily hassles and life events in major depression," *Clinical psychology & psychotherapy*, vol. 17 1, pp. 33–43, 2009.

[181] H. S. Akiskal, "Chapter 1 the scope of bipolar disorders," 2011.

[182] K. A. Pelkey, R. Chittajallu, M. T. Craig, *et al.*, "Hippocampal gabaergic inhibitory interneurons," *Physiological reviews*, vol. 97 4, pp. 1619–1747, 2017.

[183] M. Pandya, M. Altinay, D. Malone, *et al.*, "Where in the brain is depression?," *Current Psychiatry Reports*, vol. 14, pp. 634–642, 2012.

[184] M. Tastevin, L. Boyer, T. Korchia, *et al.*, "Brain spect perfusion and pet metabolism as discordant biomarkers in major depressive disorder," *EJNMMI Research*, vol. 10, 2020.

[185] E. C. Dunn, R. C. Brown, Y. Dai, *et al.*, "Genetic determinants of depression: Recent findings and future directions," *Harvard Review of Psychiatry*, vol. 23, p. 1–18, 2015.

[186] K. S. Al-Harbi, "Treatment-resistant depression: therapeutic trends, challenges, and future directions," *Patient preference and adherence*, vol. 6, pp. 369–388, 2012.

[187] B. F. Williams and R. L. Williams, "Effective programs for treating autism spectrum disorder: Applied behavior analysis models," *Routledge*, 2010.

[188] S. Ozonoff, G. S. Young, M. B. Steinfeld, *et al.*, "How early do parent concerns predict later autism diagnosis?," *Journal of Developmental & Behavioral Pediatrics*, vol. 30, pp. 367–375, 2009.

[189] T. Keller, J. L. Ramisch, and M. T. Carolan, "Relationships of children with autism spectrum disorders and their fathers," *The Qualitative Report*, vol. 19, pp. 1–15, 2014.

[190] E. J. Tenenbaum, D. Amso, B. Abar, *et al.*, "Attention and word learning in autistic, language delayed and typically developing children," *Frontiers in Psychology*, vol. 5, 2014.

[191] E. Fombonne, "The changing epidemiology of autism," *Journal of Applied Research in Intellectual Disabilities*, vol. 18, pp. 281–294, 2005.

[192] C. Lord, T. Brugha, T. Charman, *et al.*, "Autism spectrum disorder," *Nature Reviews Disease Primers*, vol. 6, pp. 1–23, 2020.

[193] L. Zwaigenbaum, M. L. Bauman, W. L. Stone, *et al.*, "Early identification of autism spectrum disorder: Recommendations for practice and research," *Pediatrics*, vol. 136, pp. S10–S40, 2015.

[194] C. Okoye, C. M. Obialo-Ibeawuchi, O. A. Obajeun, *et al.*, "Early diagnosis of autism spectrum disorder: A review and analysis of the risks and benefits," *Cureus*, vol. 15, 2023.

[195] K. Lubbers, E. M. Stijl, B. Dierckx, *et al.*, "Autism symptoms in children and young adults with fragile x syndrome, angelman syndrome, tuberous sclerosis complex, and neurofibromatosis type 1: A cross-syndrome comparison," *Frontiers in Psychiatry*, vol. 13, 2022.

[196] D. H. Geschwind, "Genetics of autism spectrum disorders," *Trends in Cognitive Sciences*, vol. 15, pp. 409–416, 2011.

[197] N. Lofthouse, L. E. Arnold, S. Hersch, *et al.*, "A review of neurofeedback treatment for pediatric adhd," *Journal of Attention Disorders*, vol. 16, pp. 351–372, 2012.

2

Therapeutic Potential of Stem Cells in Neurodegenerative Diseases

Zihni Onur Çalışkaner

Biruni University, İstanbul, Turkiye

Stem cells have been under a continuous spotlight in recent years. Stem cells have expedited countless achievements in the life sciences. The unique properties of stem cells make them fantastic cellular tools for regenerative medicine, tissue engineering, biological modeling, drug screening, and studying molecular mechanisms. Current advances in stem cell technology have also paved the way for revolutionary breakthroughs in neurodegenerative disease research at translational and clinical levels, such as developing personalized therapies, modeling disease-specific conditions to obtain deeper insights, etc. In brief, stem cells appear promising for the treatment of neurodegenerative diseases, with an increasing number of patients suffering day by day.

2.1 Introduction

Neurodegenerative diseases are characterized by the progressive deterioration or loss of neurons located in the brain and spinal cord. Neurodegenerative disorders are caused by acute or chronic neurodegeneration in the nervous system. While acute neurodegeneration can arise from acute or temporal factors, such as strong strikes, cerebral hemorrhage, infection, and inflammation, chronic neurodegeneration appears as a result of progressive loss of specific neuron types over a longer period of time and aging. Although there are several neurodegenerative diseases related to different physiological, clinical, and molecular hallmarks, advanced phases of these disorders result in severe cognitive problems with physical disabilities like memory loss, downgraded intellectual capacity, speech impediment, impaired balance, loss of reflexes, stiffness of the joints, and tremors. As reported, approximately 15% of the global human population suffers from neurodegenerative diseases, and the

DOI: 10.1201/9781003461906-2

number of cases is dramatically rising from day to day. Alzheimer's Disease (AD), Parkinson's Disease (PD), Huntington's Disease (HD), Multiple Sclerosis (MS), Amyotrophic Lateral Sclerosis (ALS), and Spinal Muscular Atrophy (SMA) are the leading and most prevalent neuropathologies worldwide that adversely affect the global economy and life quality. Despite the fact that researchers are consistently studying in this field, there are still many biological issues that need to be clarified.

Consequently, understanding the molecular mechanisms underlying the background of neurodegeneration and developing more effective strategies are indispensable. Herein, stem cells appear as alternative cellular sources to elucidate the developmental basis through disease modeling and/or to utilize them in cellular therapies. Various types of stem cells, such as embryonic stem cells, mesenchymal stem cells, and induced pluripotent stem cells, are currently the focus of many scientists and clinicians to evaluate their great potential in both modeling and therapeutic applications. That is to say that stem cells have become promising tools in translational medicine to bridge the gap between molecular pathways and a definite treatment. Within this context, prominent stem cell-based approaches for the treatment of certain neurodegenerative disorders, which advanced the investigations at pre-clinical and clinical levels to date, have been discussed in this chapter.

2.2 Stem Cells

Stem cells (SCs) are an unspecialized, unique population in multicellular organisms, holding two common characteristics: self-renewal and potency. Stem cells have enormous capability of cell division, or self-renewal capacity, to amplify and maintain the undifferentiated SC population in the body. Potency designates the ability of SCs to differentiate into particular cell lineages. In other terms, potency refers to a spectrum of potential cell fates that cells are able to commit under supporting conditions. Hereby, SCs are standing by to give rise to essential cell types when required at any time throughout the lifespan of an organism to maintain homeostasis. However, all characteristics of SCs, including self-renewal, potency, fate decision, commitment, and differentiation, are spatiotemporally orchestrated via complex internal (genetic and epigenetic mechanisms) and external (extracellular signaling, environmental conditions, etc.) factors [1].

One of the SC classification approaches is based on potency. Differentiation capacity is narrowing while going from totipotency to oligopotency. On the top, totipotency defines the capability to generate any embryonic cell type along with extraembryonic structures. Zygote is the most cult example of totipotent cells. Pluripotent stem cells (PSCs) can turn into any embryonic germ layer but not extraembryonic tissues. Embryonic stem cells and induced pluripotent stem cells represent pluripotency. Certain SCs exhibit more restricted differentiation potential and self-renewal than PSCs, differentiating into kindred cell lineages that generally originate from the same germ layer. These multipotent SCs lose their ability to specialize in miscellaneous and unrelated cell lineages. For instance, hematopoietic stem cells (HSCs) can develop into all blood cells; however, they are not able to install divergent cell lineages in practice. When multipotent cells become one step more specialized, they are henceforth called oligopotent SCs. Oligopotency conduces to form discrete cell types descended from a similar progeny. The narrowest range of differentiation is defined as unipotency. Unipotent cells can no longer be considered stem cells because they can only be sustained to constitute identical cells by dividing. Another SC classification is grounded on the specific location or origin where stem cells can be achieved. Thus, the unique character of each stem cell type, especially its ability to differentiate, makes SCs useful and precious for multiple applications in life sciences.

2.2.1 Embryonic Stem Cells (ESCs)

Following fertilization, the zygote undergoes a series of arrangements in humans. Embryonic stem cells (ESCs) in the pluripotent state migrate into the inner layer (ICM; inner cell mass) of the blastocyst, an embryonic configuration acquired by rapid cell division and mobility during early development. ESCs develop into three embryonic germ layers: the endoderm, mesoderm, and ectoderm. Subsequently, all somatic (body) cells and primordial germ cells (PGCs) arise from these ESC-derived germ layers by passing a hierarchical, multi-step course.

Human ESCs (hESCs) were first discovered and characterized by Thomson's group in 1998. They demonstrated that ESCs can be maintained in culture conditions by preserving developmental potential. Cultured ESCs were able to develop into embryonic germ layers and then various somatic cell types in vitro [2]. A great number of hESC lines were brought out of donated human embryos to study the developmental aspects of human beings and their potential in regenerative medicine. Because ESCs are embedded inside the ICM, they can be isolated by disrupting a living embryo. This is the major disadvantage and discrepancy of using ESCs for scientific research and regenerative approaches. Although the competence of ESCs in clinical studies has been documented many times [3], their creation and usage have been restricted because of legal regulations and ethical concerns in societies.

2.2.2 Adult Stem Cells (ASCs)

During the embryonic-fetal transition that orientates a body formation, some quiescent precursor cells in multipotent and oligopotent states are stored in confidential compartments, namely stem cell niches, within the tissues and organs. These niches anatomically and physiologically ensure supportive microenvironments through cell-cell and cell-extracellular matrix (ECM) interactions specific to stem cell types. Adult stem cells (ASCs) start to differentiate into related cell lineages to expand the tissue and replenish damaged or dead cells. As understood, ASCs are requisite for tissue maintenance, tissue repair, growth, and development in multicellular organisms. The main types of ASCs have been summarized below.

2.2.2.1 Mesenchymal Stem Cells (MSCs)

Mesenchymal stem cells (MSCs) are mesoderm-originated multipotent progenitors that transform into a wide range of cell types, involving osteocytes, chondrocytes, adipocytes, myoblasts, and fibroblasts. In addition to these mesodermal cells, MSCs also have transdifferentiation capacity, which means establishing somatic cells from different embryonic germ layers. Here, MSCs have been reported to give rise to neurons, glial cells, epithelial cells, hepatocytes, and so on [4]. MSCs are easily accessible from niches in various adult and neonatal tissues, such as bone marrow, adipose, dental tissues, menstrual blood, umbilical cord, placental tissues, amniotic fluid, etc. [5, 6]. Even though MSCs share common properties, but there are minor characteristic distinctions in surface markers, differentiation capacity and plasticity, self-renewal rate, survival time in the culture, and isolation procedures between cells taken from different niches [5–7].

MSCs have been proven to be safe for allogenic and autologous administration by alternative delivery routes, such as systemic injection, subcutaneous injection, intraarticular, intramuscular, surgical engraftment, intramedullary, intraperitoneal, and intracardiac [8]. In addition to the utilization of MSCs in tissue regeneration, they have versatile effects in vitro and in vivo. These biological functions may be carried out either directly by the cells themselves or by the MSC-derived secretome and exosome (extracellular vesicles; EVs) [8, 9]:

1. MSCs are able to regulate immune cell activity, proliferation, survival, infiltration, homing, and migration (immunomodulation) by secreting several cytokines and chemokines. They also exert anti-inflammatory effects.
2. MSCs regulate apoptosis in neighboring cells, usually downregulating cell death (anti-apoptosis) via paracrine or contact-dependent signaling. RNA derivatives in EVs may alter protein expression in apoptotic pathways.
3. MSCs promote the formation of blood vessels or vascularization, through the release of angiogenic factors and cytokines.
4. MSCs nurse the other stem cells and progenitor cells by modulating their proliferation, survival, activity, homing, and mobility through complex interactions.
5. MSCs can secrete antimicrobial peptides to struggle pathogens.
6. MSCs have also been reported to be resistant to several cytotoxic agents and intriguingly migrate toward the tumor microenvironment, supposing them as cellular vehicles for targeted drug delivery [10].

Ease of isolation protocols, alternative delivery routes, safety in transplanted individuals, and all these fantastic biological features above have made human MSCs and MSC-derived EVs are indispensable in cell-based therapeutic approaches for over 30 years since they were isolated in 1992 for the first time [11, 12]. For this reason, it is currently possible to come across 1621 clinical studies for the treatment of a broad range of diseases when searching for the keyword mesenchymal stem cells in the NIH Clinical Trials database (clinical.gov). Diabetic nephropathy, bronchopulmonary dysplasia, hemophilia, retinitis pigmentosa, cystic fibrosis, mandibular fractures, cardiomyopathies, diabetes mellitus, hypoxic-ischemic encephalopathy, tracheal stenosis, tendon injuries, anemias, spinal cord injury, stroke, osteoarthritis, rheumatoid arthritis, knee osteoarthritis, lupus erythematosus, cerebellar ataxia, hyposalivation, gingival recession, pneumoconiosis, cancers, Duchenne muscular dystrophy, and post-acute COVID-19 syndrome are just a minority of the samples in which MSCs have expediently been in service (clinical.gov).

2.2.2.2 Neural Stem Cells (NSCs) and Neurogenesis

Neurogenesis, first proposed by Joseph Altman in 1962 [13], is a crucial process leading to the production of nerve cells, or neurons, from neural stem cells (NSCs). Neural stem cells and neural progenitors exist in specific niches, the subventricular zone (SVZ) and the subgranular zone (SGZ), within the adult mammalian central nervous system (CNS), to provide lifelong brain plasticity [14]. NSCs are biologically more active during embryonic development; however, NSCs in adults are usually in a quiescence state [15]. Upon neural inductions, neurogenesis is triggered to allow terminal differentiation of sorts of neurons and glial cells. NSC niches in adult brains supply molecular signals, including small ligands, growth factors, systemic hormones, neurocytokines, neurotransmitters (GABA, dopamine, etc.), ECM components, and cell junction molecules, to contribute to NSC differentiation, or neurogenesis [16].

In adults, once quiescent NSCs, namely radial glia-like (RGL) cells (Type I cells) in SGZ, are activated through intrinsic and extrinsic regulators, they start to divide and generate a cell population of intermediate proliferating progenitors (IPCs). IPCs continue their differentiation course by composing neuroblasts. Neuroblasts can migrate towards certain regions of the CNS and transform into immature neurons. Finally, dentate granule cells are derived and located within the dentate gyrus in the hippocampus. On the other hand, RGL-neural stem cells (Type B cells) in SVZ first commit to transient amplifying progenitors (C cells). After dividing for multiple rounds, C cells differentiate into neuroblasts. Type B cell-derived neuroblasts then move to the olfactory bulb, where they give rise to various types of interneurons in the CNS [14, 16, 17]. Activated RGL cells (aRGL) also derive into glial cells, including astrocytes, oligodendrocytes, and ependymal cells in the human CNS [18]. Neurological diseases are essentially caused by either diminished neuronal differentiation, or the unexact functioning of the neurons. In conclusion, NSCs indispensably ensure a healthy brain by sustaining normal development and regeneration in adults. Conversely, the curation of neurodegenerative disorders also passes through neural stem cells, as reviewed in the following sections.

2.2.2.3 Hematopoietic Stem Cells (HSCs)

Hematopoietic stem cells (HSCs) are another multipotent progenitors within the human body that compose all blood cell types. HSCs mostly reside in various fetal and adult niches, including the fetal liver, umbilical cord, bone marrow, and peripheral circulation in humans [19]. HSCs go through a series of multistep differentiation processes that result in the generation of all hematological cells, called hematopoiesis. Initially, HSC (hemocytoblast) commits into common lymphoid progenitor (CLP) or common myeloid progenitor (CMP) in adult bone marrow. After CLPs further differentiate into lymphoblasts, precursors of natural killer (NK) cells, T lymphocytes, and B lymphocytes emerge. Then precursor cells complete their maturation process, in particular, hematopoietic tissues [20]. On the other hand, CMPs gradually branch into lineage-specific subfractions (MEPs and GMPs) with committed cell fate decisions. These subfractions then pursue their ripening steps in specific areas. Finally, granulocytes and monocytes (from myeloblasts), erythrocytes (from proerythroblasts), and platelets (from megakaryoblasts) arise from related precursors in a stepwise manner [21].

HSCs have been safely used as the best remedial sources for numerous hematological diseases and cancers in humans since the first allogenic HSC transplantation was practiced by Edward Donnall Thomas, a Nobel Laureate, in 1957 [22]. The rationale behind allogenic and autologous HSC transplantation is to ameliorate impaired hematopoiesis and the immune system by replacing defective HSCs with healthy or conditioned ones. Similar to MSCs, a huge number of HSC transplantations and clinical trials have been increasingly proceeding [23].

2.2.3 Induced Pluripotent Stem Cells (iPSCs)

Shinya Yamanaka (Nobel Laureate in 2012) and coworkers launched a groundbreaking milestone in the field of stem cells in 2006, proving terminally differentiated somatic cells could be reprogrammed back to the pluripotent state. Moreover, these induced pluripotent stem cells (iPSCs) that originated from human and mouse fibroblasts in laboratory conditions surprisingly repossessed all embryonic-like stem cell characteristics [24, 25]. Methodologically, ectopic overexpression of Oct4, Sox2, Klf4, and c-Myc (OSKM), a set of pluripotency-related transcription factors (Yamanaka's factors), together are able to recover ESC-like features through the reinduction of a master transcriptional regulatory network (somatic cell reprogramming). Above all, it also orchestrates the reprogramming of the epigenetic landscape, including the global DNA methylation profile, histone modification hallmarks, and miRNA expression levels, back to the pluripotent state [26, 27]. Thus, it would not be considered wrong to call iPSCs and/or somatic cell reprogramming approach "biological or cellular time machines" since they take us back to the stem cells lost in the embryonic ages of an individual. Since their discovery, many pieces of evidence have accumulated rapidly that exhibit how iPSCs are indistinguishable from ESCs in terms of differentiation capacity, differentiation range, self-renewal, spatiotemporal gene expression landscape, and epigenetic profile [27]. Thereby, iPSCs have eliminated the biological, ethical, and legal limitations because the acquisition methods of iPSCs do not interfere with a living embryo.

Conventional transgene delivery-based iPSC production methods have been reported to cause two main issues: tumorigenicity due to oncogene activation and low efficiency due to insufficient induction of genetic/epigenetic programs. These limited the usage and biological safety of iPSCs in clinical trials. However, recent advances such as transgene-free chemical cocktails, non-viral episomal vectors, miRNA delivery, and auto-erasable and replication-defective Sendai virus (SeVdp) has decimated the highlighted problems and mediated the production of clinical-grade human iPSCs [28].

As indicated, iPSCs can conveniently differentiate into various somatic cell types, particularly NSCs, neurons, MSCs, osteocytes, hematopoietic cells, fibroblasts, cardiac cells, pancreatic cells, epithelial cells, etc., by gaining whole cell-specific biological functions in vivo [29, 30]. Besides, somatic cell reprogramming lets us manufacture individual-specific embryonic-like stem cells (referred to as iPSCs) from the somatic cells, most of which are easily accessible through non-invasive methods. When altogether considered, iPSCs have come to the forefront as marvelous cellular tools for multi-task applications involving personalized disease-specific cellular therapies, tissue engineering, disease modeling, drug screening, studying developmental aspects, and so on [31]. Clinical trials in different phases continue to increase with each passing day. In total, 153 clinical studies, covering imprinted disorders, cardiovascular diseases, visual impairments, autoimmune diseases, and neurological defects, have been listed with promising outcomes in the NIH Clinical Trial database [32]. Likewise, iPSCs have been reported as feasible tools for allogenic and autologous transplantation strategies in neurodegenerative diseases [33].

2.3 Experimental and Clinical Attempts at Stem Cell Usage in Neurodegenerative Diseases

Various stem cell types are used for several clinical and research purposes within the context of neurodegenerative diseases. Certain objectives that stem cells facilitate are summarized in Table 2.1. While clinical trials are under consideration in different phases, basic research provides worthwhile knowledge. Significant insights are then progressed into translational studies that bridge the gap between basic and clinical research.

TABLE 2.1
How various stem cell types are utilized in neurodegenerative disease research

Activity	Purpose	Stem cell type
Clinical research	Cell therapy and transplantation	ESCs, iPSCs
	Neuroprotective effects	MSCs
	Modulation of neuroinflammation and immune responses	MSCs, HSCs
Basic and translational research	Neurodegenerative disease modeling	ESCs, iPSCs
	Drug screening	ESCs, iPSCs
	Understanding neurogenesis and neuronal pathways	NSCs, ESCs, iPSCs
	Activation of neurogenesis and promotion neuroregeneration	NSCs, iPSCs
	of new strategies and potential therapeutic targets in vitro/vivo	Various
	Neurotrophic effects	MSCs
	Brain organoids/spheroids	iPSCs, ESCs

The application of certain stem cell types in research activities related to widespread neurodegenerative diseases is discussed in more detail in the following titles.

2.3.1 Alzheimer's Disease (AD)

Alzheimer's disease (AD) is the leading dementia-causing brain pathology, with a rapid increase of approximately 148% in the aging population [34, 35]. AD is characterized by extracellular plaque formation and the accumulation of intracellular neurofibrillary tangles that impede brain functions, particularly memory, cognition, and learning. According to the well-accepted pathogenic mechanism, amyloid β-peptide (Aβ) is formed as a result of faulty proteolytic cleavage of amyloid precursor protein (APP), a transmembrane protein on nerve cells. Polymerized amphipathic Aβ molecules occupy synaptic space as insoluble amyloid plaques, which disrupt synaptic signaling [36, 37]. In parallel, Aβ accumulation causes hyperphosphorylation of tau protein, which normally stabilizes microtubules for a proper axonal process. This abnormal hyperphosphorylation state disrupts conformation and leads to misfolding in tau protein [38, 39]. Aberrant tau proteins aggregate as insoluble neurofibrillary tangles (NFTs) inside the neurons [39, 40]. Eventually, Aβ and tau deposition together results in neuroinflammation and neurotoxicity within the brain. While dominant inheritance of the mutations in three major genes (amyloid precursor protein (APP) gene, presenilin1 (PSEN1) gene, and presenilin

2 (PSEN2) gene) cause familial AD (FAD) [41], sporadic (SAD) or late onset AD (LOAD) originates from environmental factors and various isoforms and polymorphisms, particularly in the apolipoprotein E gene (APOE4), clusterin (CLU), complement receptor 1 (CR1), and phosphatidylinositol binding clathrin assembly protein (PICALM), bridging integrator 1 (BIN1), ATP binding cassette transporter 7 (ABCA7), membrane-spanning 4-domains subfamily A (MS4A), etc. [42, 43].

2.3.1.1 iPSCs and ESCs in AD Modeling

Recent advances in the field of induced pluripotent stem cells have enabled patient- and disease-specific embryonic-like stem cells with the potency to give several cell types, including AD-nervous system cells [44]. Hereby, iPSCs have become prominent to be used for alternative approaches. For instance, the iPSC-derived AD model has recently provided knowledge about the developmental process and pathological progress of the disorder. Secondly, iPSCs are promoted to differentiate into healthy neurons to substitute the patch of dead brain tissue in vivo [45].

Chang et al. generated iPSCs from the FAD patients carrying a heterozygous D678H mutation in the APP gene. After iPSCs were modeled into FAD-neurons, they investigated the effects of this mutation on Aβ-tau pathology and neurite formation. The study also revealed novel therapeutic targets and the indole compound NC009-1 as a promising agent for rescuing AD phenotypes [46]. Moore and colleagues examined the relationship between different PSEN1/APP mutations and Aβ/tau accumulation in an iPSC-derived human cerebral cortex model. They demonstrated that the APP mutation (V717I), APP duplication, and multiple PSEN1 mutations (Y115C, M146I) altered APP processing, resulting in increased extracellular Aβ production. The APP V717I mutation and duplication also increased neuronal tau levels and phosphorylation. Besides, pharmacological inhibition of either γ- or β-secretase alleviated extracellular Aβ peptides and tau levels with increased phosphorylation in cortical neurons of each genotype [47]. Kondo and coworkers recently developed cellular dissection of polygenicity (CDiP) technology to unravel genetic risk factors in sporadic Alzheimer's disease (SAD) [48]. In this study, researchers constituted 102 AD patient-derived iPSC lines. A genome-wide association study (GWAS) in cortical neurons that originated from iPSCs came up with 24 significant loci related to Aβ alterations. 11 of the 24 genes were associated with AD pathology for the first time. Additionally, their novel genetic analysis method (CDiP) allowed the prediction of SAD onset and hallmarks in clinical cohorts by combining GWAS iPSC-originated cells and machine learning [48, 49]. Ghatak et al. composed a cerebrocortical organoid bearing FAD-related mutations in presenilin-1 (δE9/WT, M146V/WT) and APP by differentiating iPSCs to investigate early FAD pathophysiology and mechanistic insights into hyperexcitability [50]. Remarkable evidence about the association between low-density lipoprotein receptor-related protein 1 (LRP1) and tau endocytosis and aggregation was uncovered by Rauch and coworkers. Here, comprehensive analysis in iPSC-derived AD models identified LRP1 as the main receptor that regulates tauopathy [51]. iPSCs and iPSC-originated neuron models are not only convenient for investigating AD pathophysiology but also outstanding for exploring the interaction and signaling processes between AD-neurons and microglia in a 3D microenvironment. There are also several studies representing how microglial cell behaviors, such as phagocytosis, lipogenesis, inflammatory responses, cytokine secretion, migration, and viability, dramatically underwent alterations due to Aβ/tau pathology and certain mutations related to SAD or FAD [52–56]. AD models were also created at the cellular level by using human embryonic stem cells (hESCs). For instance, mutant Presenilin1 (PSEN1 or PS1) was overexpressed in the hESC line to recapitulate AD phenotypes. Upon neural differentiation, the electrophysiological status of the synapses was extensively examined [57]. Similarly, there are plenty of studies exploring cognitive functions, genetic factors, Aβ pathophysiology, autophagy induction, neurotoxicity, and neurodegenerative hallmarks in AD models that originated from either human or mouse ESCs [58–62]. Furthermore, mouse ESCs are feasible to analyze the behaviors of AD-related cellular models in vivo by engrafting into the mice bodies.

iPSCs stand as substantial vehicles for targeted gene therapies and genome editing experimentation as well [45, 63]. As reported before, human apolipoprotein E (APOE) was identified as the most effective and most common risk factor in AD cases. While the APOE4 isoform was associated with a high risk for sporadic AD, APOE3 corresponds to a neutral risk of developing AD [64–68]. Several studies have demonstrated that the conversion of the APOE4 allele to the APOE3 allele by gene editing techniques in human iPSC-based neural models rescued the phenotypes of AD [69–72]. Trisomy 21 (Down syndrome) is known to deduce a propensity for early-onset AD due to an increased dosage of the APP gene [73–75]. Intriguingly, APP copy number was normalized via the CRISPR-Cas9 system in patient-derived iPSCs and human embryonic stem cell lines (GeneA021 and GeneA022) to observe the phenotypic effects of dosage compensation on Down syndrome-associated AD pathogenesis [76], altogether suggesting genetically manipulated iPSC-derived neurons could potentially ameliorate Aβ/tau pathophysiology-associated dementia in individuals.

Together, these and more highlight the significance and usefulness of iPSCs to interrogate the genetic events and molecular mechanisms in Alzheimer's disease.

2.3.1.2 iPSCs in Drug Screening for AD Modeling

iPSC-derived neural cells, 3D culture platforms, or organoids offer new therapeutics for Alzheimer's disease treatment before proceeding to preclinical animal tests and clinical trials. Novel pharmacological molecules are generally tested to determine how promising they are to downgrade AD symptoms.

Furthermore, candidate molecules can be evaluated for patient- or AD-type-specific conditions owing to the production method from a unique starting origin, that is, iPSC-based platforms enable the customization of drug screening studies.

A plant polyphenol, apigenin, was tested against neuroinflammation and neurotoxicity in an iPSC-derived human AD model by Balez and coworkers. When compared to healthy controls, apigenin could present neuroprotective activity in both SAD and FAD neurons by protecting iPSC-derived neurons from inflammatory stress and reducing apoptosis and hyperexcitability [77]. Another study by Yahata and colleagues exhibited a drug screening platform targeting Aβ deposition through iPS-derived neurons. Various β-/γ-secretase inhibitors, such as β-secretase inhibitor IV (BSI), γ-secretase inhibitor XXI/Compound E (GSI), non-steroidal anti-inflammatory drug (NSAID), and sulindac sulfide were found efficacious to modulate APP cleavage and Aβ production [78]. Similarly, β-secretase inhibitors were reported to regulate glycogen synthase kinase 3 (GSK3) activity and, therefore, APP-mediated tau phosphorylation in a 3D neural cell culture model with FAD mutations [79]. Hossini et al. elicited the inhibitory effects of GSI against Aβ/tau pathology through a GSK3B pathway in neurons differentiated from SAD donor-originated iPSCs as well [80]. iPSC-based neural models also proposed cholesterol metabolism as a druggable target to suppress hyperphosphorylation of tau protein. Screening a compound library composed of 1684 FDA-approved drugs revealed that cholesterol-lowering drugs reduced the aberrant tau accumulation in iPSC-derived astrocytes and neurons through a CYP46A1-Cholesterol Esters-Tau axis in Alzheimer's disease [81]. Numerous drug screening and drug repurposing platforms, including massive compound libraries, are still under evaluation in iPSC-based models to combat Aβ/tau-caused neurotoxicity and dementia in AD [82–87].

2.3.1.3 Pre-clinical or Clinical Trials of iPSCs and ESCs in AD

Due to the safety concerns about iPSCs and ethical/legal obstacles for human ESCs, cell replacement therapy does not exist at clinical grade yet. However, numerous pre-clinical attempts with human iPSCs and ESCs for the treatment of AD are still ongoing to monitor efficacy, molecular mechanisms, and biological safety in regenerative applications. Human iPSC-derived neural progenitor cells were transplanted into the hippocampus of AD mouse models in a study published in 2015. After transplantation, iPSC-derived neurons could alleviate cognitive loss and dementia in mice by allowing the spread of human-origin GABAergic neurons, choline acetyltransferase (ChAT)-positive cholinergic neurons, and alpha7 nicotinic acetylcholine receptor (α7nAChR)-positive neurons in the mouse cortex [88]. Recovery of spatial memory loss in human APP-transgenic mice after grafting neuronal precursor cells derived from human iPSCs was reported by Suzuki's research group [89]. Armijo et al. also demonstrated that the injection of mouse iPSC-derived neural precursors (iPSC-NPCs) into the hippocampus of a transgenic mouse model for AD corrected abnormalities in memory and synaptic functions [90]. Likewise, human ESC-originated cholinergic neurons were able to amend cognitive symptoms and memory deficits in mouse models with Alzheimer's disease [62, 66]. Interestingly, genetically manipulated mouse ESCs and iPSCs could attenuate AD pathophysiology. Injection of APP gene-deleted ESC- and iPSC-derived thymic epithelial progenitors ($APP^{-/-}$ ESC/iPSC-TEPs) induced an increase in anti-Aβ antibodies in the mouse serum and Aβ phagocytosing macrophages in the CNS. Thus, ESC/iPSC-TEPs resulted in the clearance of Aβ deposits in the mouse brain and counteracted AD pathology [91].

2.3.1.4 Utilization of MSCs in AD Treatment

Mesenchymal stem cells (MSCs) obtained from different tissue sources are frequently utilized in studies in vivo and in vitro for Alzheimer's disease. MSCs are closely interacting cells with their surroundings. Particularly, cell-cell contacts and paracrine factors are essential for regulating adjacent cells' functions. Herein, neurotrophic and angiogenic factors are notable for improving neural and glial cells. Babaei and colleagues elicited that autologous bone marrow mesenchymal stem cell (BM-MSC) transplantation promoted memory in age-induced Alzheimer's models of rats [92]. MSCs do not only affect the biological functions of neurons but also orchestrate immune cells in the brain, such as microglia. When BM-MSCs were grafted in mice, inflammatory microglia (M1) were inhibited and anti-inflammatory microglial cells (M2) were activated, avoiding oxidative stress and further brain damage. BM-MSCs also drive microglia cells around Aβ-accumulated sites for clearance. Thus, BM-MSCs are detected to improve spatial memory [93]. Treatment with extracellular vesicles (EVs or exosomes) of adipose tissue-derived MSCs (AD-MSCs) showed a decrease in apoptosis in the brain of the transgenic mouse model of AD. AD-MSC-derived EVs were adequate to alleviate Aβ pathology [94]. Santamaria and coworkers reported similar findings: intranasal injection of the MSC secretome into Alzheimer's mice restored brain, memory, and recognition functions by reducing amyloidosis and neuroinflammation [95]. Identically, different types of MSCs originated from the umbilical cord, Wharton's jelly, dental tissues, and the placenta, and/or their extracellular vesicles, have shown outstanding results in preclinical animal models [96–100].

Besides, there are tens of ongoing or completed clinical trials for AD patients (https://clinicaltrials.gov). For example, allogenic BM-MSC transplantation in 33 participants was reported as safe, feasible, and efficient to augment neurorecognition in patients compared to placebo. Autologous AD-MSC treatment still continues with 80 patients. Nevertheless, allogenic umbilical cord MSC (UC-MSC) transplantation is a phase I study. Although it has been reported as safe and well-tolerated, any impact on AD symptoms has not been detected so far. Most of the clinical trials with MSCs or MSC-derived extracellular vesicles safely exhibit promising results on AD treatment and the life quality of the subjected patients [97, 99, 101, 102].

2.3.1.5 Preclinical Studies of NSCs in AD Models

Neural stem cells (NSCs) are the second most prevalent stem cell type utilized in AD-related research, following MSCs. NSC transplantation is able to regulate various functions, such as attenuation of Aβ and tau pathophysiology, pacification of neuroinflammation, induction of neurogenesis, reinforcement of the cerebrovascular system, remediation of synaptic signaling, and secretion of neurotrophic factors [103]. Studies about NSCs are currently conducted on rodent models in preclinical studies. Outcomes from AD models are spectacular and predisponent for clinical trials in the near future [103–105].

2.3.2 Parkinson's Disease (PD)

Parkinson's disease (PD) is the second most widespread progressive neurodegenerative disorder that results in the deterioration of the dopaminergic (DOPA) neurons in the basal ganglia, or substantia nigra, a section of the human brain controlling movement. There are a variety of motor and non-motor dysfunctions, such as tremors, muscle stiffness, slowed movements (bradykinesia), postural deformities, cognitive deterioration, olfactory dysfunction, neuropsychiatric problems, and systemic pain [103, 106]. A characteristic molecular pathology in PD is the appearance of Lewy bodies, which are composed of aberrant α-synuclein protein. Unfolded α-synuclein deposits as stacks inside the presynaptic terminals of DOPA neurons, blocking signal transmission. Alpha-synuclein aggregation alters the phosphorylation status of tyrosine hydroxylase (TH), a main enzyme functioning in DOPA biosynthesis [107]. Furthermore, genome-wide studies elicited PD-causative genetic variations in certain genes like alpha-synuclein gene (SNCA), Parkin RBR E3 ubiquitin-protein ligase (PRKN), Parkinson protein 7 (PARK7), PTEN-induced kinase 1 (PINK1), leucine rich-repeat kinase 2 (LRRK2), prosaposin (PSAP), and glucocerebrosidase (GBA1) [103, 108].

Administration of the DOPA precursor (Levodopa) is the only applicable treatment to decelerate the disease progression and moderate the motor symptoms. However, there is still a need for effective treatment strategies that provide more permanent solutions rather than just evading symptoms. Eventually, stem cells emerge as new therapeutic tools and as satisfying PD models to understand molecular pathways in depth.

2.3.2.1 Organoids and PSCs for Modeling PD

Embryonic stem cells and patient-derived iPSCs provide a feasible platform to investigate the molecular mechanisms underlying Parkinson's disease occurrence, progression, and interruption. Additionally, pluripotent stem cells (PSCs) often facilitate cell-based drug screening [109].

One of the leading PD-derived PSC studies was published by Soldner and colleagues. Actually, they inserted the different point mutations (c.A53T (p.G209) and c.G188A (p.E46K)) into the SNCA gene and obtained modeled human ESCs to observe the pathological effects of these mutations on dopaminergic neuron differentiation. Moreover, they directly generated an iPSC line from the PD patient carrying the c.A53T mutation to validate the results in ESCs. Afterward, this mutation in ESCs and iPSCs was corrected by using zinc finger nuclease (ZFN)-mediated genome engineering. The results were significant, showing that genetically engineered PSCs could provide a basis for cell replacement therapies [110]. iPSC-derived DOPA neurons from sporadic and LRRK2-associated PD patients showed similar epigenetic alterations and an abnormal DNA methylation profile compared to healthy controls. Thus, the association between sporadic or monogenic PD pathology and the epigenomic landscape was documented for the first time in the iPSC model [111]. iPSC-derived 3D organoids are also convenient for recapitulating the complex interactions in the PD-suffered brain. A human midbrain-specific organoid comprised of iPSC-derived neural progenitor cells (from PD patients with the LRRK2-G2019S mutation) provided an efficient platform to differentiate high numbers of functional DOPA neurons. Thereby, iPSC-derived organoid mimicking complexity in the human midbrain served as a reproducible model to track neurodevelopmental defects in PD [112]. A similar human midbrain organoid was also clarified by Kim's group. They distinguished the pathological signature and expressional changes in PD patient-specific midbrain organoids bearing the LRRK2-G2019S mutation [113].

2.3.2.2 Stem Cell-based Preclinical Studies and Clinical Trials for PD

Stem cells and stem cell-differentiated neural cells serve for preclinical studies and clinical trials for the treatment of PD. A group of scientists at the Center for iPS Cell Research and Application (CiRA) in Japan has recently manufactured clinical-grade iPSC-derived DOPA neurons from a healthy individual under GMP regulations. Upon quality and safety checks for the iPSC line (QHJI01s04) via genetic and epigenetic analyses, iPSC-DOPA neurons were injected into the striatum of rat and monkey PD models. Engraftment ensured miraculous improvements in the behaviors and brain histology of subjected animals [114]. This study also received approval for a clinical trial (JMA-IIA00384, UMIN000033564) in Japan. Researchers from International Stem Cell Corporation (Carlsbad, CA, USA) commenced another clinical trial at phase I (ClinicalTrials.gov: NCT02452723). First, they manufactured GMP-level neural progenitors from human parthenogenetic pluripotent stem cells. After they ensured functionality, toxicity, tumorigenicity, and biodistribution through in vivo assays, clinical trials were started in Australia [115]. Another pre-clinical study and clinical trial subjecting clinical-grade parthenogenetic ESC-derived neurons have been conducted in China. The clinical trial

(NCT03119636) was lastly documented as standing at phase I/IIa [116]. Various pre-clinical studies are ongoing unabated to translate different kinds of PSCs to clinics, and clinical trials have been proceeding with encouraging outcomes for PD treatment [117].

2.3.3 Multiple Sclerosis (MS)

Multiple sclerosis (MS) is an inflammatory autoimmune disease targeting the CNS. Progressive MS pathology is caused by the demyelination and destruction of the axons in nerve cells. Demyelination-related neuronal damage results in atrophic lesions both in the brain and spinal cord. The main reason behind the neuronal damage is an inflammation-driven lymphocyte attack. Activated lymphocytes (B cells and T cells) infiltrate the CNS by surpassing the brain-blood barrier. Additionally, these immune cells are accumulated within the meninges. The secretion of inflammatory cytokines from T and B lymphocytes stimulates astrocytes and microglia. The secretion of autoantibodies along with cytokines from maturated B cells augments inflammation around the nerve cells [118]. Consequently, immune cells inside the CNS lead to demyelination and axonal damage. Mononuclear phagocytes gather around the demyelinating lesions to endocytose myelin remnants. Meanwhile, proinflammatory phagocytes also generate reactive oxygen and nitrogen species, cytokines, and chemokines, which expedite neuronal cell death [118, 119]. Even though iPSCs and iPSC-derived organoids are exploited for MS-specific disease modeling [120], mesenchymal stem cells (MSCs) and hematopoietic stem cells (HSCs) are broadly used for studies aimed at MS treatment.

2.3.3.1 MSCs and HSCs in MS Treatment

As mentioned above, MSCs are capable of modulating immune cell activation, inflammation, cell survival, and cell signaling via different kinds of molecules (cytokines, DNA, small RNAs, and paracrine factors) secreting directly or inside EVs. Principally, these molecules have been evidenced to have remedial impacts on autoinflammatory lesions in the CNS related to MS disease.

There has been contrary evidence about MSC utility in animal models reported in the literature. Although transplantation of mouse BM-MSCs into the MS mouse model could amend T cell ($CD4^+$ and $CD8^+$) activation, inflammatory cytokine production, and phagocytic cell functions in the secondary lymph organs, these positive outcomes were not reflected in the CNS of the experimental autoimmune encephalomyelitis (EAE) model, as expected [121]. Otherwise, intravenous administration of murine AD-MSCs illustrated therapeutic effects in the EAE model, the well-accepted platform for MS-specific preclinical studies. Injected AD-MSCs were detected as distributed in the EAE lesions in the spleen, brain, and spinal cord. Interestingly, these cells enabled neurogenesis within the lesions, besides controlling neuroinflammation and self-reactive T-cell responses and allowing remyelination and regeneration

[122]. Comparable regenerative and immunomodulatory effects of BM-MSCs were acquired in MS models as well [123, 124]. Administration of xenogenic human MSCs from different sources (umbilical cord, bone marrow, and placental tissues, etc.) in rodent EAE models also yielded promoting achievements, particularly modulation of self-reactive T lymphocytes and elimination of autoreactive B cell antibodies [118, 125]. MSC-derived EVs, or secretome, were also shown to mitigate demyelination, autoimmune reactions, and atrophic lesions within the brain and spinal cord of animal models, apart from the cells themselves [126–128]. Eventually, such preclinical investigations gave rise to numerous clinical trials for MS treatment in distinct locations worldwide (ClinicalTrials.gov). The majority of these clinical trials in phases I and II, which generally employed autologous bone marrow- and adipose tissue-originated MSCs, have been in progress with plausible outcomes and safety.

Hematopoietic stem cells (HSCs) or the whole bone marrow, where HSCs are primarily homed, are another alternative that has come out of preclinical animal studies with excellent implications. As known, autologous HSC transplantation (AHSCT) and bone marrow transplantation (BMT) have safely and efficiently been employed to cure hematopoietic disorders and autoimmune diseases in clinics for over 30 years [129]. In this regard, AHSCT and ABMT principally enforce resetting the hematopoietic system, including irregular immune cells, in multiple sclerosis. AHSCT pursues six basic steps: 1) stimulation for HSC mobilization in the bloodstream through disruption of niche interactions by chemotherapeutic agents or growth factors like cyclophosphamide, granulocyte colony-stimulating factor (G-CSF), etc.; 2) ablation or collection of mobilized HSCs from the body by apheresis; 3) reconditioning isolated HSCs in a GMP-certified laboratory; 4) wipe-out or suppression of the immune system by chemotherapy; 5) reinfusion of reconfigured HSCs into the recipient's blood circulation; and 6) patient follow-up for intended and side effects. Notably, HSC conditioning is momentous for the success of transplantation since it enables the eradication of autoreactive lymphocyte clones, restoration of self-tolerance, normalization of gene and miRNA expression, and orchestration of inflammatory actions [130].

As explained previously, AHSCT and ABMT in rodent models were able to reorchestrate T cell and B cell activity and provide concomitant therapeutic effects in EAE mice [118, 131]. Accordingly, AHSCT has steadily been administered to approximately 5000 human beings with MS based on the same rationale (clinicaltrials.gov). Most MS cases could benefit from AHSCT, with modest improvements in pathological symptoms and overall survival after transplantation [118, 132]. Nevertheless, there are still debates and issues about relapse risk, efficacy, and adverse events [132, 133]. Efforts to develop more eductive and accurate methods for HSC conditioning, patient selection, and transplantation should continue, albeit with considerable advances in HSC-based cell replacement therapy for multiple sclerosis.

2.3.4 Amyotrophic Lateral Sclerosis (ALS)

Amyotrophic lateral sclerosis (ALS) is another neurodegenerative pathology with severe defects in motor neurons and concomitantly fatal failures in multi-organ systems. ALS is the most prevalent adult neuromotor disorder, with a prevalence of 5.4 per 100,000 people in the population and an average survival time of 4 years [134, 135]. Genetic and other factors lead to devastation in upper and lower motor neurons in the motor cortex, brain stem, and spinal cord. Loss of motor control, stagnation, and weakness in voluntary muscle activity due to muscle atrophy, respiratory failure due to decay in respiratory muscles, paralysis, and difficulty in swallowing can be listed among the catastrophic symptoms of ALS. Although pathogenic variants of approximately 50 genes (involving SOD1, C9orf72, TARDBP, FUS, ATXN2, VCP, OPTN, and UBQLN2, etc.) have been associated with ALS risk so far, the non-genetic factors behind the pathological mechanisms that contribute to ALS progression have not clearly been elucidated yet [135]. Genetic variations in the alleles above correspond to the hereditary side of the disease, called familial amyotrophic lateral sclerosis (fALS). Nonetheless, glutamate neurotoxicity, oxidative stress, disruptions in axonal transport, neuroinflammation, impaired RNA metabolism, oligodendrocyte dysfunction, mitochondrial dysfunction, excitotoxicity, vesicular transport and secretion defects, and faults in DNA repair are some of the common proposed cellular mechanisms [136]. Therefore, lack of knowledge is accompanied by the unavailability and ineffectiveness of the medication. Herein, stem cells again come to the forefront as potential instruments for ALS modeling and cell replacement therapy.

2.3.4.1 Drug Screening in iPSC/ESC-based ALS Models

Ignorance of the molecular background has urged researchers to discover ALS-related mechanisms and then find therapeutics targeting these pathways. Moreover, creating preclinical ALS models in vivo is challenging, and attempted animal models remain inadequate to mimic the pathological features of ALS. Hence, iPSCs have contributed to troubleshooting and have overcome the obstacles in this context via reprogramming the cells derived from the ALS patients themselves. Human motor neurons differentiated from patient iPSCs have established an in vitro platform for ALS-specific drug testing. Firstly, the anti-epileptic drug Ezogabine (Retigabine), a voltage-gated potassium (K^+) channel activator, was repurposed for the treatment of fALS-dependent neuronal hyperexcitability [137]. Ezogabine then proceeded to a phase II trial (NCT02450552) involving 65 fALS patients. Secondly, Ropinirole was distinguished as a result of screening a panel including FDA-approved drugs in an iPSC-derived sporadic ALS model. ALS-related phenotypes could be relatively reversed in motor neurons from FUS/TARDBP-ALS iPSCs exposed to Ropinirole [138]. This drug has been self-tolerated and safe for 29 enrolled participants in a phase 1/2a randomized trial [139]. Meanwhile, drug screening assay in the iPSC-derived SOD1-fALS model suggested Bosutinib, a src tyrosine kinase inhibitor, as a potent agent, rescuing motor neuron deterioration and inducing motor neuron survival [140]. Following to Ropinirole, it underwent a phase I trial in 2019 [141]. Tauroursodeoxycholic acid (TUDCA), a hydrophilic bile acid, was also reported to prevent the degeneration of motor neurons derived from mouse and human ESC lines carrying SOD1 mutations. TUDCA also promoted neurite outgrowth in vitro and lessened muscle denervation in a mouse model [142]. These neuroprotective findings led to distinct clinical trials in phases II and III (NCT00877604, NCT03127514, and NCT03800524). Lastly, screening with 160 bioactive small molecules in human ESC- and iPSC-derived motor neurons yielded the Rho kinase inhibitor Y-27632 as an anti-ALS medication. As shown, administration of Y-27632, or Fasudil, induced neural proliferation, amplified neuron number, and enhanced response to neurotrophic factors compared to vehicle control [143]. Subsequently, Fasudil has also been subjected to a phase II clinical trial recently (NCT03792490).

It is obvious that each clinical trial has been initiated as a consequence of drug testing using pluripotent stem cell-based platforms. So, the success of repurposed drugs in clinical trials has also authenticated the reliability, adaptability, and truth of pluripotent stem cells in ALS research, from the laboratory to the clinic.

2.3.4.2 NSCs and MSCs in ALS Precision Cell Therapies

Numerous preclinical investigations have been deducing the victory of translational stem cell therapy for ALS [144, 145]. In 2012, pioneering clinical research published that autologous transplantation of CD133-positive NSCs within the frontal motor cortex of 67 ALS patients was deemed safe and well-tolerated with mild adverse effects [146]. Another phase I study conducted on a cohort of six sporadic ALS patients illustrated that surgical implantation of fetal NSCs into the anterior of the spinal cord halted disease progression with no severe side effects [147]. Similarly, MSC administration in participants within the scope of phase 1/2 (NCT01051882) and 2a (NCT01777646) clinical trials resulted in an upturn in ALS-related scores and in muscle atrophy progression owing to neurotrophic factors secreted by transplanted MSCs [148]. Since drawbacks and limitations of current stem cell therapies for ALS treatment exist, developing safer and more convenient methods is indispensable.

2.4 Conclusion

Even though there is a great variety of neurodegenerative diseases in humans, loss and/or dysfunction of certain neuron types in the nervous system underlie the basis of all. Replacement of the lost or faulty neurons with properly functioning cells appears as the most plausible, efficient, and well-tolerated treatment strategy. In this sense, various stem cell types have been shown to fulfill this task very well by maintaining disease-targeted neuronal differentiation in the affected individuals' CNS. Despite the fact that some are still under in vitro evaluation, a nonignorable number of stem cell lineages have started to elicit successful and promising results in patients with neurodegenerative defects such as Alzheimer's disease, Parkinson's disease, multiple sclerosis, and much more that was not reviewed in this chapter. In conclusion, recent developments in stem cell technologies have paved the way for personalized neurodegenerative disease treatment. The studies still continue unabated, with great hopes.

2.5 Acknowledgment

I express my great gratitude to Dr. Uygar Şaşmaz (Biruni University, İstanbul, Türkiye) for his kind support in typesetting the manuscript using the LaTex document editor.

Bibliography

[1] N. Smith, S. Shirazi, D. Cakouros, *et al.*, "Impact of environmental and epigenetic changes on mesenchymal stem cells during aging," *International Journal of Molecular Sciences*, vol. 24, p. 6499, 3 2023.

[2] J. A. Thomson, J. Itskovitz-Eldor, S. S. Shapiro, *et al.*, "Embryonic stem cell lines derived from human blastocysts," *Science*, vol. 282, pp. 1145–1147, 11 1998.

[3] A. Golchin, A. Chatziparasidou, P. Ranjbarvan, *et al.*, *Embryonic Stem Cells in Clinical Trials: Current Overview of Developments and Challenges*, pp. 19–37. 2020.

[4] C. Krabbe, J. Zimmer, and M. Meyer, "Neural transdifferentiation of mesenchymal stem cells – a critical review," *APMIS*, vol. 113, pp. 831–844, 11 2005.

[5] S. Poliwoda, N. Noor, E. Downs, *et al.*, "Stem cells: a comprehensive review of origins and emerging clinical roles in medical practice," *Orthopedic Reviews*, vol. 14, 8 2022.

[6] H. Ren, Y. Sang, F. Zhang, *et al.*, "Comparative analysis of human mesenchymal stem cells from umbilical cord, dental pulp, and menstrual blood as sources for cell therapy," *Stem Cells International*, vol. 2016, pp. 1–13, 2016.

[7] R. Hass, C. Kasper, S. Böhm, *et al.*, "Different populations and sources of human mesenchymal stem cells (msc): A comparison of adult and neonatal tissue-derived msc," *Cell Communication and Signaling*, vol. 9, p. 12, 12 2011.

[8] P. Saeedi, R. Halabian, and A. A. I. Fooladi, "A revealing review of mesenchymal stem cells therapy, clinical perspectives and modification strategies," *Stem Cell Investigation*, vol. 6, pp. 34–34, 9 2019.

[9] L. Giovannelli, E. Bari, C. Jommi, *et al.*, "Mesenchymal stem cell secretome and extracellular vesicles for neurodegenerative diseases: Risk-benefit profile and next steps for the market access," *Bioactive Materials*, vol. 29, pp. 16–35, 11 2023.

[10] L. S. Litvinova, V. V. Shupletsova, O. G. Khaziakhmatova, *et al.*, "Human mesenchymal stem cells as a carrier for a cell-mediated drug delivery," *Frontiers in Bioengineering and Biotechnology*, vol. 10, 2 2022.

[11] S. Haynesworth, J. Goshima, V. Goldberg, *et al.*, "Characterization of cells with osteogenic potential from human marrow," *Bone*, vol. 13, pp. 81–88, 1992.

[12] H. M. Lazarus, S. E. Haynesworth, S. L. Gerson, *et al.*, "Ex vivo expansion and subsequent infusion of human bone marrow-derived stromal progenitor cells (mesenchymal progenitor cells): implications for therapeutic use.," *Bone marrow transplantation*, vol. 16, pp. 557–64, 10 1995.

[13] J. Altman, "Are new neurons formed in the brains of adult mammals?," *Science*, vol. 135, pp. 1127–1128, 3 1962.

[14] A. Rodríguez-Bodero and J. M. Encinas-Pérez, "Does the plasticity of neural stem cells and neurogenesis make them biosensors of disease and damage?," *Frontiers in Neuroscience*, vol. 16, 9 2022.

[15] N. Urban and F. Guillemot, "Neurogenesis in the embryonic and adult brain: same regulators, different roles," *Frontiers in Cellular Neuroscience*, vol. 8, 11 2014.

[16] A. M. Bond, G. li Ming, and H. Song, "Adult mammalian neural stem cells and neurogenesis: Five decades later," *Cell Stem Cell*, vol. 17, pp. 385–395, 10 2015.

[17] H. S. Ghosh, "Adult neurogenesis and the promise of adult neural stem cells," *Journal of Experimental Neuroscience*, vol. 13, p. 117906951985687, 1 2019.

[18] S. Falk and M. Götz, "Glial control of neurogenesis," *Current Opinion in Neurobiology*, vol. 47, pp. 188–195, 12 2017.

[19] X. Gao, C. Xu, N. Asada, *et al.*, "The hematopoietic stem cell niche: from embryo to adult.," *Development (Cambridge, England)*, vol. 145, 1 2018.

[20] A. Y. Lai and M. Kondo, "T and b lymphocyte differentiation from hematopoietic stem cell," *Seminars in Immunology*, vol. 20, pp. 207–212, 8 2008.

[21] K. Weiskopf, P. J. Schnorr, W. W. Pang, *et al.*, "Myeloid cell origins, differentiation, and clinical implications," *Microbiology Spectrum*, vol. 4, 10 2016.

[22] E. D. Thomas, H. L. Lochte, W. C. Lu, *et al.*, "Intravenous infusion of bone marrow in patients receiving radiation and chemotherapy," *New England Journal of Medicine*, vol. 257, pp. 491–496, 9 1957.

[23] I. Henig and T. Zuckerman, "Hematopoietic stem cell transplantation—50 years of evolution and future perspectives," *Rambam Maimonides Medical Journal*, vol. 5, p. e0028, 10 2014.

[24] K. Takahashi and S. Yamanaka, "Induction of pluripotent stem cells from mouse embryonic and adult fibroblast cultures by defined factors," *Cell*, vol. 126, pp. 663–676, 8 2006.

[25] K. Takahashi, K. Tanabe, M. Ohnuki, *et al.*, "Induction of pluripotent stem cells from adult human fibroblasts by defined factors," *Cell*, vol. 131, pp. 861–872, 11 2007.

[26] K. Nishino, K. Takasawa, K. Okamura, *et al.*, "Identification of an epigenetic signature in human induced pluripotent stem cells using a linear machine learning model," *Human Cell*, vol. 34, pp. 99–110, 1 2021.

[27] M. van den Hurk, G. Kenis, C. Bardy, *et al.*, "Transcriptional and epigenetic mechanisms of cellular reprogramming to induced pluripotency," *Epigenomics*, vol. 8, pp. 1131–1149, 8 2016.

[28] J. Mao, Q. Saiding, S. Qian, *et al.*, "Reprogramming stem cells in regenerative medicine," *Smart Medicine*, vol. 1, 12 2022.

[29] J. Gorecka, V. Kostiuk, A. Fereydooni, *et al.*, "The potential and limitations of induced pluripotent stem cells to achieve wound healing," *Stem Cell Research and Therapy*, vol. 10, p. 87, 12 2019.

[30] Y. Oh and J. Jang, "Directed differentiation of pluripotent stem cells by transcription factors," *Molecules and cells*, vol. 42, pp. 200–209, 3 2019.

[31] V. K. Singh, M. Kalsan, N. Kumar, *et al.*, "Induced pluripotent stem cells: applications in regenerative medicine, disease modeling, and drug discovery," *Frontiers in cell and developmental biology*, vol. 3, p. 2, 2015.

[32] D. Ilic and C. Ogilvie, "Pluripotent stem cells in clinical setting—new developments and overview of current status," *Stem Cells*, vol. 40, pp. 791–801, 9 2022.

[33] A. Ebrahimi, E. Keske, A. Mehdipour, *et al.*, "Somatic cell reprogramming as a tool for neurodegenerative diseases," *Biomedicine and Pharmacotherapy*, vol. 112, p. 108663, 4 2019.

[34] X. Li, X. Feng, X. Sun, *et al.*, "Global, regional, and national burden of alzheimer's disease and other dementias, 1990–2019," *Frontiers in Aging Neuroscience*, vol. 14, p. 937486, 10 2022.

[35] Y. Y. Wang, S. F. Yu, H. Y. Xue, *et al.*, "Effectiveness and safety of acupuncture for the treatment of alzheimer's disease: A systematic review and meta-analysis," *Frontiers in Aging Neuroscience*, vol. 12, p. 519485, 5 2020.

[36] C. Y. Ewald and C. Li, "Understanding the molecular basis of alzheimer's disease using a caenorhabditis elegans model system," *Brain Structure and Function*, vol. 214, pp. 263–283, 3 2010.

[37] Y. Gong, L. Chang, K. L. Viola, *et al.*, "Alzheimer's disease-affected brain: Presence of oligomeric aβ ligands (addls) suggests a molecular basis for reversible memory loss," *Proceedings of the National Academy of Sciences of the United States of America*, vol. 100, pp. 10417–10422, 9 2003.

[38] M. Kolarova, F. García-Sierra, A. Bartos, *et al.*, "Structure and pathology of tau protein in alzheimer disease," *International Journal of Alzheimer's Disease*, 2012.

[39] J. A. Trejo-Lopez, A. T. Yachnis, and S. Prokop, "Neuropathology of alzheimer's disease," *Neurotherapeutics*, vol. 19, 2022.

[40] M. Ahani-Nahayati, A. Shariati, M. Mahmoodi, *et al.*, "Stem cell in neurodegenerative disorders; an emerging strategy," *International Journal of Developmental Neuroscience*, vol. 81, pp. 291–311, 6 2021.

[41] I. Piaceri, B. Nacmias, and S. Sorbi, "Genetics of familial and sporadic alzheimer's disease," *Frontiers in Bioscience - Elite*, vol. 5 E, 2013.

[42] C. Bellenguez, F. Küçükali, I. E. Jansen, *et al.*, "New insights into the genetic etiology of alzheimer's disease and related dementias," *Nature Genetics*, vol. 54, 2022.

[43] T. König and E. Stögmann, "Genetics of alzheimer's disease," *Wiener Medizinische Wochenschrift*, vol. 171, 2021.

[44] F. J. Rodriguez-Jimenez, J. Ureña-Peralta, P. Jendelova, *et al.*, "Alzheimer's disease and synapse loss: What can we learn from induced pluripotent stem cells? hipscs and alzheimer's disease modeling," *Journal of Advanced Research*, vol. 54, 2023.

[45] H. E. Marei, M. U. A. Khan, and A. Hasan, "Potential use of ipscs for disease modeling, drug screening, and cell-based therapy for alzheimer's disease," *Cellular and Molecular Biology Letters*, vol. 28, p. 98, 11 2023.

[46] K. H. Chang, G. J. Lee-Chen, C. C. Huang, *et al.*, "Modeling alzheimer's disease by induced pluripotent stem cells carrying app d678h mutation," *Molecular Neurobiology*, vol. 56, 2019.

[47] S. Moore, L. D. Evans, T. Andersson, *et al.*, "App metabolism regulates tau proteostasis in human cerebral cortex neurons," *Cell Reports*, vol. 11, pp. 689–696, 5 2015.

[48] T. Kondo, Y. Yada, T. Ikeuchi, *et al.*, "Cdip technology for reverse engineering of sporadic alzheimer's disease," *Journal of Human Genetics*, vol. 68, pp. 231–235, 3 2023.

[49] T. Kondo, N. Hara, S. Koyama, *et al.*, "Dissection of the polygenic architecture of neuronal aβ production using a large sample of individual ipsc lines derived from alzheimer's disease patients," *Nature Aging*, vol. 2, pp. 125–139, 2 2022.

[50] S. Ghatak, N. Dolatabadi, D. Trudler, *et al.*, "Mechanisms of hyperexcitability in alzheimer's disease hipsc-derived neurons and cerebral organoids vs isogenic controls," *eLife*, vol. 8, 11 2019.

[51] J. N. Rauch, G. Luna, E. Guzman, *et al.*, "Lrp1 is a master regulator of tau uptake and spread," *Nature*, vol. 580, pp. 381–385, 4 2020.

[52] E. M. Abud, R. N. Ramirez, E. S. Martinez, *et al.*, "ipsc-derived human microglia-like cells to study neurological diseases," *Neuron*, vol. 94, pp. 278–293.e9, 4 2017.

[53] B. J. Andreone, L. Przybyla, C. Llapashtica, *et al.*, "Alzheimer's-associated plcγ2 is a signaling node required for both trem2 function and the inflammatory response in human microglia," *Nature Neuroscience*, vol. 23, pp. 927–938, 8 2020.

[54] N. Fattorelli, A. Martinez-Muriana, L. Wolfs, *et al.*, "Stem-cell-derived human microglia transplanted into mouse brain to study human disease," *Nature Protocols*, vol. 16, pp. 1013–1033, 2 2021.

[55] J. Hasselmann, M. A. Coburn, W. England, *et al.*, "Development of a chimeric model to study and manipulate human microglia in vivo," *Neuron*, vol. 103, pp. 1016–1033.e10, 9 2019.

[56] R. Sims, S. J. van der Lee, A. C. Naj, *et al.*, "Rare coding variants in plcg2, abi3, and trem2 implicate microglial-mediated innate immunity in alzheimer's disease," *Nature Genetics*, vol. 49, pp. 1373–1384, 9 2017.

[57] M. Honda, I. Minami, N. Tooi, *et al.*, "The modeling of alzheimer's disease by the overexpression of mutant presenilin 1 in human embryonic stem cells," *Biochemical and Biophysical Research Communications*, vol. 469, pp. 587–592, 1 2016.

[58] B. Foveau, A. S. Correia, S. S. Hébert, *et al.*, "Stem cell-derived neurons as cellular models of sporadic alzheimer's disease," *Journal of Alzheimer's Disease*, vol. 67, pp. 893–910, 2 2019.

[59] D. Y. Kim, S. H. Choi, J. S. Lee, *et al.*, "Feasibility and efficacy of intra-arterial administration of embryonic stem cell derived-mesenchymal stem cells in animal model of alzheimer's disease," *Journal of Alzheimer's Disease*, vol. 76, pp. 1281–1296, 8 2020.

[60] Y. Shi, P. Kirwan, J. Smith, *et al.*, "A human stem cell model of early alzheimer's disease pathology in down syndrome," *Science Translational Medicine*, vol. 4, 3 2012.

[61] T. Ubina, M. Magallanes, S. Srivastava, *et al.*, "A human embryonic stem cell model of aβ-dependent chronic progressive neurodegeneration," *Frontiers in Neuroscience*, vol. 13, 9 2019.

[62] W. Yue, Y. Li, T. Zhang, *et al.*, "Esc-derived basal forebrain cholinergic neurons ameliorate the cognitive symptoms associated with alzheimer's disease in mouse models," *Stem Cell Reports*, vol. 5, pp. 776–790, 11 2015.

[63] A. McTague, G. Rossignoli, A. Ferrini, *et al.*, "Genome editing in ipsc-based neural systems: From disease models to future therapeutic strategies," *Frontiers in Genome Editing*, vol. 3, 3 2021.

[64] J. F. Arboleda-Velasquez, F. Lopera, M. O'Hare, *et al.*, "Resistance to autosomal dominant alzheimer's disease in an apoe3 christchurch homozygote: a case report," *Nature Medicine*, vol. 25, pp. 1680–1683, 11 2019.

[65] Y. L. Guen, M. E. Belloy, B. Grenier-Boley, *et al.*, "Association of rare <i>apoe</i> missense variants v236e and r251g with risk of alzheimer disease," *JAMA Neurology*, vol. 79, p. 652, 7 2022.

[66] C.-C. Liu, T. Kanekiyo, H. Xu, *et al.*, "Apolipoprotein e and alzheimer disease: risk, mechanisms and therapy," *Nature Reviews Neurology*, vol. 9, pp. 106–118, 2 2013.

[67] A.-C. Raulin, S. V. Doss, Z. A. Trottier, *et al.*, "Apoe in alzheimer's disease: pathophysiology and therapeutic strategies," *Molecular Neurodegeneration*, vol. 17, p. 72, 11 2022.

[68] W. J. Strittmatter, A. M. Saunders, D. Schmechel, *et al.*, "Apolipoprotein e: high-avidity binding to beta-amyloid and increased frequency of type 4 allele in late-onset familial alzheimer disease," *Proceedings of the National Academy of Sciences*, vol. 90, pp. 1977–1981, 3 1993.

[69] Y.-T. Lin, J. Seo, F. Gao, *et al.*, "Apoe4 causes widespread molecular and cellular alterations associated with alzheimer's disease phenotypes in human ipsc-derived brain cell types," *Neuron*, vol. 98, p. 1294, 6 2018.

[70] K. Meyer, H. M. Feldman, T. Lu, *et al.*, "Rest and neural gene network dysregulation in ipsc models of alzheimer's disease," *Cell Reports*, vol. 26, pp. 1112–1127.e9, 1 2019.

[71] S. Raman, N. Brookhouser, and D. A. Brafman, "Using human induced pluripotent stem cells (hipscs) to investigate the mechanisms by which apolipoprotein e (apoe) contributes to alzheimer's disease (ad) risk," *Neurobiology of Disease*, vol. 138, p. 104788, 5 2020.

[72] C. Wang, R. Najm, Q. Xu, *et al.*, "Gain of toxic apolipoprotein e4 effects in human ipsc-derived neurons is ameliorated by a small-molecule structure corrector," *Nature Medicine*, vol. 24, pp. 647–657, 5 2018.

[73] E. Doran, D. Keator, E. Head, *et al.*, "Down syndrome, partial trisomy 21, and absence of alzheimer's disease: The role of app," *Journal of Alzheimer's Disease*, vol. 56, pp. 459–470, 1 2017.

[74] L. N. Geller and H. Potter, "Chromosome missegregation and trisomy 21 mosaicism in alzheimer's disease," *Neurobiology of Disease*, vol. 6, pp. 167–179, 6 1999.

[75] H. Potter, A. Granic, and J. Caneus, "Role of trisomy 21 mosaicism in sporadic and familial alzheimer's disease," *Current Alzheimer Research*, vol. 13, pp. 7–17, 12 2015.

[76] D. A. Ovchinnikov, O. Korn, I. Virshup, *et al.*, "The impact of app on alzheimer-like pathogenesis and gene expression in down syndrome ipsc-derived neurons," *Stem Cell Reports*, vol. 11, pp. 32–42, 7 2018.

[77] R. Balez, N. Steiner, M. Engel, *et al.*, "Neuroprotective effects of apigenin against inflammation, neuronal excitability and apoptosis in an induced pluripotent stem cell model of alzheimer's disease," *Scientific Reports*, vol. 6, p. 31450, 8 2016.

[78] N. Yahata, M. Asai, S. Kitaoka, *et al.*, "Anti-aβ drug screening platform using human ips cell-derived neurons for the treatment of alzheimer's disease," *PLoS ONE*, vol. 6, p. e25788, 9 2011.

[79] S. H. Choi, Y. H. Kim, M. Hebisch, *et al.*, "A three-dimensional human neural cell culture model of alzheimer's disease," *Nature*, vol. 515, pp. 274–278, 11 2014.

[80] A. M. Hossini, M. Megges, A. Prigione, *et al.*, "Induced pluripotent stem cell-derived neuronal cells from a sporadic alzheimer's disease donor as a model for investigating ad-associated gene regulatory networks," *BMC Genomics*, vol. 16, p. 84, 12 2015.

[81] R. van der Kant, V. F. Langness, C. M. Herrera, *et al.*, "Cholesterol metabolism is a druggable axis that independently regulates tau and amyloid-β in ipsc-derived alzheimer's disease neurons," *Cell Stem Cell*, vol. 24, pp. 363–375.e9, 3 2019.

[82] C. Arber, C. Lovejoy, and S. Wray, "Stem cell models of alzheimer's disease: progress and challenges," *Alzheimer's Research and Therapy*, vol. 9, p. 42, 12 2017.

[83] F. Fanizza, L. Boeri, F. Donnaloja, *et al.*, "Development of an induced pluripotent stem cell-based liver-on-a-chip assessed with an alzheimer's disease drug," *ACS Biomaterials Science and Engineering*, vol. 9, pp. 4415–4430, 7 2023.

[84] T. Kondo, K. Imamura, M. Funayama, *et al.*, "ipsc-based compound screening and in vitro trials identify a synergistic anti-amyloid β combination for alzheimer's disease," *Cell Reports*, vol. 21, pp. 2304–2312, 11 2017.

[85] H. Park, J. Kim, and C. Ryou, "A three-dimensional spheroid co-culture system of neurons and astrocytes derived from alzheimer's disease patients for drug efficacy testing," *Cell Proliferation*, vol. 56, 6 2023.

[86] J.-C. Park, S.-Y. Jang, D. Lee, *et al.*, "A logical network-based drug-screening platform for alzheimer's disease representing pathological features of human brain organoids," *Nature Communications*, vol. 12, p. 280, 1 2021.

[87] G. Williams, A. Gatt, E. Clarke, *et al.*, "Drug repurposing for alzheimer's disease based on transcriptional profiling of human ipsc-derived cortical neurons," *Translational Psychiatry*, vol. 9, p. 220, 9 2019.

[88] N. Fujiwara, J. Shimizu, K. Takai, *et al.*, "Cellular and molecular mechanisms of the restoration of human app transgenic mouse cognitive dysfunction after transplant of human ips cell-derived neural cells," *Experimental Neurology*, vol. 271, pp. 423–431, 9 2015.

[89] N. Fujiwara, J. Shimizu, K. Takai, *et al.*, "Restoration of spatial memory dysfunction of human app transgenic mice by transplantation of neuronal precursors derived from human ips cells," *Neuroscience Letters*, vol. 557, pp. 129–134, 12 2013.

[90] E. Armijo, G. Edwards, A. Flores, *et al.*, "Induced pluripotent stem cell-derived neural precursors improve memory, synaptic and pathological abnormalities in a mouse model of alzheimer's disease," *Cells*, vol. 10, p. 1802, 7 2021.

[91] J. Zhao, M. Su, Y. Lin, *et al.*, "Administration of amyloid precursor protein gene deleted mouse esc-derived thymic epithelial progenitors attenuates alzheimer's pathology," *Frontiers in Immunology*, vol. 11, 8 2020.

[92] P. Babaei, B. S. Tehrani, and A. Alizadeh, "Transplanted bone marrow mesenchymal stem cells improve memory in rat models of alzheimer's disease," *Stem Cells International*, vol. 2012, pp. 1–8, 2012.

[93] K. Yokokawa, N. Iwahara, S. Hisahara, *et al.*, "Transplantation of mesenchymal stem cells improves amyloid-β pathology by modifying microglial function and suppressing oxidative stress," *Journal of Alzheimer's Disease*, vol. 72, pp. 867–884, 11 2019.

[94] M. Lee, J.-J. Ban, S. Yang, *et al.*, "The exosome of adipose-derived stem cells reduces β-amyloid pathology and apoptosis of neuronal cells derived from the transgenic mouse model of alzheimer's disease," *Brain Research*, vol. 1691, pp. 87–93, 7 2018.

[95] G. Santamaria, E. Brandi, P. L. Vitola, *et al.*, "Intranasal delivery of mesenchymal stem cell secretome repairs the brain of alzheimer's mice," *Cell Death and Differentiation*, vol. 28, pp. 203–218, 1 2021.

[96] Y. Duan, L. Lyu, and S. Zhan, "Stem cell therapy for alzheimer's disease: A scoping review for 2017–2022," *Biomedicines*, vol. 11, p. 120, 1 2023.

[97] J. Hu and Xiaochuan, "Alzheimer's disease: From pathogenesis to mesenchymal stem cell therapy – bridging the missing link," *Frontiers in Cellular Neuroscience*, vol. 15, 2 2022.

[98] M. Jeyaraman, R. L. Rajendran, S. Muthu, *et al.*, "An update on stem cell and stem cell-derived extracellular vesicle-based therapy in the management of alzheimer's disease," *Heliyon*, vol. 9, p. e17808, 7 2023.

[99] S. Regmi, D. D. Liu, M. Shen, *et al.*, "Mesenchymal stromal cells for the treatment of alzheimer's disease: Strategies and limitations," *Frontiers in Molecular Neuroscience*, vol. 15, 10 2022.

[100] Z.-H. Xie, Z. Liu, X.-R. Zhang, *et al.*, "Wharton's jelly-derived mesenchymal stem cells alleviate memory deficits and reduce amyloid-β deposition in an app/ps1 transgenic mouse model," *Clinical and Experimental Medicine*, vol. 16, pp. 89–98, 2 2016.

[101] Y. Fang, T. Gao, B. Zhang, *et al.*, "Recent advances: Decoding alzheimer's disease with stem cells," *Frontiers in Aging Neuroscience*, vol. 10, 3 2018.

[102] R. Srivastava, A. Li, T. Datta, *et al.*, "Advances in stromal cell therapy for management of alzheimer's disease," *Frontiers in Pharmacology*, vol. 13, 10 2022.

[103] X. Chen, S. Jiang, R. Wang, *et al.*, "Neural stem cells in the treatment of alzheimer's disease: Current status, challenges, and future prospects," *Journal of Alzheimer's Disease*, vol. 94, pp. S173–S186, 7 2023.

[104] Y. Hayashi, H.-T. Lin, C.-C. Lee, *et al.*, "Effects of neural stem cell transplantation in alzheimer's disease models," *Journal of Biomedical Science*, vol. 27, p. 29, 12 2020.

[105] Z. Zhou, B. Shi, Y. Xu, *et al.*, "Neural stem/progenitor cell therapy for alzheimer disease in preclinical rodent models: a systematic review and meta-analysis," *Stem Cell Research and Therapy*, vol. 14, p. 3, 1 2023.

[106] M. Mamelak, "Parkinson's disease, the dopaminergic neuron and gammahydroxybutyrate," *Neurology and Therapy*, vol. 7, pp. 5–11, 6 2018.

[107] T. N. Alerte, A. A. Akinfolarin, E. E. Friedrich, *et al.*, "α-synuclein aggregation alters tyrosine hydroxylase phosphorylation and immunoreactivity: Lessons from viral transduction of knockout mice," *Neuroscience Letters*, vol. 435, pp. 24–29, 4 2008.

[108] M. Funayama, K. Nishioka, Y. Li, *et al.*, "Molecular genetics of parkinson's disease: Contributions and global trends," *Journal of Human Genetics*, vol. 68, pp. 125–130, 3 2023.

[109] E. Ferrari, A. Cardinale, B. Picconi, *et al.*, "From cell lines to pluripotent stem cells for modelling parkinson's disease," *Journal of Neuroscience Methods*, vol. 340, p. 108741, 7 2020.

[110] F. Soldner, J. Laganière, A. W. Cheng, *et al.*, "Generation of isogenic pluripotent stem cells differing exclusively at two early onset parkinson point mutations," *Cell*, vol. 146, pp. 318–331, 7 2011.

[111] R. Fernández-Santiago, I. Carballo-Carbajal, G. Castellano, *et al.*, "Aberrant epigenome in ipsc-derived dopaminergic neurons from parkinson's disease patients," *EMBO Molecular Medicine*, vol. 7, pp. 1529–1546, 12 2015.

[112] L. M. Smits, L. Reinhardt, P. Reinhardt, *et al.*, "Modeling parkinson's disease in midbrain-like organoids," *npj Parkinson's Disease*, vol. 5, p. 5, 4 2019.

[113] H. Kim, H. J. Park, H. Choi, *et al.*, "Modeling g2019s-lrrk2 sporadic parkinson's disease in 3d midbrain organoids," *Stem Cell Reports*, vol. 12, pp. 518–531, 3 2019.

[114] D. Doi, H. Magotani, T. Kikuchi, *et al.*, "Pre-clinical study of induced pluripotent stem cell-derived dopaminergic progenitor cells for parkinson's disease," *Nature Communications*, vol. 11, p. 3369, 7 2020.

[115] I. Garitaonandia, R. Gonzalez, T. Christiansen-Weber, *et al.*, "Neural stem cell tumorigenicity and biodistribution assessment for phase i clinical trial in parkinson's disease," *Scientific Reports*, vol. 6, p. 34478, 9 2016.

[116] Y.-K. Wang, W.-W. Zhu, M.-H. Wu, *et al.*, "Human clinical-grade parthenogenetic esc-derived dopaminergic neurons recover locomotive defects of nonhuman primate models of parkinson's disease," *Stem Cell Reports*, vol. 11, pp. 171–182, 7 2018.

[117] Y. Cha, T.-Y. Park, P. Leblanc, *et al.*, "Current status and future perspectives on stem cell-based therapies for parkinson's disease," *Journal of Movement Disorders*, vol. 16, pp. 22–41, 1 2023.

[118] J. A. Smith, A. M. Nicaise, R.-B. Ionescu, *et al.*, "Stem cell therapies for progressive multiple sclerosis," *Frontiers in Cell and Developmental Biology*, vol. 9, 7 2021.

[119] E. Grajchen, J. J. A. Hendriks, and J. F. J. Bogie, "The physiology of foamy phagocytes in multiple sclerosis," *Acta Neuropathologica Communications*, vol. 6, p. 124, 12 2018.

[120] J. Martínez-Larrosa, C. Matute-Blanch, X. Montalban, *et al.*, "Modelling multiple sclerosis using induced pluripotent stem cells," *Journal of Neuroimmunology*, vol. 349, p. 577425, 12 2020.

[121] Y. Xin, J. Gao, R. Hu, *et al.*, "Changes of immune parameters of t lymphocytes and macrophages in eae mice after bm-mscs transplantation," *Immunology Letters*, vol. 225, pp. 66–73, 9 2020.

[122] G. Constantin, S. Marconi, B. Rossi, *et al.*, "Adipose-derived mesenchymal stem cells ameliorate chronic experimental autoimmune encephalomyelitis," *Stem Cells*, vol. 27, pp. 2624–2635, 10 2009.

[123] Y. Liu, Y. Ma, B. Du, *et al.*, "Mesenchymal stem cells attenuated blood-brain barrier disruption via downregulation of aquaporin-4 expression in eae mice," *Molecular Neurobiology*, vol. 57, pp. 3891–3901, 9 2020.

[124] M. M. Mahfouz, R. M. Abdelsalam, M. A. Masoud, *et al.*, "The neuroprotective effect of mesenchymal stem cells on an experimentally induced model for multiple sclerosis in mice," *Journal of Biochemical and Molecular Toxicology*, vol. 31, p. e21936, 9 2017.

[125] A. Gugliandolo, P. Bramanti, and E. Mazzon, "Mesenchymal stem cells in multiple sclerosis: Recent evidence from pre-clinical to clinical studies," *International Journal of Molecular Sciences*, vol. 21, p. 8662, 11 2020.

[126] M. Jafarinia, F. Alsahebfosoul, H. Salehi, *et al.*, "Therapeutic effects of extracellular vesicles from human adipose-derived mesenchymal stem cells on chronic experimental autoimmune encephalomyelitis," *Journal of Cellular Physiology*, vol. 235, pp. 8779–8790, 11 2020.

[127] Z. Li, F. Liu, X. He, *et al.*, "Exosomes derived from mesenchymal stem cells attenuate inflammation and demyelination of the central nervous system in eae rats by regulating the polarization of microglia," *International Immunopharmacology*, vol. 67, pp. 268–280, 2 2019.

[128] F. H. Shamili, M. Alibolandi, H. Rafatpanah, *et al.*, "Immunomodulatory properties of msc-derived exosomes armed with high affinity aptamer toward mylein as a platform for reducing multiple sclerosis clinical score," *Journal of Controlled Release*, vol. 299, pp. 149–164, 4 2019.

[129] T. Alexander, R. Greco, and J. A. Snowden, "Hematopoietic stem cell transplantation for autoimmune disease," *Annual Review of Medicine*, vol. 72, pp. 215–228, 1 2021.

[130] F. Collins, M. Kazmi, and P. A. Muraro, "Progress and prospects for the use and the understanding of the mode of action of autologous hematopoietic stem cell transplantation in the treatment of multiple sclerosis," *Expert Review of Clinical Immunology*, vol. 13, pp. 611–622, 6 2017.

[131] M. M. Bakhuraysah, C. Siatskas, and S. Petratos, "Hematopoietic stem cell transplantation for multiple sclerosis: is it a clinical reality?," *Stem Cell Research and Therapy*, vol. 7, p. 12, 12 2016.

[132] F. Nabizadeh, K. Pirahesh, N. Rafiei, *et al.*, "Autologous hematopoietic stem-cell transplantation in multiple sclerosis: A systematic review and meta-analysis," *Neurology and Therapy*, vol. 11, pp. 1553–1569, 12 2022.

[133] A. Mariottini, E. D. Matteis, and P. A. Muraro, "Haematopoietic stem cell transplantation for multiple sclerosis: Current status," *BioDrugs*, vol. 34, pp. 307–325, 6 2020.

[134] K. A. Jellinger, "Understanding depression with amyotrophic lateral sclerosis: a short assessment of facts and perceptions," *Journal of Neural Transmission*, vol. 131, pp. 107–115, 2 2024.

[135] R. Mejzini, L. L. Flynn, I. L. Pitout, *et al.*, "Als genetics, mechanisms, and therapeutics: Where are we now?," *Frontiers in Neuroscience*, vol. 13, 12 2019.

[136] S. Najafi, P. Najafi, N. K. Farkhad, *et al.*, "Mesenchymal stem cell therapy in amyotrophic lateral sclerosis (als) patients: A comprehensive review of disease information and future perspectives," *Iranian journal of basic medical sciences*, vol. 26, pp. 872–881, 2023.

[137] B. J. Wainger, E. Kiskinis, C. Mellin, *et al.*, "Intrinsic membrane hyperexcitability of amyotrophic lateral sclerosis patient-derived motor neurons," *Cell Reports*, vol. 7, pp. 1–11, 4 2014.

[138] K. Fujimori, M. Ishikawa, A. Otomo, *et al.*, "Modeling sporadic als in ipsc-derived motor neurons identifies a potential therapeutic agent," *Nature Medicine*, vol. 24, pp. 1579–1589, 10 2018.

[139] S. Morimoto, S. Takahashi, D. Ito, *et al.*, "Phase 1/2a clinical trial in als with ropinirole, a drug candidate identified by ipsc drug discovery," *Cell Stem Cell*, vol. 30, pp. 766–780.e9, 6 2023.

[140] K. Imamura, Y. Izumi, A. Watanabe, *et al.*, "The src/c-abl pathway is a potential therapeutic target in amyotrophic lateral sclerosis," *Science Translational Medicine*, vol. 9, 5 2017.

[141] K. Imamura, Y. Izumi, M. Nagai, *et al.*, "Safety and tolerability of bosutinib in patients with amyotrophic lateral sclerosis (idream study): A multicentre, open-label, dose-escalation phase 1 trial," *eClinicalMedicine*, vol. 53, p. 101707, 11 2022.

[142] S. Thams, E. R. Lowry, M.-H. Larraufie, *et al.*, "A stem cell-based screening platform identifies compounds that desensitize motor neurons to endoplasmic reticulum stress," *Molecular Therapy*, vol. 27, pp. 87–101, 1 2019.

[143] N. J. Lamas, B. Johnson-Kerner, L. Roybon, *et al.*, "Neurotrophic requirements of human motor neurons defined using amplified and purified stem cell-derived cultures," *PLoS ONE*, vol. 9, p. e110324, 10 2014.

[144] E. Abati, N. Bresolin, G. Comi, *et al.*, "Advances, challenges, and perspectives in translational stem cell therapy for amyotrophic lateral sclerosis," *Molecular Neurobiology*, vol. 56, pp. 6703–6715, 10 2019.

[145] A. Aljabri, A. Halawani, G. B. Lajdam, *et al.*, "The safety and efficacy of stem cell therapy as an emerging therapy for als: A systematic review of controlled clinical trials," *Frontiers in Neurology*, vol. 12, 12 2021.

[146] H. R. Martínez, J. F. Molina-Lopez, M. T. González-Garza, *et al.*, "Stem cell transplantation in amyotrophic lateral sclerosis patients: Methodological approach, safety, and feasibility," *Cell Transplantation*, vol. 21, pp. 1899–1907, 9 2012.

[147] L. Mazzini, M. Gelati, D. Profico, *et al.*, "Human neural stem cell transplantation in als: initial results from a phase i trial," *Journal of Translational Medicine*, vol. 13, p. 17, 2015.

[148] P. Petrou, Y. Gothelf, Z. Argov, *et al.*, "Safety and clinical effects of mesenchymal stem cells secreting neurotrophic factor transplantation in patients with amyotrophic lateral sclerosis," *JAMA Neurology*, vol. 73, p. 337, 3 2016.

3

Tissue Engineered Models of Brain Tumors and Their Applications

Tugba Bal

Üsküdar University, İstanbul, Türkiye

Diverse physiological processes are dictated and contributed by the brain. Thus, any pathological state such as tumors adversely modifies the brain and exerts disadvantageous effects throughout the body. Among such tumors, especially glioblastoma (GBM) is the deadliest due to its aggressiveness, invasive capacity and late diagnosis which recall advanced bio-technologies to address these issues. Today, clinics are submerged into a diverse set of GBM diagnosis and treatment strategies, yet it demands the advancement of current treatment. Tissue engineering can be a powerful tool for researchers and clinicians in various aspects and scenarios of this disease to decode the nature of this tumor and prolong patient survival.

3.1 Introduction

Brain tumors are a heterogenous group of diseases mainly classified with unique histopathology and molecular signatures. In general, different tools including staining, microscopy, molecular genetics, and profiling have been fundamental for diagnosis and classification leading to more than 50 subgroups of cancer in the central nervous system (CNS). Among brain tumors, glioblastoma (GBM), a subgroup of adult-type diffuse glioma defined as WHO grade IV brain tumor [1] will be the focus of the analysis of tissue-engineered models in this chapter. GBM is the most aggressive brain tumor with 14.6-month survival and it constitutes 50% of the malignant brain tumors. Surgical removal, radiation- and chemo-therapy remain the current routes to achieve better prognosis, yet they require significant improvement for patient survival [2]. As survival rate is low and new treatment strategies are required, analysis of tumor environment along with tissue-engineered models for personalized

DOI: 10.1201/9781003461906-3

medicine, mathematical modeling, dissecting the cellular and molecular nature of the tumor for basic research are keys to address challenges to find a cure.

Since diversity and changes in cellular and extracellular environments are primary mediators between pre-clinical tissue engineering models and clinical trials for brain tumors, GBM microenvironment will be highlighted to understand the sources and contribution of cellular and molecular heterogeneity in this chapter. Non-cellular components of this 3D network will also be summarized, as they are key players to develop innovative *in vitro* mimics of tumor tissue. A detailed analysis will further be performed on GBM models in tissue engineering with their current applications.

3.2 Glioblastoma (GBM) Microenvironment

In GBM, tumor and its growth are not isolated, as they include a complex interplay between cellular and non-cellular components contributed by significant changes in tissue organization, interactions and signaling. This environment is assembled with cancer cells and cancer stem cells, tissue resident cells, infiltrating immune system cells and vasculature. Besides, non-cellular components are crucial, as they play a pivotal role in tumor progression and therapy. Thus, our current understanding of this crosstalk is of utmost importance to the onset, progression and prognosis of GBM as well as is a key hallmark to establish diverse treatment and tissue-engineered model strategies to improve clinical outcomes. This 3D non-cellular network of tumor environment is built with extracellular matrix (ECM), soluble signals and their gradients [3, 4]. In this section, an overview of these cellular and non-cellular constituents of GBM microenvironment, as well as their essential tasks for tumor and tumor-model reconstruction will be provided.

3.2.1 Cellular Environment and Signals of GBM

GBM onset and progression modify the content of the relevant brain tissue in a unique pattern. In this tumor, cancer cells, cancer stem cells, tissue-resident cells, resident and migrating immune system cells, and brain vasculature are the major cells/cell sources in tumor mass or in the surrounding tissue. Additionally, interface between brain and blood circulation is built with blood-brain barrier (BBB) that contributes to both healthy brains as well as the development of related diseases [3, 4].

3.2.1.1 Cancer Cells, Cancer Stem Cells (CSCs)

Currently, cell of origin for GBM is largely unknown, but it has been considered that neural stem cells, astrocytes, oligodendrocyte precursor cells and glial precursor cells have potential to give rise to GBM cancer cells. Continual uncontrolled cell growth and genomic instability of these cells contribute to the hallmarks of GBM during tumor development. To undergo transformation into a GBM cancer cell, these cells accumulate various characteristic genetic alterations influencing cell behavior and metabolism. Activating or inactivating mutations in cellular cascades such as growth factor signaling, tumor suppressor pathways (p53, PTEN and retinoblastoma) and telomerase activity, cyclin-dependent kinases and their inhibitors mediate global modifications in the cellular network [5]. However, it has been revealed that GBM has genetic and epigenetic heterogeneity. For example, of 367 GBM patients analyzed by Ma et al., 62% of GBM tissue samples showed CDKN2A/B mutation and 43% were positive for EGFR mutations [6]. GBM also shows distinct patterning in DNA methylation within and between tumors [7].

Unlike a healthy brain, this tumor microenvironment is the home for GBM stem cells which have self-renewal and differentiation capacity, as well as interact with cellular and non-cellular elements of GBM to direct cell behavior, resist therapy, remodel ECM, invade and suppress immune screening [8, 9]. Within this space, nano-sized lipid bilayer-enclosed structures called cancer-derived extracellular vesicles are basic links to deliver important factors that are essential for various stages of GBM. These vesicles contain growth factors, receptors, RNAs, diverse set of enzymes and other proteins to mediate expansion of the tumor. After release, activity of the vesicles goes beyond primary tissue, and they can even leave the extracellular environment of the primary tumor and travel through biofluids exerting effects in distant regions (Figure 3.1) [10–13]. These vesicles also alter the immune activity where they mediate inactivation and death of immune system cells. For example, PDL-1 delivered through extracellular vesicles promote PD-L1—PD1 interaction of T cells and thereby, driving their inactivation and death. Thus, PDL-1 containing vesicles contribute immunosuppressive niche of GBM [14]. Further, extracellular vesicles containing TGF-β inactivate T cells so that granzyme and perforin secretion is inhibited and IFN-γ secretion is prevented [15]. Other factors include IL-10 and PGE2, as well as cell-cell contact mediated death through Fas—FasL, PD-L1—PD1 interaction [16, 17].

3.2.1.2 Tissue Resident Cell Landscape of GBM: Neurons, Astrocytes, Microglia, and Oligodendrocytes

Neurons in the brain are affected by impaired functioning and these cells are under dynamic bidirectional interaction with glioma cells. In an example study of molecular program modification of neurons by GBM, tumor-adjacent brain tissue neurons were shown to express PD-L1 under IFN-β based control to trigger proliferation arrest and apoptosis of tumor cells in patient tissue sections and mouse isograft model [18]. Yet, GBM tumor cells adapt an unfavorable status for neurons. They can secrete sCD44 that links tau hyperphosphorylation and pathology of neurodegenerative diseases such as Alzheimer's disease

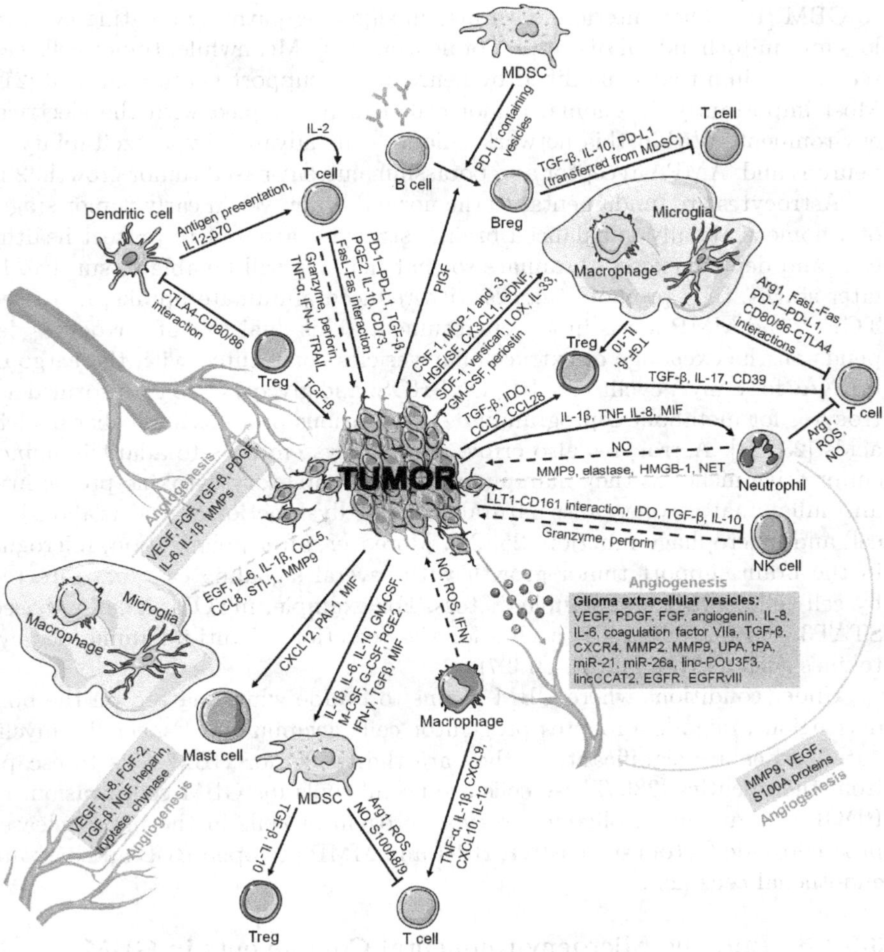

FIGURE 3.1
Selected examples of soluble molecules and membrane-associated proteins in invasive, immunosuppressive and angiogenic networks of immune system cells and tumors. BLACK arrows mark the activation of target cells with relevant factors. BLUNT BLACK arrows point out inhibitory activity through the mentioned factors. GREY arrows indicate factors involved in angiogenesis. DASHED arrows represent immune activity against the tumor. DASHED GREY arrows show factors in direct effect on tumor cells to promote invasion. The figure was generated using Servier Medical Art, provided by Servier, licensed under a Creative Commons Attribution 4.0 unported license.

to GBM [19]. They interfere with insulin signaling pathway creating synapse loss and mitochondrial disruption of neurons [20]. Meanwhile, tumor cells can secrete laminin that is modified by neurons and support neuron survival [21]. Most importantly, in glioma, tumor cells can be coupled with the electrical environment. Within this network, glioma cells advance hyperexcitability of neurons and, AMPA-receptor and potassium current-based tumor growth [22].

Astrocytes are fundamental to the normal brain, yet in early tumor stages of a homeostatically imbalanced brain, astrocytes attempt to protect healthy cells and deplete excess glutamate so that neurons will be able to survive. In later stages, they promote tumors with reduced glutamate uptake, increased TGF-β and MMP levels in the environment. This dual role of astrocytes depends on the exchange of extracellular vesicles constituted with the cargo of mRNAs for c-myc, cyclin-D3, RP, OXPHOS, and glycolysis to transformed astrocytes for metabolic reprogramming, and various proteins and other nucleic acids [23, 24]. Astrocytes also criple immune system cells to adapt immunosuppressive niche, as they manipulate pro-inflammatory cytokine profile into anti-inflammatory one, cause natural killer cell dysfunction as well as abolish T cell and macrophage function [25, 26]. Moreover, after polarization, microglia in the brain support tumor growth with several signaling cascades directed by cell-cell contact and soluble factors. For example, mTOR signaling-based STAT3 phosphorylation is a clue for the secretion of anti-inflammatory cytokines such as IL-6 and IL-10 [27].

Under conditions where GBM begins to invade white matter, on the border regions, oligodendrocytes progenitor cells accumulate. Especially, myelinated axons are significant, as they are the tracks for GBM cells to escape from therapeutics [28]. These cells are useful tools for GBM cell invasion, as PDGF-C signaling of oligodendrocytes progenitor cells in the brain releases proangiogenic factors such as IGFBP-1 and MMP9 to open BBB and activate endothelial cells [29].

3.2.1.3 Immune Microenvironmental Components in GBM

Among cellular components in GBM, tumor associated macrophages/microglia (TAMs) are one of the most abundant cells, as they usually constitute up to 50% of the cells in tumor tissue. Sources of TAMs are macrophages infiltrating into the brain and tissue-resident microglia. In healthy brain, microglia are considered as effector macrophages of the CNS. However, in brain tumors, critical roles of TAM rely on immunosuppression, support of invasion, proliferation as well as angiogenesis. Soluble factors and certain enzymes are secreted by glioma cells to recruit TAMs to the area of tumor mass to promote growth (Figure 3.1) [30, 31]. TAMs secrete various factors to boost GBM invasiveness such as EGF to increase proliferation and motility [32], TIMP-1, IL-6, and CCL5 induced by GBM cell extracellular vesicles for ECM degradation and tumor growth [33], CCL8 for invasion and stem-cell like characteristic of

GBM cells [34], MMP-9 to degrade ECM [35], STI-1 in glioma proliferation and migration [36], IL-1β for stemness and chemo-resistance [37].

Macrophages need to be polarized to M1 and M2 lineages to operate as anti-tumor and pro-tumor macrophages. This conversion is dictated by, for example, IFN-γ/LPS/GM-CSF cues for polarization into M1 macrophages whereas M2 macrophages rely on IL-4/IL-13/M-CSF signaling [38]. In anti-cancer surveillance strategy of macrophages, oxidative stress prompted by NO and ROS, and IFN-γ derived from M1 macrophages are directed to kill GBM cells [39, 40]. This class of macrophages also secretes a wide range of other cytokines to activate T cells for targeted tumor cell destruction, as M1 macrophage factors of TNF-α, IL-1β, CXCL9, CXCL10, and IL-12 activate T cells to target tumor cell for destruction [41–43]. In contrast, contributed by alternative activation of M2 macrophages, TAMs suppress cytotoxic T cell activity by PD-L1—PD1, and Fas—FasL dependent cell-cell contact as well as CTLA-4—CD80/86 engagement [31, 44]. Their capability of arginase-1 expression depletes a critical amino acid, L-arginine, in extracellular space resulting in impairment of metabolism and co-receptor expression, thus lowered proliferation and function of T cells [45]. In addition to immunosuppression and invasion, these cells produce considerable amount of factors to push angiogenesis of GBM. So far, it has been demonstrated that well-known stimulating factors such as VEGF, TGF-β, and FGF elicit signals for pericytes and endothelial cells in tumor vascularization [46, 47].

Neutrophils are other member of immune myeloid lineage migrated to the brain and they communicate with GBM cells and vascular network of brain through diverse set of soluble factors. Once recruited by GBM, presence of HGF in tumor microenvironment leads to production of tumor cell-killing NO from neutrophils. However, neutrophils support tumor invasion by degrading ECM with elastase [48, 49]. Their accumulation in brain tumors is correlated with glioma grade and parallel to T cell suppresion and high levels of Arg1, ROS, and NO by migrating bone-marrow derived neutrophils [50]. Their potential to induce secretion of S1004A protein from CSCs, thereby activation of epithelial-to-mesenchymal transition and tumor invasion are confirmed *in vivo*, as reported by Liang et al., depletion of S1004A and anti-VEGF therapy were shown to be effective against glioma progression [51]. As supporters, HMGB-1 and neutrophil extracellular traps (NET) are tumor-promoting factors acting through cancer cell proliferation and invasion. Tumor infiltrating neutrophil-derived HMGB-1 binds to RAGE of glioma cells and stimulates NF-$\kappa\beta$ transcription pathway factor and, leads to secretion of IL-8 that results in poor prognosis [52]. S100A8 and 9, VEGF and MMP9 are other proteins expressed by neutrophils for ECM degradation, endothelial cell activation and angiogenesis in tumors [53, 54].

As a part of innate immune system, natural killer (NK) cells attack the brain tumor through perforin and granzyme creating a lytic pore and activating caspases. Pro-inflammatory cytokines such as TNF-α and IFN-γ of NK cells attract and activate antigen-presenting cells and T cells. Yet as counterattack, signaling through released molecules such as IDO, TGF-β, and IL-10, as well as cell-cell contact with GBM cells disable NK cells. For instance, glioma cells express LLT1 as a protection mechanism against NK-mediated lysis. This molecule interacts with CD161 receptor on NK cells to block cytotoxicity and diminish IFN-γ expression [55–57].

When normal brain switches into tumor-promoting environment, anti-tumor activity of dendritic cells and T cells are severely affected. Dendritic cells mainly function in antigen presentation to T cells and secrete IFN-γ [58]. Combination of secreted IL-2 by CD4+ T cells with antigen presentation provokes CD8+ T cells to begin anti-tumor attack through perforin and granzyme, as well as by secreting TNF-α, IFN-γ, and TRAIL [59, 60]. However, CTLA-4 of Tregs interacts with CD80/86 coreceptor of dendritic cells to deplete it by trogocytosis so that these cells can no longer activate T cells leading to escape of tumor cells from immune-screening [61]. Other Treg-based mechanisms committed to tumor survival include inhibition of T cells by lL-17 [62] and management of glioma stemness through TGF-β–NF-κB–IL6–STAT3 pathway [63]. TGF-β also diminishes effector T cell survival and function, as it has been reported that especially TGF-β-based immunoregulation halts expression of the soluble or membrane-bound proteins such as perforin, granzyme, Fas-L, IFN-γ, and IL-2 [64, 65]. Another favorable aspect of Treg activity depends on CD39 enzyme on Treg membrane in which this enzyme converts ATP to AMP starting the cascade of adenosine formation by CD73 of glioma cells. This adenosine binds to Aa2R on T cells to inhibit its activity, directs macrophage fate to M2 phenotype and switches on Treg production [66]. To do so, recruitment of Tregs to the site of brain tumors is contributed by soluble factors such as CCL2 [67, 68], IDO [69], CCL28 [70], and TGF-β [71]. Activation of Tregs through TGF-β and IL-10 by MDSC also advances pro-tumor status [72]. By conferring aforementioned tumor promoting actions in GBM development, Tregs are reported to be associated with poor glioma patient survival [67].

Under physiological conditions, mast cells recruit and stimulate neutrophils, promote wound healing and fibrosis, react against allergens, carry neuroimmune interactions and, function in blood coagulation and vascular permeability [73]. In GBM, mast cells are mobilized towards tumor mass by CXCL12, PAI-1 and MIF of tumor cells [74, 75]. Upon trigger, mast cells cause inflammation and apoptosis of tumors, but also promote immunosuppression and produce representative factors in Figure 3.1 to guide blood vessel cells and promote angiogenesis in cancer [76, 77].

The existence of other cell groups such as myeloid derived suppressor cells (MDSCs) also determines whether pro- or anti-tumor course will progress. MDSCs are mixed population of bone-marrow derived immune system cells accumulating in blood and tumor of glioma patients. These cells are reported to be drawn to and activated by the tumors where they proliferate and exert many activities including suppression of effector T cells, development of Tregs, induction M2 phenotype of macrophages and control of NK cell function [71, 78–80]. They suppress T cells with several mechanisms by relying on the production of certain proteins and other chemicals. For instance, MDSCs can deplete T cell survival and function inducer amino acid, L-arginine, in the environment by arginase 1 and promote tumor with S100A8/9 [72, 81]. Another important issue is the transfer of MDSC vesicles containing PD-L1 to convert B cells into immunosuppressive Bregs. After uptaking the vesicles, these cells begin to express CD155, IL-10, and TGF-β, and have capability to suppress effector CD8+ T cell activation and function [82]. Additionally, PIGF signal changes naive B cells to TGF-β expressing Bregs to control T cell behavior [83].

3.2.2 Extracellular Matrix (ECM) of Brain and GBM

Apart from cells, soft tissue of brain is contributed by interstitial system that fills the gap between the cells. This system is composed of interstitial fluid that bathes the surface of cells and an ECM for cellular functions necessary for development, maintenance, and treatment efficiency. In GBM, important features of this network are altered to serve for the tumor growth [84].

3D network of brain is primarily built on the arrangements of nonfibrillar and fibrillar proteins and composition differs within brain regions [85]. Besides, certain ECM structures are present in the brain: Neural interstitial matrix, perineuronal nets (PNNs) and basement membrane of BBB (Figure 3.2). Neural interstitial matrix is a proteinous network occupying the space of brain parenchyma. It is assembled into the interconnected web of ECM through mainly hyaluronic acid, chondroitin sulfate proteoglycans (CSPGs), tenascins and link proteins, at a small quantity of collagen, laminin, fibronectin and elastin [86]. PNNs are a proteinous web covering neurons as physical barrier managing diverse functions at neuron-neuron, neuron-ECM interface [87]. They manage distribution of receptors such as AMPAR on the cell surface at synaptic cleft and inhibit juvenile plasticity [88, 89], protect against oxidative stress [90], act as reservoirs for cations [91], as well as sequester plasticity-related (e.g. Sema3A) and PNN assembly-related (e.g.Nptx2) molecules [92, 93]. These nets are rich in hyaluronic acid, proteoglycans, tenascins and link proteins [87, 94]. In contrast, basement membrane is a sheet-like structure wrapping around the blood vessels and assists formation of BBB for strict permeability control in/out of brain. This layer has a distinct composition enriched with collagen, laminin, fibronectin, perlecan, nidogen/entactin, and agrin [95, 96].

Considering the distribution of each protein and polysaccharide, their roles in (patho)physiology of development and adults have taken significant attention in basic research and clinics. It is proven non-cellular microenvironment goes under significant modifications which eventually impose tumor-promoting course in the prognosis and treatment for many brain diseases. For instance, as a physical barrier, hyaluronic acid coating hinders GBM cells so that it restricts immune surveillance and, therefore, halts immune attack.

CD44 interaction with hyaluronic acid also triggers expression of certain pathways implicated in GBM migration and survival [97]. Another significant brain ECM protein group is chondroitin sulfate proteoglycans (CSPGs) that reveal robust changes in function and level in healthy and diseased state [98]. With increased but uneven expression in GBM, collagen IV contributes disrupted basement membrane in tissue sections and allows migration of tumor cells as previously demonstrated [99, 100]. Moreover, laminin-411 is highly expressed in GBM patients resulting in poor survival and high risk of recurrence of tumor by driving invasion and potentially supporting angiogenesis [101]. In GBM, fibronectin interactions direct tumor growth via cell migration, differentiation, and contributes tumor angiogenesis [102]. Additionally, investigation of the mechanism of action of elastin in brain tumors indicate that GBM cells express tropoelastin (soluble form of elastin) and a cell surface receptor called elastin binding protein to adhere elastin and to invade [103].

3.2.3 Vasculature in Brain and GBM

A dynamic network of vessels supplies blood to meet the metabolic demands of the brain. However, transport processes are far more strictly controlled due to the presence of blood-brain barrier (BBB) which is one of the prominent reasons for the failure of drug delivery into the brain (Figure 3.2). As an interface between blood and brain tissue, BBB is present on different types of vessels providing a unique pathway for cellular activity. Function of the barrier is not limited to be a physical barrier, but it is also essential for ion homeostasis, neurotransmitter and growth factor level control, prevention of leakage into the brain and protection against neurotoxins. However, modifications in this interface are observed as clinical signature events in GBM [104–106].

The microenvironmental background of the BBB in capillaries is shaped by multiple factors. A continuous layer of endothelial cells is held together thoroughly by mainly cell-cell junctions and attached to extracellular space with various cell surface receptors. This blood-contacting layer is coated by the basement membrane and is supported by pericytes and astrocytes [107, 108]. The junctions and their components as active mediators of endothelial layer integrity are summarized in Figure 3.2. These junctions mediate cell-cell connection, transfer, transendothelial leukocyte migration, and signaling. Although BBB dictates the flow of substances between the blood and the brain, each molecule has a distinct pathway through endothelium to route themselves in and out of the brain [109–111].

BBB undergoes transformation into the blood-tumor barrier in GBM. Blood-tumor barrier features are heterogeneous and, reduced junctions, nonuniform pericyte localization, astrocyte end-feet displacement result in permeable vessels thereby advancing fluid pressure and accessibility into the brain [112]. In brain tumors, the profile of the endothelial cells differs within the tumor and from the surrounding tissue. In these distinct regions, endothelial transporters and carriers are differentially expressed in the endothelial cells

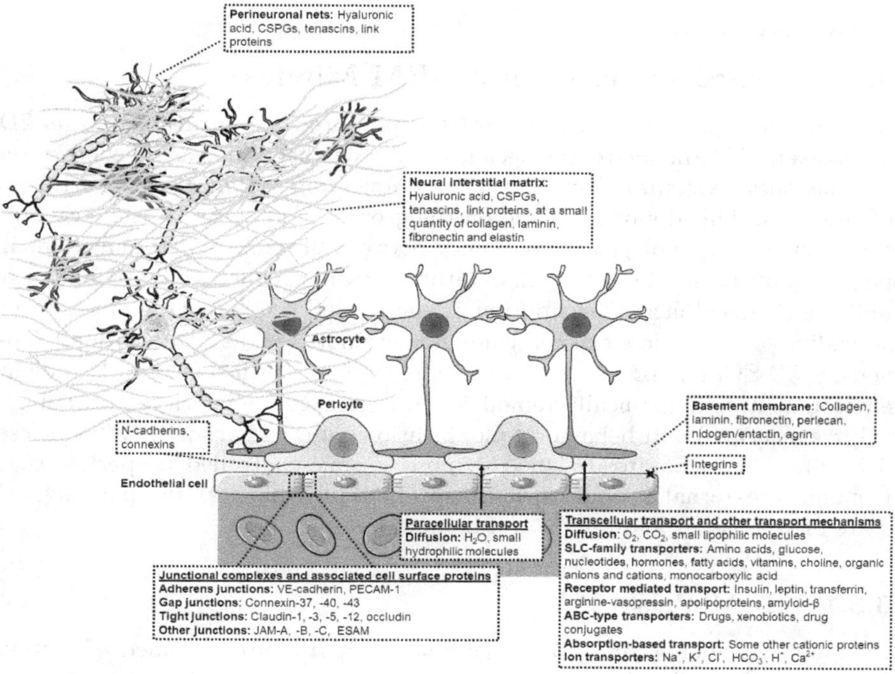

FIGURE 3.2
BBB of capillaries and ECM in the brain. The figure was partly generated using Servier Medical Art, provided by Servier, licensed under a Creative Commons Attribution 4.0 unported license.

populating tumor core and periphery resulting in the alteration of the fundamental transport mechanisms. SLC2A1, ABCG2, ABCB1, SLCO1A2, and MFSD2A are some of the examples carriers with lowered expression in the tumor core. Of the note, LRP-1 and, fenestration and permeability-associated protein, PLVAP are overexpressed in GBM [107, 113, 114]. Moreover, morphological abnormalities of endothelial cells are reported in the blood-tumor barrier. Phenotype of endothelial cells presumes a flattened morphology with an enlarged nucleus that has a boost in migration potential in contrast to the cobblestone phenotype of a healthy state [115]. Besides, once quiescent endothelial cells are activated by tumor cells, they undergo transcriptional reprogramming. Within this network, activated growth loops sustain and push for angiogenesis [116, 117]. In GBM, pericytes play protective roles for the tumor and contribute invasion process [118]. Associated with hyperdilated and thin-walled blood vessels of GBM, CSC-derived pericyte coverage of blood vessels determines prognosis, as high pericyte coverage in GBM establishes low patient survival. Results of ablation of these pericytes manifest as increased vascular permeability and chemotherapeutic efficiency of etoposide [119].

3.3 *In vitro* Experimental GBM Mimics

In traditional practice, cells are isolated, cultured and manipulated as 2D monolayers. Yet, in the recent decades, there has been increasing concern on whether these systems reflect the native organization or they are mere artifacts of the body. This doubt has risen on the ground of analysis on the mechanical, chemical and biological discrepancy between 2D culture and multicellular body organization. Typically, 2D culture presents higher stiffness and near uniform chemical factor distribution, induces cellular polarity with monolayer spreading, and restricts cell-cell communication as well as organization. Conversely, 3D ECM accommodates for various interactions in a chemical-gradient environment, is dynamically remodeled and manages cellularity, morphological, translational and behavioral modifications of cells harbored. When these 3D culture systems are designed to possess time-controlled properties that respond to external stimuli, various aspects of physiological and pathological state of the tissues and organs can be uncovered [120, 121].

3.3.1 2D Models

Although 2D monolayer systems as gold standards are devoided of certain features of the body, they significantly contributed to the advancement of today's research. This approach is still in practice and invaluable tool to meet the demand to supply specific amount of cells for diverse set of applications. Their common utilization as pre-clinical models is attributed to their low cost, simplicity, and ease of maintenance [122], yet they fail to sustain important characteristics such as cellular and genetic heterogeneity, and microenvironment of tumors. These drawbacks led to unreliable drug efficacy and modeling data in clinics [123, 124].

3.3.2 2.5D Models

Standard bare tissue culture polystyrene surfaces were dominant in cancer studies in pre-clinical research for several decades, but biomaterial coated-plastic or -glass surfaces are increasingly employed to study tumors as pre-clinical 2.5D models. These coated surfaces can be modified with ECM derived proteins such as collagen I and laminin, with ECM mimics such as matrigel and decellularized ECM, or with adhesion ligands such as RGD [125–129].

In 2.5D models, micropatterned and nanofiber substrates can provide physiologically relevant topological ECM cues as described in previous reports. In a recent study, electrospun polystyrene fibers were tuned to analyze directionality of U87 single cell migration in motility assays [130]. Additionally, U87 cells on electrospun suspended gelatin mesofibers displayed aggregation, deformation, and migration dynamics [131] and poly(vinyl alcohol) coated silicon wafer with an altered strip width and complex design provided important insights on cell adhesion and migration [132]. U251 cells on STEP fibers and C6 cells on laminin coated linear grooves have serviced to exercise the impact of geometry on the migration speed and dimensions, and cytoskeletal modeling [133, 134]. Aside from the role of topographic information on migration and mechanisms behind, it can still be applied to proliferation, invasion, and investigation of driving factors of gene expresssion pattern [135, 136].

3.3.3 3D Models

After 2.5D models, 3D models gained popularity as versatile tools to address the bottlenecks of conventional 2D models on the simulation of the GBM complexity. Currently, 3D models are formulated as scaffold-free, scaffold-based, and hybrid strategies. Additionally, microfluidic/chip systems and organotypic slices are of current interest, especially to harness native tumor tissue properties.

Scaffold-free models (Figure 3.3 and Table 3.1) in GBM are constructed as organizations of (hetero)spheroids and organoids. During this process, cell-cell cohesion is amplified by driving minimum interaction with any non-cell surface. Thereby, it leads to spontaneous cell arrangements in 3D configurations. This assembly is considered superior over 2D monolayer culture, as it can imitate various features of solid tumors. Even certain aspects of the animal models of the disease cannot match the development stages of humans where patient-derived organoids can be preferable to model disease and even to discover patient-specific responses. The possibility of real-time imaging, biobanking and high-throughput analysis are other benefits of these technologies [137–139]. Besides, *in vitro* culture creates development of three distinct zones (proliferative, quiescent and necrotic zones) within especially spheroids with larger than 500 μm in diameter. Non-uniform features of pH, gases, nutrients, and other soluble factors are further posed by 3D organization of spheroids with high similarity to native tumor [140]. An organoid is also 3D assembly of cells, but it is composed of different cell types mimicking the cellular composition, function and physiology of the tissue/organ they originate, as well as better imitate genetics and phenotype of tumor tissue. Conversely, they require growth factor cocktails to sustain tissue architecture and, tissue procurement and processing alterations hamper standardization [122, 123, 141].

In hanging drop (Figure 3.3A), 20–40 μl drops of cell suspension stay on the lid by surface tension and, gravity leads to aggregation and compaction of cells into spheroids. This technique is relatively simple, cost-effective, provides control over spheroid size and content, but it is labor-intensive, challenging in scale-up and traditionally does not support the addition of a fresh medium or soluble factors during the incubation period [122, 142, 143]. 384 well-hanging drop arrays can overcome these major drawbacks, as they allow time-lapse imaging, on-site staining and drug treatment, and culture of distinct types

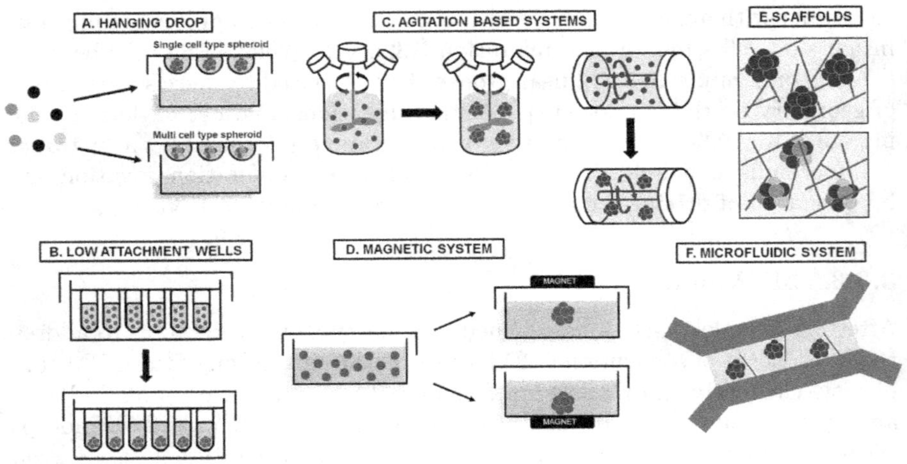

FIGURE 3.3
Summary of the most common GBM (hetero)spheroid formation techniques. **A.** Hanging drop, **B.** Low attachment wells, **C.** Agitation-based systems, **D.** Magnetic systems, **E.** Scaffolds, **F.** Microfluidic systems.

of spheroids in one drop [144, 145]. Other two main methods to prevent cell-surface binding, thus, forcing cell-cell adherence and the growth of spheroids in suspension are low attachment surfaces and agitation-based strategies. In low attachment surfaces (Figure 3.3B), treatment with polymers such as agarose or commercially available ultra-low attachment well plate systems are commonly utilized. In these systems, shaking can serve as an external factor to facilitate spontaneous spheroid manufacture. Homogenous size distribution of spheroids in each round/flat bottom well with high viability can be achieved with this method [146–149], but the application of this system on non-coated surfaces such as petri dishes results in a wide range of size distribution of spheroids and low throughput [150]. Agitation based strategies such as shakers and rotating wall-based NASA HARV bioreactor system harness the capability of continuous stirring to prevent cell adhesion (Figure 3.3C). Thus, single-cell suspension is restricted to cell-cell adhesion resulting in aggregation and spheroid formation. Although large-scale production and ease of access to spheroid are advantageous, requirement of the specialized equipment, heterogeneity of spheroid size and shape, and risk of cell disruption due to shear during stirring create complications when this method is applied [142, 151]. In another strategy, magnetic levitation (Figure 3.3D) uses magnetized cells and, gravity is overcome by magnetic force mostly located at the top of the cells. Magnetic systems/agents such as iron oxide can be applied to serve this purpose [152, 153]. Although fast spheroid formation is obtained in this method, preparation of magnetic particles is essential before levitation and the number of cells produced will be limited [142].

Alternatively, single cell suspensions can be encapsulated in synthetic or natural porous scaffolds such as matrigel which allow cell-matrix and/or cell-cell interaction, and emergence of spheroids (Figure 3.3E). These systems can be altered on application basis, but diffusion limitation and confinement can amplify cell death [142, 154, 155]. For survival and clonal expansion of cells, growth factor supplement such as EGF and bFGF can also be added to the medium for patient-derived cells/tissues [156, 157].

Given those facts, spheroids/organoids are remarkable to reproduce certain features of GBM. Through this strategy, they can offer an alternative route for the development of tumor substitutes to minimize animal experiments and cost, time, and labor-related issues to discover new treatments or improve current therapeutic efficacy. But they should be modified to incorporate biological and chemical criteria such as cell composition and ECM, biochemical and biophysical cues related to drug resistance, malignancy and perivascular niche. These drawbacks led to the emergence of biocompatible natural and/or synthetic biomaterial scaffold-based models with tunable properties and diverse cell composition. Scaffold-based methods not only create GBM models to study disease and therapy but also are ideal alternatives to certain assays such as scratch assay [151, 158–160]. Finally, a combination of scaffold-based and scaffold-free strategies offer a unique platform for GBM in macro-scale and in micro-scale changes, as non-cellular and cellular environment can be reshaped accordingly [159, 161–165].

Currently, microfluidic devices stand as one of recent techniques established for various applications in biomedical sciences from diagnosis to molecular studies. In GBM applications, modeling of a wide range of aspects including tumor biology, drug discovery, on-site analysis and real-time monitoring of therapeutic efficiency can be devised on microfluidic devices (Figure 3.3F). Polydimethylsiloxane (PDMS) is the most common material to design diverse shapes, chambers and channels, and it can be modified with natural or synthetic materials such as collagen I and decellularized ECM [172–176].

Organotypic brain slice culture experiments have been successfully practiced in neuroscience and are adapted to GBM modeling as well. These platforms offer access to *in vivo* brain sections to manipulate and study *ex vivo.* These slices are 200-350 μm in thickness and can be derived from mouse, rat and human biopsies. The sections can carry tumor or cells (patient-derived, commercially available)/spheroids associated with the tumor which can be cultured on/injected into healthy slices. This technique is promising to fill the experimental gap between *in vivo* and *in vitro* in cell behavior analysis, drug screening, and cell therapy and to study the impact of tumor mass on healthy regions [177–181]. Although brain slice culture decreases study duration from months to weeks compared to animal models, major limitations include the cost, source of slices, inability to recapitulate effect of BBB and hypoxia [182, 183].

TABLE 3.1
Scaffold-free approaches of GBM models.

Technique	Cell source/cell line	Ref.
Hanging drop	DBTRG, U251	[166]
Inverted hanging drop chips	LN229, patient-derived mouse xenograft cells	[167]
Methylcellulose modified hanging drops	Patient derived GBM cells, NCH82, HUVEC combinations	[162]
Medium in oil	UVW	[168]
Magnetic levitation	LN229, U251 (combined with) human astrocytes	[152]
NASA HARV bioreactor	GBM patient derived cells	[169]
Uncoated or agarose coated well plate	CSCs and umbilical cord MSCs	[146]
Agar coated flask	GBM patient derived cells, primary PDX-derived cells	[170]
Encapsulation in matrigel drops with shaking culture in growth factor (EGF, FGF-2) enriched, serum-free culture medium	GBM patient derived cells	[155]
Round bottom ultra-low attachment microplate (liquid overlay technique)	U87, C8D1A astrocytes and HUVEC combination	[148]
Processing human GBM tissue followed by culture in ultra low attachment plates with shaking in serum-free culture medium	Human GBM tissue	[156]
Processing into pieces and culture in nontreated, flat bottom well plate on orbital shaker	Human GBM tissue	[157]
Growth factor (EGF, FGF-2) enriched, serum-free culture medium and ultra-low attachment plates	U87, U251, A172, SF767, primary GBM cells	[171]

3.4 Applications of GBM Models in Basic and Clinical Research

As described in previous sections, scaffold-based, scaffold-free and hybrid models of GBM have been developed with diverse techniques. This section involves application of such technologies in preclinics and clinics pointing out the promise of dimensional and other manipulations for the future of GBM treatment and research.

3.4.1 Tumor Biology

In vitro GBM models play a pivotal role in decoding the tumor considering microenvironment, communication and heterogeneity, and omics knowledge. This dynamic environment dictates permissive conditions for various natural processes. Eventually, not only the cellularity of tumor and blood vessel network change but also an escape route to other possible habitats is established to harbor a metastatic niche. In spheroid and organoid systems, the establishment of hypoxic core, proliferation and packaging zones [155, 168], GSC interaction with MSCs [146], differentiation [184], surfaceome and endocytome [185] were researched and also, they are combined with scaffold-based and microfluidic systems. In these approaches, ECM analogs with various scaffolds provide invaluable aspects of tumor biology.

In general, physical properties of substrates/scaffolds have been reported to control diverse mechanisms. To delineate role of these properties on malignancy, Pedron et al. encapsulated U87 cells in gelatin hydrogels and manipulated stiffness with monomer concentration and degree of functionalization. They observed that U87 tumor cell proliferation and spreading were promoted in stiff gelatin gels with greater steric hindrance. Moreover, thicker and more crosslinked gels interfered with diffusivity largely and cells in such gels, expressed elevated levels of HIF1 and VEGF due to hypoxia [186]. Likewise, changes in stiffness guide migration and morphological switches [187]. Characteristics of network microstructure such as porosity, spatial organization, and degradability are among the other main factors dictating invasion of cells, as more ordered networks are also linked to spreading and migratory phenotype. For this purpose, a recent comparison between a collagen gel and hyaluronic acid gel provided that single tumor cells remained rounded with a tendency to form aggregates in compact hyaluronic gels with curled fibers whereas in porous collagen gels, cells were more isolated, elongated with a larger motility. Spheroid invasion assays further confirmed superiority of the ordering in networks [163]. Furthermore, degradation of scaffolds is crucial for especially pore sizes smaller than cellular dimensions, as cells in natural ECM pave their migration and trajectory by mainly enzymatic degradation of the ECM. Transition into a biomimetic system generally follows the same rule for migration and invasion of healthy or tumor cells. To represent this mechanism in a preclinical model, Hill et al. designed tunable PEG hydrogels and degradability was a major determinant of invasion supported by adhesion ligand, RGDS. Non-degradable gels were reported to be not infiltrated by GBM tumor cells whereas invasion increased throughout the culture period for degradable ones being higher with adhesive hydrogels [164]. Presentation of cell adhesion sites is equally important for a scaffold to sustain migration of encapsulated cells.

For instance, agarose in collagen gels is reported to increase stiffness and create an intercalating matrix accompanied with significant retardation of cell invasion suggesting critical result of sterical hinderance and loss of cell binding sites in collagen [188].

In tumor environment, stromal cells interact with CSCs by cell-cell interactions and soluble factors. In an effort to confirm this, McCoy et al. previously described that endothelial cells encapsulated with GSC spheroids stimulated stemness markers, limited the loss of Nestin+ cells and advanced the migration distance of these cells through contribution of endothelial signal of IL-8 [189]. Additionally, various gene expressions were enriched in a bioprinted tetra-culture of GSCs, macrophages, astrocytes, and neural progenitor cells. This system promoted invasion, polarized macrophages into TAM and partially differentiated neural progenitor cells to retaliate against immune suppression [190] highlighting the requirement of dynamic interplay between CSCs, tissue-resident, and immune system cells in a unique microenvironment.

As one of the final aspects of tumor biology, angiogenesis is a key for survival of tumor mass, to direct migration of immune system cells to the brain as well as to establish metastatic niche. In literature, scaffold-based and microfluidic systems are constructed to investigate role and mechanisms behind for *in vitro presence of pericytes and astrocytes with* angiogenesis. In one of such applications, endothelial cells in gelation hydrogels increased average branch and total network length, as well as production of laminin, ZO-1 and GLUT1 featuring onset of intact BBB formation. Co-encapsulation of GBM spheroids with brain vascular cells enhanced outgrowth area and number of invasion distance, promoted expression of certain GBM signature proteins (e.g., MMP9, PGDFAA, OPN, IL-8), yet no significant advancement was observed when only endothelial cells were used in GBM spheroids addressing the requirement of supporting cells for the stability of vessels [159].

3.4.2 Drug Response

Today's clinics is overcome by drugs mainly failing due to incompatibility in transition from bench to bedside. So far, many drug candidates offered limited clinical success heavily depending on 2D cell culture of immortalized cell lines such as U87 as first-line approach [191]. Later, pharmacokinetics and pharmacodynamics are investigated on mainly ectopically or orthotopically transplanted or genetically engineered murine models. However, lifespan, anatomical, physiological, and metabolic differences between humans and especially mice are main shortcomings for *in vivo* modeling. Further, mutation mechanism, possible lack of immune cell-tumor cell interaction in immunocompromised mice, inability to provide communications between tumor cell-stromal cells of primary tumors in mouse xenograft models adversely affect the utilization of these animals as pre-clinical models. Large animal models such as primates, canine, and pigs are also under research to shorten the gap between pre-clinical and clinical applications, but not well-documented as in murine models [191–194].

In recent years, GBM models are recreated to improve and facilitate the drug discovery, screening, and patient specific therapeutic strategies. In these studies, cell source (immortalized or patient-derived), cellular and environmental heterogeneity, communication, variation of omics information, resistance mechanisms as well as BBB characteristics have been the central interest to achieve significant advancement in clinical translation. In one of the example studies, Han et al. reported the emergence of DOX-resistant U87 cell phenotype in a GBM microfluidic device. After DOX treatment, GBM cells that repopulated the empty chambers led to emergence of DOX-resistant cells with an IC50 value 30-fold larger than wild-type cells. In these resistant cells, mutations in genes of DOX transport, metabolism, and signaling were reported as major contributors for DOX resistance [195].

More readily, first step to 3D has been linked to (hetero)spheroids and organoids models, and these approaches provided influential results for drug screening. These models can replicate collection of intratumoral cell type and cycle dynamics, as GBM solid tumor is constituted by proliferating and quiescent subpopulations that are linked to tumor recurrence after treatment. As it is previously reported, both quiescent and proliferative GBM cells have potential to form spheres but size is measured to be small in quiescent ones. In this model, quiescent GBM cell organoids were more resistant to temozolomide treatment and radiotherapy with distinct gene expression profile such as increased expression of ECM proteins of FN1, laminins, collagens, and tenascin C [154]. Cellular heterogeneity in terms of tumor cell subpopulations further extents the range of drug response. In one of such studies, Sivakumar et al. arranged spheroid models with four types of GBM cells with mainly distinct EGFR mutations to address effects of tumor population. During culture, drug treatments reshaped the spheroid composition highlighting the dominant contribution of genetic heterogeneity of tumor cells [196].

In chemotherapy, although main target is the tumor cells for the sake of prognosis, all remaining patient cells are also exposed to deleterious effects of the drugs and may present the potential side effects. For this reason, especially 3D models are great to analyze overall toxicity risks associated with the treatment. For instance, in GBM patient heterospheroids of tumor cells and iPSC-derived neural progenitor cells, selective induction of tumor cell apoptosis by temozolomide can be modeled [197]. However, chemotherapy drugs used for GBM patients often exert toxic effects on astrocytes and, 2D systems have been limited to uncover such effects. As an innovative approach for the establishment of clinical relevance, the micro-pillar based chips devised with GBM or astrocytes allowed spheroid formation and were promising to screen accuracy of various chemotherapeutic drugs [198]. Besides, as a probable role to cure GBM, selective targeting tumor cells and immune system cells can be advantageous. To illustrate this effect, in a recent study, targeting GBM cells and TAMs by PD-1 and CSF1R dual inhibition was shown to be effective by promoting T cell extravasation and GBM cell apoptosis, especially in mesenchymal GBM [199]. Another substantial evidence is provided by Heinrich et al. in paracrine model of GBM where GL261 glioblastoma cells and RAW264.7 macrophages have provided the opportunity to implement detailed expression analysis of GBM markers, and genes related epithelial-to-mesenchymal transition of tumor cells, ECM remodeling enzymes, and many other genes that were considerably upregulated in contrast to 2D surfaces. The results were comparable with GBM patient samples lessening the contradictions between *in vitro* models and clinical trials [200]. Further, CSCs are identified as major connection to poor prognosis [201]. Thus, they are promising to be additional novel targets to eradicate tumor population as such function of the epigenetic suppressor called polycomb repressive complex 2 was diminished with S-adenosyl methionine competitive inhibitor (GSK343) to invoke potent tumor killing effects [202] and by also considering communication with stromal cells [203]. The physical barrier of ECM is also critical for substantial improvement of clinical success, as it hinders diffusion of drugs reaching tumor cells, as well as provides cues that alter tumor cell behavior against the drug. In one of example studies, Hermida et al. demonstrated that significant resistance to cisplatin was observed in RGDS-alginate gels in contrast to 2D culture confirming clinical trial failure of this drug [203].

In analysis of drug response, BBB is a key issue for both drug penetration and distribution towards tumor cells. As such, patient-derived GBM cells co-encapsulated with stromal cells in gelatin gels were discovered to be affected differentially, as temozolomide treatment increased cPARP+ apoptotic tumor cell number, but within 10 μm distance of microvascular network, number of cPARP- tumor cells were higher when all vascular cell types were encapsulated with GBM cells [159]. Likewise, status of integrity and density of blood vessels in GBM are subject to modifications depending on the stage of tumor, invasion and location. In an attempt to study this effect, a biomimetic microfluidic system of GBM-22 and pericyte heterospheroids surrounded with endothelial cells, pericytes, and astrocytes in fibrin addresses to the challenge of intact BBB with functional cell-cell junctions. Instead of naked drugs, a carrier system is also current interest for cancer treatment and even if a drug delivery vehicle is chosen as a core strategy, still targeting GBM will be limited by penetration through BBB. For targeted drug delivery to overcome adverse effects of toxicity and poor BBB penetration, chemotherapy drug carriers can be functionalized with ligands of cell surface receptors [204].

Moreover, these scaffold systems are utilized to fabricate microwell-based chip systems to benefit from the continual drug capture and release, and gradient establishment even if single injection was performed [205]. Similarly, tumor tissue architecture serves as solid ground to imitate the necrotic region of GBM and can be targeted for drug delivery. In an effort to show corresponding role of this microenvironment, GBM cells in collagen gel constituted mid-section of the central chamber to create a region with high number of dead cells (necrotic core) was successfully formed. In a trial of hypoxia-activated pro-drug, tirapazamine, therapy was more effective in the core of the central chamber where the development of hypoxia and necrotic core were located, as outer layers were more oxygenated [174]. To translate into clinics, these drug screening platforms can be manufactured as patient-on-chip systems by a combination of scaffolds with patient-derived GBM cells which ultimately aim to predict patient-specific prognosis and to choose the best course of treatment unique to each patient [206].

3.4.3 Immunotherapy

Since the extensive information on the development and microenvironment of tumors have been uncovered, these mechanisms are actively targeted to eradicate tumor cells within the body. As explained above, tumor microenvironment has significant impact on the growth and metastasis of the tumors especially by immunosuppression. Therefore, addressing to the possible routes of the inference of immunosuppression and firing the immune reaction can be benefited to achieve good prognosis. In this strategy, activation of immune system and exploitation of the immune activity are harnessed in the cancer immunotherapy as a potential alternative to traditional therapy to eliminate tumors cells from the body as well as to prevent relapse [207]. For this purpose, vaccines, oncolytic viruses, immune check-point blockade, and adoptive cell transfer can be combined with primary treatments of chemo- and radiotherapy to overcome the barrier of the cancer immunosuppression [208–210]. Currently, some of these strategies are under clinical trials for GBM [211, 212]. For these therapies, *in vivo* models are commonly investigated and further, clues derived from *in vitro* GBM models have provided profitable data in the area to discover therapeutic targets and engineered immune system cells [213]. As a recent evidence of promise of this approach, in clinical trials, genetically engineered T cells (CAR-T) have been investigated to direct and amplify T cell cytotoxicity towards GBM cells [214]. These T cells are engineered to carry surface proteins that can recognize tumor antigens so that their tumor-killing efficacy is improved. To achieve this, Jacob et al. co-cultured patient-derived GBM organoids with anti-EGFRvIII CAR-T cells and, activated T cells secreted amplified levels of IL-2, IFN-γ, and TNF-α, they effectively killed tumor cells upon antigen recognition and proliferated at the periphery of the organoids [157]. Combinatorial application of this therapy also holds potential for patient and tumor-infiltrating T cell survival, as B7H3-CAR-T cells combined with IL-7 expressing oncolytic adenovirus provided promising activity both *in vitro* and *in vivo* [215].

3.4.4 Response to Radiotherapy

In clinics, it is often impossible to remove whole tumor mass and outcome remains to be poor, as unresected cancer cells continue to grow causing recurrence. This issue highlights the necessity and influence of chemotherapy and radiotherapy on the mortality due to GBM. Thus, a platform to investigate the efficiency of any therapy has utmost importance to determine the course of the treatment. Various 3D systems are applied as models in the analysis of radiation dosage and resistance mechanisms for tumors [168, 216]. In order to achieve this goal, McMillan et al. investigated the effect of radiation dosage on UWV spheroid setting and concluded that 8 Gy dose sufficiently impaired tumor growth and size both in large and small spheroids compared to 4 Gy dose. Size is not the only limiting factor, as quiescent tumor cells within the population alter the potency of irradiation-induced toxicity on tumors. As reported, dormant UWV spheroids were more aggressive and resistant to radiation probably due to their ability to respond fast to repair DNA damage compared nutrient rich ones [168].

3.4.5 Biobanking

Biobanking is another area of interest for GBM models as it serves as a source of biological material and related medical data with systematic information. This collection of samples and other data have been stored to create patient-like models in personalized medicine, to model diseases, to obtain omics data for various conditions and other applications in information technologies to revolutionize current translational oncology [217, 218]. Frozen GBM tissue, formalin-fixed, and paraffin-embedded block of GBM tissue [217, 219], single cell lines from tumors [220] or patient-derived organoid biobanks [156, 157] are developed for GBM biobanking during research and as a component of national clinical database. Single cell and tissue biobanking are desirable, as they provide comparable profile with public datasets, and they can be used as drug test platforms for screening and designing effective treatment methods for personalized medicine [220–222].

3.5 Concluding Remarks

Uncontrolled growth of cells with diverse genotypic and phenotypic collection in the CNS has been one of the deadliest cases for patient survival. So far, many research has been directed to improve the prognosis of GBM patients and, to achieve success in clinics, well-suited *in vitro* models have been recognized as necessity to develop various treatment strategies. During this process, tumor biology has been dissected and critical role of both soluble factors and ECM and, tumor residing and infiltrating cells were delineated. This led to acknowledgement of the potential models with dimensional, cellular, physical, and chemical differences to lessen the gap between *in vitro* and *in vivo*. Today, these systems have been investigated in a wide array of applications including the discovery of different treatments, possibility of personalized medicine, to elucidate diverse aspects of the tumor biology and to create biobanks. This extensive effort expanded the survival of patients about two years, yet promising results can be achieved with the development of more realistic models for clinics and the area is gradually expanding with encouraging outcomes. In the current state, we still search for the discovery of the cure for GBM and there is an urgent need to address not only tumor eradication, but also metastasis and recurrence. New designs contributed by computational models (molecular docking, disease models) and single-cell analysis can be future of GBM modeling and perhaps, pre-clinical drug test environment. Obtained information is an opportunity to analyze the applicability and reliability of these treatments to recurrent or metastatic carcinoma and other groups of cancer.

Bibliography

[1] D. N. Louis, A. Perry, and P. Wesseling et al., "The 2021 WHO classification of tumors of the central nervous system: a summary," *Neuro-Oncology*, vol. 23, no. 8, pp. 1231–1251, 2021.

[2] S. DeCordova, A. Shastri, and A. G. Tsolaki et al., "Molecular heterogeneity and immunosuppressive microenvironment in glioblastoma," *Frontiers in Immunology*, vol. 11, p. 1402, 2020.

[3] K. J. Wolf, J. Chen, and J. D. Coombes et al., "Dissecting and rebuilding the glioblastoma microenvironment with engineered materials," *Nature Reviews Materials*, vol. 4, no. 10, pp. 651–668, 2019.

[4] D. F. Quail and J. A. Joyce, "The microenvironmental landscape of brain tumors," *Cancer Cell*, vol. 31, no. 3, pp. 326–341, 2017.

[5] H. J. Kim, J. W. Park, and J. H. Lee, "Genetic architectures and cell-of-origin in glioblastoma," *Frontiers in Oncology*, vol. 10, p. 615400, 2021.

[6] S. Ma, S. Rudra, and J. L. Campian et al., "Prognostic impact of CDKN2A/B deletion, TERT mutation, and EGFR amplification on histological and molecular IDH-wildtype glioblastoma," *Neuro-Oncology Advances*, vol. 2, no. 1, p. vdaa126, 2020.

[7] A. Wenger, S. Ferreyra Vega, and T. Kling et al., "Intratumor DNA methylation heterogeneity in glioblastoma: implications for DNA methylation-based classification," *Neuro-Oncology*, vol. 21, no. 5, pp. 616–627, 2019.

[8] K. Biserova, A. Jakovlevs, and R. Uljanovs et al., "Cancer stem cells: significance in origin, pathogenesis and treatment of glioblastoma," *Cells*, vol. 10, no. 3, p. 621, 2021.

[9] B. C. Prager, S. Bhargava, and V. Mahadev et al., "Glioblastoma stem cells: driving resilience through chaos," *Trends in Cancer*, vol. 6, no. 3, pp. 223–235, 2020.

[10] M. Del Bene, D. Osti, and S. Faletti et al., "Extracellular vesicles: the key for precision medicine in glioblastoma," *Neuro-Oncology*, vol. 24, no. 2, pp. 184–196, 2021.

[11] T. Simon, E. Jackson, and G. Giamas, "Breaking through the glioblastoma micro-environment via extracellular vesicles," *Oncogene*, vol. 39, no. 23, pp. 4477–4490, 2020.

[12] A. Yekula, A. Yekula, and K. Muralidharan et al., "Extracellular vesicles in glioblastoma tumor microenvironment," *Frontiers in Immunology*, vol. 10, p. 3137, 2020.

[13] D. M. Mallawaaratchy, S. Hallal, and B. Russell et al., "Comprehensive proteome profiling of glioblastoma-derived extracellular vesicles identifies markers for more aggressive disease," *Journal of Neuro-oncology*, vol. 131, pp. 233–244, 2017.

[14] F. L. Ricklefs, Q. Alayo, and H. Krenzlin et al., "Immune evasion mediated by PD-L1 on glioblastoma-derived extracellular vesicles," *Science Advances*, vol. 4, no. 3, p. eaar2766, 2018.

[15] A. Yekula, V. R. Minciacchi, and M. Morello et al., "Large and small extracellular vesicles released by glioma cells *in vitro* and *in vivo*," *Journal of Extracellular Vesicles*, vol. 9, no. 1, p. 1689784, 2020.

[16] J. Tang, P. Flomenberg, and L. Harshyne et al., "Glioblastoma patients exhibit circulating tumor-specific CD8+ T Cells," *Clinical Cancer Research*, vol. 11, no. 14, pp. 5292–5299, 2005.

[17] J. Litak, M. Mazurek, and C. Grochowski et al., "PD-L1/PD-1 axis in glioblastoma multiforme," *International Journal of Molecular Sciences*, vol. 20, no. 21, p. 5347, 2019.

[18] Y. Liu, R. Carlsson, and M. Ambjørn et al., "PD-L1 expression by neurons nearby tumors ındicates better prognosis in glioblastoma patients," *Journal of Neuroscience*, vol. 33, no. 35, pp. 14231–14245, 2013.

[19] S. Lim, D. Kim, and S. Ju et al., "Glioblastoma-secreted soluble CD44 activates tau pathology in the brain," *Experimental & Molecular Medicine*, vol. 50, no. 4, pp. 1–11, 2018.

[20] P. Jarabo, C. de Pablo, and H. Herranz et al., "Insulin signaling mediates neurodegeneration in glioma," *Life Science Alliance*, vol. 4, no. 3, p. e202000693, 2021.

[21] J. Faria, L. Romão, and S. Martins et al., "Interactive properties of human glioblastoma cells with brain neurons in culture and neuronal modulation of glial laminin organization," *Differentiation*, vol. 74, no. 9-10, pp. 562–572, 2006.

[22] H. S. Venkatesh, W. Morishita, and A. C. Geraghty et al., "Electrical and synaptic integration of glioma into neural circuits," *Nature*, vol. 573, no. 7775, pp. 539–545, 2019.

[23] L. Nieland, L. M. Morsett, and M. L. D. Broekman et al., "Extracellular vesicle-mediated bilateral communication between glioblastoma and astrocytes," *Trends in Neurosciences*, vol. 44, no. 3, pp. 215–226, 2021.

[24] A. Zeng, Z. Wei, and R. Rabinovsky et al., "Glioblastoma-derived extracellular vesicles facilitate transformation of astrocytes via reprogramming oncogenic metabolism," *Iscience*, vol. 23, no. 8, p. 101420, 2020.

[25] D. Henrik Heiland, V. M. Ravi, and S. P. Behringer et al., "Tumor-associated reactive astrocytes aid the evolution of immunosuppressive environment in glioblastoma," *Nature Communications*, vol. 10, no. 1, p. 2541, 2019.

[26] H. Zhang, Y. Zhou, and B. Cui et al., "Novel insights into astrocyte-mediated signaling of proliferation, invasion and tumor immune microenvironment in glioblastoma," *Biomedicine & Pharmacotherapy*, vol. 126, p. 110086, 2020.

[27] A. A. Dumas, N. Pomella, and G. Rosser et al., "Microglia promote glioblastoma via mTOR-mediated immunosuppression of the tumour microenvironment," *The EMBO Journal*, vol. 39, no. 15, p. e103790, 2020.

[28] T. Hide, I. Shibahara, and T. Kumabe, "Novel concept of the border niche: glioblastoma cells use oligodendrocytes progenitor cells (GAOs) and microglia to acquire stem cell-like features," *Brain Tumor Pathology*, vol. 36, pp. 63–73, 2019.

[29] Y. Huang, C. Hoffman, and P. Rajappa et al., "Oligodendrocyte progenitor cells promote neovascularization in glioma by disrupting the blood–brain barrier," *Cancer Research*, vol. 74, no. 4, pp. 1011–1021, 2014.

[30] D. Hambardzumyan, D. H. Gutmann, and H. Kettenmann, "The role of microglia and macrophages in glioma maintenance and progression," *Nature Neuroscience*, vol. 19, no. 1, pp. 20–27, 2016.

[31] A. Buonfiglioli and D. Hambardzumyan, "Macrophages and microglia: the cerberus of glioblastoma," *Acta Neuropathologica Communications*, vol. 9, no. 1, p. 54, 2021.

[32] M. Pudełek, K. Król, and J. Catapano et al., "Epidermal growth factor (EGF) augments the invasive potential of human glioblastoma multiforme cells via the activation of collaborative EGFR/ROS-dependent signaling," *International Journal of Molecular Sciences*, vol. 21, no. 10, p. 3605, 2020.

[33] K. E. van der Vos, E. R. Abels, and X. Zhang et al., "Directly visualized glioblastoma-derived extracellular vesicles transfer RNA to microglia/macrophages in the brain," *Neuro-Oncology*, vol. 18, no. 1, pp. 58–69, 2015.

[34] X. Zhang, L. Chen, and W.-q. Dang et al., "CCL8 secreted by tumor-associated macrophages promotes invasion and stemness of glioblastoma cells via ERK1/2 signaling," *Laboratory Investigation*, vol. 100, no. 4, pp. 619–629, 2020.

[35] F. Hu, M.-C. Ku, and D. Markovic et al., "Glioma-associated microglial MMP9 expression is upregulated by TLR2 signaling and sensitive to minocycline," *International Journal of Cancer*, vol. 135, no. 11, pp. 2569–2578, 2014.

[36] A. C. C. da Fonseca, H. Wang, and H. Fan et al., "Increased expression of stress inducible protein 1 in glioma-associated microglia/macrophages," *Journal of Neuroimmunology*, vol. 274, no. 1-2, pp. 71–77, 2014.

[37] T. Hide, Y. Komohara, and Y. Miyasato et al., "Oligodendrocyte progenitor cells and macrophages/microglia produce glioma stem cell niches at the tumor border," *EBioMedicine*, vol. 30, pp. 94–104, 2018.

[38] H. Grégoire, L. Roncali, and A. Rousseau et al., "Targeting tumor associated macrophages to overcome conventional treatment resistance in glioblastoma," *Frontiers in Pharmacology*, vol. 11, p. 368, 2020.

[39] R. K. Tiwari, S. Singh, and C. L. Gupta et al., "Repolarization of glioblastoma macrophage cells using non-agonistic Dectin-1 ligand encapsulating TLR-9 agonist: plausible role in regenerative medicine against brain tumor," *International Journal of Neuroscience*, vol. 131, no. 6, pp. 591–598, 2021.

[40] K. Kashfi, J. Kannikal, and N. Nath, "Macrophage reprogramming and cancer therapeutics: role of INOS-derived NO," *Cells*, vol. 10, no. 11, p. 3194, 2021.

[41] I. G. House, P. Savas, and J. Lai, et al., "Macrophage-derived CXCL9 and CXCL10 are required for antitumor immune responses following immune checkpoint blockade," *Clinical Cancer Research*, vol. 26, no. 2, pp. 487–504, 2020.

[42] A. Xiong, J. Zhang, and Y. Chen et al., "Integrated single-cell transcriptomic analyses reveal that GPNMB-high macrophages promote PN-MES transition and impede T cell activation in GBM," *EBioMedicine*, vol. 83, p. 104239, 2022.

[43] K. Hattermann, S. Sebens, and O. Helm et al., "Chemokine expression profile of freshly isolated human glioblastoma-associated macrophages/microglia," *Oncology Reports*, vol. 32, no. 1, pp. 270–276, 2014.

[44] Z. Zhu, H. Zhang, and B. Chen et al., "PD-L1-mediated immunosuppression in glioblastoma is associated with the infiltration and M2-polarization of tumor-associated macrophages," *Frontiers in Immunology*, vol. 11, p. 588552, 2020.

[45] I. Zhang, D. Alizadeh, and J. Liang et al., "Characterization of arginase expression in glioma-associated microglia and macrophages," *PLOS ONE*, vol. 11, no. 12, p. e0165118, 2016.

[46] S. Roesch, C. Rapp, and S. Dettling et al., "When immune cells turn bad—tumor-associated microglia/macrophages in glioma," *International Journal of Molecular Sciences*, vol. 19, no. 2, p. 436, 2018.

[47] Y. Chen, Y. Song, and W. Du et al., "Tumor-associated macrophages: an accomplice in solid tumor progression," *Journal of Biomedical Science*, vol. 26, no. 1, p. 78, 2019.

[48] G. Wang, J. Wang, and C. Niu et al., "Neutrophils: new critical regulators of glioma," *Frontiers in Immunology*, vol. 13, p. 927233, 2022.

[49] Y.-J. Lin, K.-C. Wei, and P.-Y. Chen et al., "Roles of neutrophils in glioma and brain metastases," *Frontiers in Immunology*, vol. 12, p. 701383, 2021.

[50] P. Magod, I. Mastandrea, and L. Rousso-Noori et al., "Exploring the longitudinal glioma microenvironment landscape uncovers reprogrammed pro-tumorigenic neutrophils in the bone marrow," *Cell Reports*, vol. 36, no. 5, p. 109480, 2021.

[51] J. Liang, Y. Piao, and L. Holmes et al., "Neutrophils promote the malignant glioma phenotype through S100A4," *Clinical Cancer Research*, vol. 20, no. 1, pp. 187–198, 2014.

[52] C. Zha, X. Meng, and L. Li at al., "Neutrophil extracellular traps mediate the crosstalk between glioma progression and the tumor microenvironment via the HMGB1/RAGE/IL-8 axis," *Cancer Biology & Medicine*, vol. 17, no. 1, pp. 154–168, 2020.

[53] J. Jablonska, S. Leschner, and K. Westphal et al., "Neutrophils responsive to endogenous IFN-β regulate tumor angiogenesis and growth in a mouse tumor model," *The Journal of Clinical Investigation*, vol. 120, no. 4, pp. 1151–1164, 2010.

[54] I. Ozel, I. Duerig, and M. Domnich et al., "The good, the bad, and the ugly: neutrophils, angiogenesis, and cancer," *Cancers*, vol. 14, no. 3, p. 536, 2022.

[55] A. J. Sedgwick, N. Ghazanfari, and P. Constantinescu et al., "The role of NK cells and innate lymphoid cells in brain cancer," *Frontiers in Immunology*, vol. 11, p. 1549, 2020.

[56] M. Wang, Z. Zhou, and X. Wang et al., "Natural killer cell awakening: unleash cancer-immunity cycle against glioblastoma," *Cell Death & Disease*, vol. 13, no. 7, p. 588, 2022.

[57] P. Roth, M. Mittelbronn, and W. Wick et al., "Malignant glioma cells counteract antitumor immune responses through expression of lectin-like transcript-1," *Cancer Research*, vol. 67, no. 8, pp. 3540–3544, 2007.

[58] U. Johansson, L. Walther-Jallow, and A. Hofmann et al., "Dendritic cells are able to produce IL-12p70 after uptake of apoptotic cells," *Immunobiology*, vol. 216, no. 1, pp. 251–255, 2011.

[59] A. Karachi, F. Dastmalchi, and S. Nazarian et al., "Optimizing T cell-based therapy for glioblastoma," *Frontiers in Immunology*, vol. 12, p. 705580, 2021.

[60] J. Dörr, S. Waiczies, and U. Wendling et al., "Induction of TRAIL-mediated glioma cell death by human T cells," *Journal of Neuroimmunology*, vol. 122, no. 1-2, pp. 117–124, 2002.

[61] M. Tekguc, J. B. Wing, and M. Osaki et al., "Treg-expressed CTLA-4 depletes CD80/CD86 by trogocytosis, releasing free PD-L1 on antigen-presenting cells," *Proceedings of the National Academy of Sciences*, vol. 118, no. 30, p. e2023739118, 2021.

[62] H. Liang, L. Yi, and X. Wang et al., "Interleukin-17 facilitates the immune suppressor capacity of high-grade glioma-derived CD4 (+) CD25 (+) Foxp3 (+) T cells via releasing transforming growth factor beta," *Scandinavian Journal of Immunology*, vol. 80, no. 2, pp. 144–150, 2014.

[63] S. Liu, C. Zhang, and B. Wang et al., "Regulatory T cells promote glioma cell stemness through TGF-β–NF-κB–IL6–STAT3 signaling," *Cancer Immunology, Immunotherapy*, pp. 2601–2616, 2021.

[64] D. A. Thomas and J. Massagué, "TGF-β directly targets cytotoxic T cell functions during tumor evasion of immune surveillance," *Cancer Cell*, vol. 8, no. 5, pp. 369–380, 2005.

[65] K. I. Woroniecka, K. E. Rhodin, and P. Chongsathidkiet et al., "T-cell dysfunction in glioblastoma: applying a new framework," *Clinical Cancer Research*, vol. 24, no. 16, pp. 3792–3802, 2018.

[66] M. Ott, K.-H. Tomaszowski, and A. Marisetty et al., "Profiling of patients with glioma reveals the dominant immunosuppressive axis is refractory to immune function restoration," *JCI Insight*, vol. 5, no. 17, p. e134386, 2020.

[67] J. F. M. Jacobs, A. J. Idema, and K. F. Bol et al., "Prognostic significance and mechanism of Treg infiltration in human brain tumors," *Journal of Neuroimmunology*, vol. 225, no. 1-2, pp. 195–199, 2010.

[68] J. T. Jordan, W. Sun, and S. F. Hussain et al., "Preferential migration of regulatory T cells mediated by glioma-secreted chemokines can be blocked with chemotherapy," *Cancer Immunology, Immunotherapy*, vol. 57, pp. 123–131, 2008.

[69] D. A. Wainwright, I. V. Balyasnikova, and A. L. Chang et al., "IDO expression in brain tumors increases the recruitment of regulatory T cells and negatively impacts survival," *Clinical Cancer Research*, vol. 18, no. 22, pp. 6110–6121, 2012.

[70] A. Facciabene, X. Peng, and I. S. Hagemann et al., "Tumour hypoxia promotes tolerance and angiogenesis via CCL28 and Treg cells," vol. 475, pp. 226–230, 2011.

[71] M. M. Grabowski, E. W. Sankey, and K. J. Ryan et al., "Immune suppression in gliomas," *Journal of Neuro-oncology*, vol. 151, pp. 3–12, 2021.

[72] Y. Yang, C. Li, and T. Liu et al., "Myeloid-derived suppressor cells in tumors: from mechanisms to antigen specificity and microenvironmental regulation," *Frontiers in Immunology*, vol. 11, 2020.

[73] S. C. Bischoff, "Role of mast cells in allergic and non-allergic immune responses: comparison of human and murine data," *Nature Reviews Immunology*, vol. 7, no. 2, pp. 93–104, 2007.

[74] J. Põlajeva, A. M. Sjösten, and N. Lager et al., "Mast cell accumulation in glioblastoma with a potential role for stem cell factor and chemokine CXCL12," *PLOS ONE*, vol. 6, no. 9, p. e25222, 2011.

[75] A. Roy, A. Coum, and V. D. Marinescu et al., "Glioma-derived plasminogen activator inhibitor-1 (PAI-1) regulates the recruitment of LRP1 positive mast cells," *Oncotarget*, vol. 6, no. 27, pp. 23647–23661, 2015.

[76] S. Attarha, A. Roy, and B. Westermark et al., "Mast cells modulate proliferation, migration and stemness of glioma cells through downregulation of GSK3β expression and inhibition of STAT3 activation," *Cellular Signalling*, vol. 37, pp. 81–92, 2017.

[77] D. E. A. Komi and F. A. Redegeld, "Role of mast cells in shaping the tumor microenvironment," *Clinical Reviews in Allergy & Immunology*, vol. 58, no. 3, pp. 313–325, 2020.

[78] B. Otvos, D. J. Silver, and E. E. Mulkearns-Hubert et al., "Cancer stem cell-secreted macrophage migration inhibitory factor stimulates myeloid derived suppressor cell function and facilitates glioblastoma immune evasion," *Stem Cells*, vol. 34, no. 8, pp. 2026–2039, 2016.

[79] C. Groth, X. Hu, and R. Weber et al., "Immunosuppression mediated by myeloid-derived suppressor cells (MDSCs) during tumour progression," *British Journal of Cancer*, vol. 120, no. 1, pp. 16–25, 2019.

[80] Z. Ye, X. Ai, and L. Zhao et al., "Phenotypic plasticity of myeloid cells in glioblastoma development, progression, and therapeutics," *Oncogene*, vol. 40, no. 42, pp. 6059–6070, 2021.

[81] P. Gielen, B. M. Schulte, and E. D. Kers-Rebel et al., "Elevated levels of polymorphonuclear myeloid-derived suppressor cells in patients with glioblastoma highly express S100A8/9 and arginase and suppress T cell function," *Neuro-Oncology*, vol. 18, no. 9, pp. 1253–1264, 2016.

[82] C. Lee-Chang, A. Rashidi, and J. Miska et al., "Myeloid-derived suppressive cells promote B cell–mediated immunosuppression via transfer of PDL-1 in glioblastoma," *Cancer Immunology Research*, vol. 7, no. 12, pp. 1928–1943, 2019.

[83] S. Han, S. Feng, and M. Ren et al., "Glioma cell-derived placental growth factor induces regulatory B cells," *The International Journal of Biochemistry & Cell Biology*, vol. 57, pp. 63–68, 2014.

[84] Y. Lei, H. Han, and F. Yuan et al., "The brain interstitial system: anatomy, modeling, *in vivo* measurement, and applications," *Progress in Neurobiology*, vol. 157, pp. 230–246, 2017.

[85] S. Dauth, T. Grevesse, and H. Pantazopoulos, et al., "Extracellular matrix protein expression is brain region dependent," *Journal of Comparative Neurology*, vol. 524, no. 7, pp. 1309–1336, 2016.

[86] L. W. Lau, R. Cua, and M. B. Keough et al., "Pathophysiology of the brain extracellular matrix: a new target for remyelination," *Nature Reviews Neuroscience*, vol. 14, no. 10, pp. 722–729, 2013.

[87] D. Testa, A. Prochiantz, and D. A. A, "Perineuronal nets in brain physiology and disease," *Seminars in Cell & Developmental Biology*, vol. 89, pp. 125–135, 2019.

[88] R. Frischknecht, M. Heine, and D. Perrais et al., "Brain extracellular matrix affects AMPA receptor lateral mobility and short-term synaptic plasticity," *Nature Neuroscience*, vol. 12, no. 7, pp. 897–904, 2009.

[89] K. K. Lensjø, M. E. Lepperød, and G. Dick et al., "Removal of perineuronal nets unlocks juvenile plasticity through network mechanisms of decreased inhibition and increased gamma activity," *Journal of Neuroscience*, vol. 37, no. 5, pp. 1269–1283, 2017.

[90] J.-H. Cabungcal, P. Steullet, and H. Morishita et al., "Perineuronal nets protect fast-spiking interneurons against oxidative stress," *Proceedings of the National Academy of Sciences*, vol. 110, no. 22, pp. 9130–9135, 2013.

[91] M. Morawski, T. Reinert, and W. Meyer-Klaucke et al., "Ion exchanger in the brain: quantitative analysis of perineuronally fixed anionic binding sites suggests diffusion barriers with ion sorting properties," *Scientific Reports*, vol. 5, no. 1, p. 16471, 2015.

[92] F. De Winter, J. C. F. Kwok, and J. W. Fawcett et al., "The chemorepulsive protein semaphorin 3A and perineuronal net-mediated plasticity," *Neural Plasticity*, vol. 2016, p. 3679545, 2016.

[93] H. M. Van't Spijker, D. Rowlands, and J. Rossier et al., "Neuronal pentraxin 2 binds PNNs and enhances PNN formation," *Neural Plasticity*, vol. 2019, p. 6804575, 2019.

[94] J. W. Fawcett, T. Oohashi, and T. Pizzorusso, "The roles of perineuronal nets and the perinodal extracellular matrix in neuronal function," *Nature Reviews Neuroscience*, vol. 20, no. 8, pp. 451–465, 2019.

[95] N. J. Abbott, L. Rönnbäck, and E. Hansson, "Astrocyte–endothelial interactions at the blood–brain barrier," *Nature Reviews Neuroscience*, vol. 7, no. 1, pp. 41–53, 2006.

[96] M. S. Thomsen, L. J. Routhe, and T. Moos, "The vascular basement membrane in the healthy and pathological brain," *Journal of Cerebral Blood Flow & Metabolism*, vol. 37, no. 10, pp. 3300–3317, 2017.

[97] M. A. Pibuel, D. Poodts, and M. Díaz et al., "The scrambled story between hyaluronan and glioblastoma," *Journal of Biological Chemistry*, vol. 296, p. 100549, 2021.

[98] D. Carulli, T. Pizzorusso, and J. C. F. Kwok et al., "Animals lacking link protein have attenuated perineuronal nets and persistent plasticity," *Brain*, vol. 133, no. 8, pp. 2331–2347, 2010.

[99] H. Wang, Z. Liu, and A. Li et al., "COL4A1 as a novel oncogene associated with the clinical characteristics of malignancy predicts poor prognosis in glioma," *Experimental and Therapeutic Medicine*, vol. 22, no. 5, p. 1224, 2021.

[100] G. P. Cribaro, E. Saavedra-López, and L. Romarate et al., "Three-dimensional vascular microenvironment landscape in human glioblastoma," *Acta Neuropathologica Communications*, vol. 9, no. 1, p. 24, 2021.

[101] T. Sun, R. Patil, and A. Galstyan et al., "Blockade of a laminin-411–Notch axis with CRISPR/Cas9 or a nanobioconjugate inhibits glioblastoma growth through tumor-microenvironment cross-talk," *Cancer Research*, vol. 79, no. 6, pp. 1239–1251, 2019.

[102] L. Dzikowski, R. Mirzaei, and S. Sarkar et al., "Fibrinogen in the glioblastoma microenvironment contributes to the invasiveness of brain tumor-initiating cells," *Brain Pathology*, vol. 31, no. 5, p. e12947, 2021.

[103] B. Coquerel, F. Poyer, and F. Torossian et al., "Elastin-derived peptides: matrikines critical for glioblastoma cell aggressiveness in a 3-D system," *Glia*, vol. 57, no. 16, pp. 1716–1726, 2009.

[104] J. M. Ross, C. Kim, and D. Allen et al., "The expanding cell diversity of the brain vasculature," *Frontiers in Physiology*, vol. 11, 2020.

[105] J. Guyon, C. Chapouly, and L. Andrique et al., "The normal and brain tumor vasculature: morphological and functional characteristics and therapeutic targeting," *Frontiers in Physiology*, vol. 12, p. 622615, 2021.

[106] H. Kadry, B. Noorani, and L. Cucullo, "A blood–brain barrier overview on structure, function, impairment, and biomarkers of integrity," *Fluids and Barriers of the CNS*, vol. 17, no. 1, p. 69, 2020.

[107] Z. Zhao, A. R. Nelson, and C. Betsholtz et al., "Establishment and dysfunction of the blood-brain barrier," *Cell*, vol. 163, no. 5, pp. 1064–1078, 2015.

[108] P. S. Steeg, "The blood–tumour barrier in cancer biology and therapy," *Nature Reviews Clinical Oncology*, vol. 18, no. 11, pp. 696–714, 2021.

[109] M. D. Sweeney, A. P. Sagare, and B. V. Zlokovic, "Blood–brain barrier breakdown in Alzheimer disease and other neurodegenerative disorders," *Nature Reviews Neurology*, vol. 14, no. 3, pp. 133–150, 2018.

[110] E. Belykh, K. V. Shaffer, and C. Lin et al., "Blood-brain barrier, blood-brain tumor barrier, and fluorescence-guided neurosurgical oncology: delivering optical labels to brain tumors," *Frontiers in Oncology*, vol. 10, p. 739, 2020.

[111] M. D. Sweeney, Z. Zhao, and A. Montagne et al., "Blood-brain barrier: from physiology to disease and back," *Physiological Reviews*, vol. 99, no. 1, pp. 21–78, 2019.

[112] C. D. Arvanitis, G. B. Ferraro, and R. K. Jain, "The blood–brain barrier and blood–tumour barrier in brain tumours and metastases," *Nature Reviews Cancer*, vol. 20, no. 1, pp. 26–41, 2020.

[113] Y. Xie, L. He, and R. Lugano et al., "Key molecular alterations in endothelial cells in human glioblastoma uncovered through single-cell RNA sequencing," *JCI Insight*, vol. 6, no. 15, p. e150861, 2021.

[114] F. Yang, Y. Xie, and J. Tang et al., "Uncovering a distinct gene signature in endothelial cells associated with contrast enhancement in glioblastoma," *Frontiers in Oncology*, vol. 11, p. 683367, 2021.

[115] C. Charalambous, T. C. Chen, and F. M. Hofman, "Characteristics of tumor-associated endothelial cells derived from glioblastoma multiforme," *Neurosurgical Focus FOC*, vol. 20, no. 4, p. E22, 2006.

[116] N. N. Khodarev, J. Yu, and E. Labay et al., "Tumour-endothelium interactions in co-culture: coordinated changes of gene expression profiles and phenotypic properties of endothelial cells," *Journal of Cell Science*, vol. 116, no. 6, pp. 1013–1022, 2003.

[117] S. Kenig, M. B. D. Alonso, and M. M. Mueller et al., "Glioblastoma and endothelial cells cross-talk, mediated by SDF-1, enhances tumour invasion and endothelial proliferation by increasing expression of cathepsins B, S, and MMP-9," *Cancer Letters*, vol. 289, no. 1, pp. 53–61, 2010.

[118] L. Cheng, Z. Huang, and W. Zhou et al., "Glioblastoma stem cells generate vascular pericytes to support vessel function and tumor growth," *Cell*, vol. 153, no. 1, pp. 139–152, 2013.

[119] W. Zhou, C. Chen, and Y. Shi et al., "Targeting glioma stem cell-derived pericytes disrupts the blood-tumor barrier and improves chemotherapeutic efficacy," *Cell Stem Cell*, vol. 21, no. 5, pp. 591–603.e4, 2017.

[120] G. S. Hussey, J. L. Dziki, and S. F. Badylak, "Extracellular matrix-based materials for regenerative medicine," *Nature Reviews Materials*, vol. 3, no. 7, pp. 159–173, 2018.

[121] G. Huang, F. Li, and X. Zhao et al., "Functional and biomimetic materials for engineering of the three-dimensional cell microenvironment," *Chemical Reviews*, vol. 117, no. 20, pp. 12764–12850, 2017.

[122] S. Gunti, A. T. K. Hoke, and K. P. Vu et al., "Organoid and spheroid tumor models: techniques and applications," *Cancers*, vol. 13, no. 4, p. 874, 2021.

[123] Z. Gilazieva, A. Ponomarev, and C. Rutland et al., "Promising applications of tumor spheroids and organoids for personalized medicine," *Cancers*, vol. 12, no. 10, p. 2727, 2020.

[124] B. W. S. Phon, M. N. A. Kamarudin, and S. Bhuvanendran et al., "Transitioning pre-clinical glioblastoma models to clinical settings with biomarkers identified in 3d cell-based models: a systematic scoping review," *Biomedicine & Pharmacotherapy*, vol. 145, p. 112396, 2022.

[125] S. Rao, R. Sengupta, and E. J. Choe et al., "CXCL12 mediates trophic interactions between endothelial and tumor cells in glioblastoma," *PLOS ONE*, vol. 7, no. 3, p. e33005, 2012.

[126] C. Wang, Q. Zhao, and X. Zheng et al., "Decellularized brain extracellular matrix slice glioblastoma culture model recapitulates the interaction between cells and the extracellular matrix without a nutrient-oxygen gradient interference," *Acta Biomaterialia*, vol. 158, pp. 132–150, 2023.

[127] K. Pogoda, R. Bucki, and F. J. Byfield et al., "Soft substrates containing hyaluronan mimic the effects of increased stiffness on morphology, motility, and proliferation of glioma cells," *Biomacromolecules*, vol. 18, no. 10, pp. 3040–3051, 2017.

[128] B. Ananthanarayanan, Y. Kim, and S. Kumar, "Elucidating the mechanobiology of malignant brain tumors using a brain matrix-mimetic hyaluronic acid hydrogel platform," *Biomaterials*, vol. 32, no. 31, pp. 7913–7923, 2011.

[129] S. A. Langhans, "Three-dimensional *in vitro* cell culture models in drug discovery and drug repositioning," *Frontiers in Pharmacology*, vol. 9, p. 6, 2018.

[130] N. Hashimoto, R. Kitai, and S. Fujita et al., "Single-cell analysis of unidirectional migration of glioblastoma cells using a fiber-based scaffold," *ACS Applied Bio Materials*, vol. 6, no. 2, pp. 765–773, 2023.

[131] E. L. Gill, S. Willis, and M. Gerigk et al., "Fabrication of designable and suspended microfibers via low-voltage 3D micropatterning," *ACS Applied Materials & Interfaces*, vol. 11, no. 22, pp. 19679–19690, 2019.

[132] A. Bourkoula, E. Mavrogonatou, and P. Pavli et al., "Guided cell adhesion, orientation, morphology and differentiation on silicon substrates photolithographically micropatterned with a cell-repellent cross-linked poly(vinyl alcohol) film," *Biomedical Materials*, vol. 14, no. 1, p. 014101, 2018.

[133] H. M. Estabridis, A. Jana, and A. Nain et al., "Cell migration in 1D and 2D nanofiber microenvironments," *Annals of Biomedical Engineering*, vol. 46, pp. 392–403, 2018.

[134] P. Monzo, Y. K. Chong, and C. Guetta-Terrier et al., "Mechanical confinement triggers glioma linear migration dependent on formin FHOD3," *Molecular Biology of the Cell*, vol. 27, no. 8, pp. 1246–1261, 2016.

[135] A. Erickson, P. A. Chiarelli, and J. Huang et al., "Electrospun nanofibers for 3-D cancer models, diagnostics, and therapy," *Nanoscale Horizons*, vol. 7, pp. 1279–1298, 2022.

[136] S. S. Rao, M. T. Nelson, and R. Xue et al., "Mimicking white matter tract topography using core–shell electrospun nanofibers to examine migration of malignant brain tumors," *Biomaterials*, vol. 34, no. 21, pp. 5181–5190, 2013.

[137] S.-j. Kim, E. M. Kim, and M. Yamamoto et al., "Engineering multicellular spheroids for tissue engineering and regenerative medicine," *Advanced Healthcare Materials*, vol. 9, no. 23, p. 2000608, 2020.

[138] M. Li and J. C. Izpisua Belmonte, "Organoids—preclinical models of human disease," *New England Journal of Medicine*, vol. 380, no. 6, pp. 569–579, 2019.

[139] T. J. Grundy, E. De Leon, and K. R. Griffin et al., "Differential response of patient-derived primary glioblastoma cells to environmental stiffness," *Scientific Reports*, vol. 6, no. 1, p. 23353, 2016.

[140] I. Mó, I. J. Sabino, and D. d. Melo-Diogo et al., "The importance of spheroids in analyzing nanomedicine efficacy," *Nanomedicine*, vol. 15, no. 15, pp. 1513–1525, 2020.

[141] B. L. LeSavage, R. A. Suhar, and N. Broguiere et al., "Next-generation cancer organoids," *Nature Materials*, vol. 21, no. 2, pp. 143–159, 2022.

[142] B. Pinto, A. C. Henriques, and P. M. A. Silva et al., "Three-dimensional spheroids as *in vitro* preclinical models for cancer research," *Pharmaceutics*, vol. 12, no. 12, p. 1186, 2020.

[143] T. Bal, D. C. Oran, and Y. Sasaki et al., "Sequential coating of insulin secreting beta cells within multilayers of polysaccharide nanogels," *Macromolecular Bioscience*, vol. 18, no. 5, p. e1800001, 2018.

[144] A. Y. Hsiao, Y.-C. Tung, and X. Qu et al., "384 hanging drop arrays give excellent Z-factors and allow versatile formation of co-culture spheroids," *Biotechnology and Bioengineering*, vol. 109, no. 5, pp. 1293–1304, 2012.

[145] Y.-C. Tung, A. Y. Hsiao, and S. G. Allen et al., "High-throughput 3D spheroid culture and drug testing using a 384 hanging drop array," *Analyst*, vol. 136, pp. 473–478, 2011.

[146] A. Bajetto, A. Pattarozzi, and A. Corsaro et al., "Different effects of human umbilical cord mesenchymal stem cells on glioblastoma stem cells by direct cell interaction or via released soluble factors," *Frontiers in Cellular Neuroscience*, vol. 11, p. 312, 2017.

[147] F. Mirab, Y. J. Kang, and S. Majd, "Preparation and characterization of size-controlled glioma spheroids using agarose hydrogel microwells," *PLOS ONE*, vol. 14, no. 1, p. e0211078, 2019.

[148] P. S. Nakod, Y. Kim, and S. S. Rao, "The impact of astrocytes and endothelial cells on glioblastoma stemness marker expression in multicellular spheroids," *Cellular and Molecular Bioengineering*, vol. 14, no. 6, p. 639—651, 2021.

[149] M. Vinci, S. Gowan, and F. Boxall et al., "Advances in establishment and analysis of three-dimensional tumor spheroid-based functional assays for target validation and drug evaluation," *BMC Biology*, vol. 10, p. 29, 2012.

[150] J. M. Kelm, N. E. Timmins, and C. J. Brown et al., "Method for generation of homogeneous multicellular tumor spheroids applicable to a wide variety of cell types," *Biotechnology and Bioengineering*, vol. 83, no. 2, pp. 173–180, 2003.

[151] A. S. Nunes, A. S. Barros, and E. C. Costa et al., "3D tumor spheroids as *in vitro* models to mimic *in vivo* human solid tumors resistance to therapeutic drugs," *Biotechnology and Bioengineering*, vol. 116, no. 1, pp. 206–226, 2019.

[152] G. R. Souza, J. R. Molina, and R. M. Raphael et al., "Three-dimensional tissue culture based on magnetic cell levitation," *Nature Nanotechnology*, vol. 5, no. 4, pp. 291–296, 2010.

[153] E. Türker, N. Demirçak, and A. Arslan-Yildiz, "Scaffold-free three-dimensional cell culturing using magnetic levitation," *Biomaterials Science*, vol. 6, pp. 1745–1753, 2018.

[154] R. Tejero, Y. Huang, and I. Katsyv et al., "Gene signatures of quiescent glioblastoma cells reveal mesenchymal shift and interactions with niche microenvironment," *EBioMedicine*, vol. 42, pp. 252–269, 2019.

[155] C. G. Hubert, M. Rivera, and L. C. Spangler et al., "A three-dimensional organoid culture system derived from human glioblastomas recapitulates the hypoxic gradients and cancer stem cell heterogeneity of tumors found *in vivo*," *Cancer Research*, vol. 76, no. 8, pp. 2465–2477, 2016.

[156] F. Jacob, R. D. Salinas, and D. Y. Zhang et al., "A patient-derived glioblastoma organoid model and biobank recapitulates inter- and intratumoral heterogeneity," *Cell*, vol. 180, no. 1, pp. 188–204.e22, 2020.

[157] F. Jacob, G.-l. Ming, and H. Song, "Generation and biobanking of patient-derived glioblastoma organoids and their application in CAR T cell testing," *Nature Protocols*, vol. 15, no. 12, pp. 4000–4033, 2020.

[158] M. Tang, Q. Xie, and R. C. Gimple et al., "Three-dimensional bioprinted glioblastoma microenvironments model cellular dependencies and immune interactions," *Cell Research*, vol. 30, no. 10, pp. 833–853, 2020.

[159] M. T. Ngo, J. N. Sarkaria, and B. A. C. Harley, "Perivascular stromal cells instruct glioblastoma invasion, proliferation, and therapeutic response within an engineered brain perivascular niche model," *Advanced Science*, vol. 9, no. 31, p. 2201888, 2022.

[160] E. Bakirci, N. Schaefer, and O. Dahri et al., "Melt electrowritten *in vitro* radial device to study cell growth and migration," *Advanced Biosystems*, vol. 4, no. 10, p. 2000077, 2020.

[161] J. Cha, S.-G. Kang, and P. Kim, "Strategies of mesenchymal invasion of patient-derived brain tumors: microenvironmental adaptation," *Scientific Reports*, vol. 6, no. 1, p. 24912, 2016.

[162] A. S. Tatla, A. W. Justin, and C. Watts et al., "A vascularized tumoroid model for human glioblastoma angiogenesis," *Scientific Reports*, vol. 11, no. 1, p. 19550, 2021.

[163] R. C. Pereira, R. Santagiuliana, and L. Ceseracciu et al., "Elucidating the role of matrix porosity and rigidity in glioblastoma type IV progression," *Applied Sciences*, vol. 10, no. 24, p. 9076, 2020.

[164] L. Hill, J. Bruns, and S. P. Zustiak, "Hydrogel matrix presence and composition influence drug responses of encapsulated glioblastoma spheroids," *Acta Biomaterialia*, vol. 132, pp. 437–447, 2021.

[165] I. Koh, J. Cha, and J. Park et al., "The mode and dynamics of glioblastoma cell invasion into a decellularized tissue-derived extracellular matrix-based three-dimensional tumor model," *Scientific Reports*, vol. 8, no. 1, p. 4608, 2018.

[166] S. Wang, Y. Wang, and J. Xiong et al., "Novel brain-stiffness-mimicking matrix gel enables comprehensive invasion analysis of 3D cultured GBM cells," *Frontiers in Molecular Biosciences*, vol. 9, p. 588, 2022.

[167] A. Ganguli, A. Mostafa, and C. Saavedra et al., "Three-dimensional microscale hanging drop arrays with geometric control for drug screening and live tissue imaging," *Science Advances*, vol. 7, no. 17, p. eabc1323, 2021.

[168] K. S. McMillan, A. G. McCluskey, and A. Sorensen et al., "Emulsion technologies for multicellular tumour spheroid radiation assays," *Analyst*, vol. 141, pp. 100–110, 2016.

[169] M. Ingram, G. B. Techy, and R. Saroufeem et al., "Three-dimensional growth patterns of various human tumor cell lines in simulated microgravity of a NASA bioreactor," *In Vitro Cellular & Developmental Biology-Animal*, vol. 33, pp. 459–466, 1997.

[170] S. A. Abdul Rahim, A. Dirkse, and A. Oudin et al., "Regulation of hypoxia-induced autophagy in glioblastoma involves ATG9A," *British Journal of Cancer*, vol. 117, no. 6, pp. 813–825, 2017.

[171] D. Fanfone, A. Idbaih, and J. Mammi et al., "Profiling anti-apoptotic BCL-xL protein expression in glioblastoma tumorspheres," *Cancers*, vol. 12, no. 10, p. 2853, 2020.

[172] X. Cai, R. G. Briggs, and H. B. Homburg et al., "Application of microfluidic devices for glioblastoma study: current status and future directions," *Biomedical Microdevices*, vol. 22, p. 60, 2020.

[173] J. Ma, N. Li, and Y. Wang et al., "Engineered 3D tumour model for study of glioblastoma aggressiveness and drug evaluation on a detachably assembled microfluidic device," *Biomedical microdevices*, vol. 20, no. 3, p. 80, 2018.

[174] J. M. Ayuso, M. Virumbrales-Muñoz, and A. Lacueva et al., "Development and characterization of a microfluidic model of the tumour microenvironment," *Scientific Reports*, vol. 6, no. 1, p. 36086, 2016.

[175] H.-G. Yi, Y. H. Jeong, and Y. Kim et al., "A bioprinted human-glioblastoma-on-a-chip for the identification of patient-specific responses to chemoradiotherapy," *Nature Biomedical Engineering*, vol. 3, no. 7, pp. 509–519, 2019.

[176] L. Neufeld, E. Yeini, and N. Reisman et al., "Microengineered perfusable 3D-bioprinted glioblastoma model for *in vivo* mimicry of tumor microenvironment," *Science Advances*, vol. 7, no. 34, p. eabi9119, 2021.

[177] N. Minami, Y. Maeda, and S. Shibao et al., "Organotypic brain explant culture as a drug evaluation system for malignant brain tumors," *Cancer Medicine*, vol. 6, no. 11, pp. 2635–2645, 2017.

[178] M. A. Marques-Torrejon, E. Gangoso, and S. M. Pollard, "Modelling glioblastoma tumour-host cell interactions using adult brain organotypic slice co-culture," *Disease Models & Mechanisms*, vol. 11, no. 2, p. dmm031435, 2018.

[179] A. B. Satterlee, D. E. Dunn, and D. C. Lo et al., "Tumoricidal stem cell therapy enables killing in novel hybrid models of heterogeneous glioblastoma," *Neuro-Oncology*, vol. 21, no. 12, pp. 1552–1564, 2019.

[180] J. J. Parker, P. Canoll, and L. Niswander et al., "Intratumoral heterogeneity of endogenous tumor cell invasive behavior in human glioblastoma," *Scientific Reports*, vol. 8, no. 1, p. 18002, 2018.

[181] T. Eisemann, B. Costa, and J. Strelau et al., "An advanced glioma cell invasion assay based on organotypic brain slice cultures," *BMC Cancer*, vol. 18, no. 1, p. 103, 2018.

[182] H. Pineau and V. Sim, "POSCAbilities: the application of the prion organotypic slice culture assay to neurodegenerative disease research," *Biomolecules*, vol. 10, no. 7, p. 1079, 2020.

[183] R. Gómez-Oliva, S. Domínguez-García, and L. Carrascal et al., "Evolution of experimental models in the study of glioblastoma: toward finding efficient treatments," *Frontiers in Oncology*, vol. 10, p. 614295, 2021.

[184] K. S. Sung, J.-K. Shim, and J.-H. Lee et al., "Success of tumorsphere isolation from WHO grade IV gliomas does not correlate with the weight of fresh tumor specimens: an immunohistochemical characterization of tumorsphere differentiation," *Cancer Cell International*, vol. 16, no. 1, p. 75, 2016.

[185] V. Governa, H. Talbot, and K. Gonçalves de Oliveira et al., "Landscape of surfaceome and endocytome in human glioma is divergent and depends on cellular spatial organization," *Proceedings of the National Academy of Sciences*, vol. 119, no. 9, p. e2114456119, 2022.

[186] S. Pedron and B. A. C. Harley, "Impact of the biophysical features of a 3D gelatin microenvironment on glioblastoma malignancy," *Journal of Biomedical Materials Research Part A*, vol. 101, no. 12, pp. 3404–3415, 2013.

[187] S. S. Rao, J. DeJesus, and A. R. Short et al., "Glioblastoma behaviors in three-dimensional collagen-hyaluronan composite hydrogels," *ACS Applied Materials & Interfaces*, vol. 5, no. 19, pp. 9276–9284, 2013.

[188] T. A. Ulrich, A. Jain, and K. Tanner et al., "Probing cellular mechanobiology in three-dimensional culture with collagen–agarose matrices," *Biomaterials*, vol. 31, no. 7, pp. 1875–1884, 2010.

[189] M. G. McCoy, D. Nyanyo, and C. K. Hung et al., "Endothelial cells promote 3D invasion of GBM by IL-8-dependent induction of cancer stem cell properties," *Scientific Reports*, vol. 9, no. 1, p. 9069, 2019.

[190] M. Tang, S. K. Tiwari, and K. Agrawal et al., "Rapid 3D bioprinting of glioblastoma model mimicking native biophysical heterogeneity," *Small*, vol. 17, no. 15, p. 2006050, 2021.

[191] S. A. Patil, A. Hosni-Ahmed, and T. S. Jones et al., "Novel approaches to glioma drug design and drug screening," *Expert Opinion on Drug Discovery*, vol. 8, no. 9, pp. 1135–1151, 2013.

[192] W. H. Hicks, C. E. Bird, and M. N. Pernik et al., "Large animal models of glioma: current status and future prospects," *Anticancer Research*, vol. 41, no. 11, pp. 5343–5353, 2021.

[193] F. L. Robertson, M.-A. Marqués-Torrejón, and G. M. Morrison et al., "Experimental models and tools to tackle glioblastoma," *Disease Models & Mechanisms*, vol. 12, no. 9, p. dmm040386, 2019.

[194] P. Liu, S. Griffiths, and D. Veljanoski et al., "Preclinical models of glioblastoma: limitations of current models and the promise of new developments," *Expert Reviews in Molecular Medicine*, vol. 23, p. e20, 2021.

[195] J. Han, Y. Jun, and S. H. Kim et al., "Rapid emergence and mechanisms of resistance by U87 glioblastoma cells to doxorubicin in an *in vitro* tumor microfluidic ecology," *Proceedings of the National Academy of Sciences*, vol. 113, no. 50, pp. 14283–14288, 2016.

[196] H. Sivakumar, M. Devarasetty, and D. E. Kram et al., "Multi-cell type glioblastoma tumor spheroids for evaluating sub-population-specific drug response," *Frontiers in Bioengineering and Biotechnology*, vol. 8, p. 538663, 2020.

[197] S. Plummer, S. Wallace, and G. Ball et al., "A human iPSC-derived 3D platform using primary brain cancer cells to study drug development and personalized medicine," *Scientific Reports*, vol. 9, no. 1, p. 1407, 2019.

[198] S.-Y. Lee, Y. Teng, and M. Son et al., "High-dose drug heat map analysis for drug safety and efficacy in multi-spheroid brain normal cells and GBM patient-derived cells," *PLOS ONE*, vol. 16, no. 12, p. e0251998, 2021.

[199] X. Cui, C. Ma, and V. Vasudevaraja et al., "Dissecting the immunosuppressive tumor microenvironments in glioblastoma-on-a-chip for optimized PD-1 immunotherapy," *eLife*, vol. 9, p. e52253, 2020.

[200] M. A. Heinrich, R. Bansal, and T. Lammers et al., "3D-Bioprinted minibrain: a glioblastoma model to study cellular interactions and therapeutics," *Advanced Materials*, vol. 31, no. 14, p. 1806590, 2019.

[201] K. Wang, F. M. Kievit, and A. E. Erickson et al., "Culture on 3D chitosan-hyaluronic acid scaffolds enhances stem cell marker expression and drug resistance in human glioblastoma cancer stem cells," *Advanced Healthcare Materials*, vol. 5, no. 24, pp. 3173–3181, 2016.

[202] T. Yu, Y. Wang, and Q. Hu et al., "The EZH2 inhibitor GSK343 suppresses cancer stem-like phenotypes and reverses mesenchymal transition in glioma cells," *Oncotarget*, vol. 8, no. 58, pp. 98348–98539, 2017.

[203] M. A. Hermida, J. D. Kumar, and D. Schwarz et al., "Three dimensional *in vitro* models of cancer: bioprinting multilineage glioblastoma models," *Advances in Biological Regulation*, vol. 75, p. 100658, 2020.

[204] J. P. Straehla, C. Hajal, and H. C. Safford, "A predictive microfluidic model of human glioblastoma to assess trafficking of blood–brain barrier-penetrant nanoparticles," *Proceedings of the National Academy of Sciences*, vol. 119, no. 23, p. e2118697119, 2022.

[205] Y. Fan, D. T. Nguyen, and Y. Akay et al., "Engineering a brain cancer chip for high-throughput drug screening," *Scientific Reports*, vol. 6, no. 1, p. 25062, 2016.

[206] M. Ratliff, H. Kim, and H. Qi et al., "Patient-derived tumor organoids for guidance of personalized drug therapies in recurrent glioblastoma," *International Journal of Molecular Sciences*, vol. 23, no. 12, p. 6572, 2022.

[207] S. Han and J. Wu, "Three-dimensional (3D) scaffolds as powerful weapons for tumor immunotherapy," *Bioactive Materials*, vol. 17, pp. 300–319, 2022.

[208] L. Barros, M. A. Pretti, and L. Chicaybam et al., "Immunological-based approaches for cancer therapy," *Clinics*, vol. 73, p. e429s, 2018.

[209] P. Mu, S. Zhou, and T. Lv et al., "Newly developed 3D *in vitro* models to study tumor–immune interaction," *Journal of Experimental & Clinical Cancer Research*, vol. 42, no. 1, p. 81, 2023.

[210] M. W. Yu and D. F. Quail, "Immunotherapy for glioblastoma: current progress and challenges," *Frontiers in Immunology*, vol. 12, p. 676301, 2021.

[211] M. Yang, I. Y. Oh, and A. Mahanty et al., "Immunotherapy for glioblastoma: current state, challenges, and tuture perspectives," *Cancers*, vol. 12, no. 9, 2020.

[212] X. Xu, F. Stockhammer, and M. Schmitt et al., "Cellular-based immunotherapies for patients with glioblastoma multiforme," *Journal of Immunology Research*, vol. 2012, p. 764213, 2012.

[213] M. Bausart, V. Préat, and A. Malfanti, "Immunotherapy for glioblastoma: the promise of combination strategies," *Journal of Experimental & Clinical Cancer Research*, vol. 41, no. 1, p. 35, 2022.

[214] M. Lim, Y. Xia, and C. Bettegowda et al., "Current state of immunotherapy for glioblastoma," *Nature Reviews Clinical Oncology*, vol. 15, no. 7, pp. 422–442, 2018.

[215] J. Huang, M. Zheng, and Z. Zhang et al., "Interleukin-7-loaded oncolytic adenovirus improves CAR-T cell therapy for glioblastoma," *Cancer Immunology, Immunotherapy*, vol. 70, pp. 2453–2465, 2021.

[216] J. M. Heffernan, J. B. McNamara, and S. Borwege et al., "PNIPAAm-co-Jeffamine® (PNJ) scaffolds as *in vitro* models for niche enrichment of glioblastoma stem-like cells," *Biomaterials*, vol. 143, pp. 149–158, 2017.

[217] A. Clavreul, G. Soulard, and J.-M. Lemée et al., "The French glioblastoma biobank (FGB): a national clinicobiological database," *Journal of Translational Medicine*, vol. 17, no. 1, p. 133, 2019.

[218] L. Annaratone, G. De Palma, and G. Bonizzi et al., "Basic principles of biobanking: from biological samples to precision medicine for patients," *Virchows Archiv*, vol. 479, pp. 233–246, 2021.

[219] L. Wang, J. Jung, and H. Babikir et al., "A single-cell atlas of glioblastoma evolution under therapy reveals cell-intrinsic and cell-extrinsic therapeutic targets," *Nature Cancer*, vol. 3, no. 12, pp. 1534–1552, 2022.

[220] P. Johansson, C. Krona, and S. Kundu et al., "A patient-derived cell atlas informs precision targeting of glioblastoma," *Cell Reports*, vol. 32, no. 2, p. 107897, 2020.

[221] A. Clavreul, L. Autier, and J.-M. Lemée et al., "Management of recurrent glioblastomas: what can we learn from the French glioblastoma biobank?," *Cancers*, vol. 14, no. 22, p. 5510, 2022.

[222] A. C. Fuentes-Fayos, M. E. G-García, and J. M. Pérez-Gómez et al., "Metformin and simvastatin exert additive antitumour effects in glioblastoma via senescence-state: clinical and translational evidence," *EBioMedicine*, vol. 90, p. 104484, 2023.

4

Brain Tumor Detection Using Image Processing Techniques

Kristin Surpuhi Benli
Üsküdar University, İstanbul, Türkiye

A brain tumor impairs the body's ability to operate normally and is a potentially fatal condition. Early diagnosis and effective treatment planning are contingent upon the early detection of brain tumors. The role of MRI scanning in medical research has become increasingly prominent over the past few years. Medical image analysis heavily relies on digital image processing. The image segmentation process is of paramount importance in image processing, as it facilitates the extraction of data from intricate medical images. The segmentation of brain tumors involves the separation of abnormal brain tissue (tumor) from the healthy brain tissue. Several researchers have previously proposed techniques for detecting and segmenting brain tumors. An overview of the techniques to detect brain tumors through MRI image segmentation is provided in this book chapter. This book chapter is composed of five sections: Section I gives a brief introduction about the brain tumor detection study. Section II explains magnetic resonance imaging. Section III describes the brain tumor detection stages; pre-processing, skull stripping, and various segmentation techniques. Section IV discusses an overview of prior researches and Section IV concludes the book chapter.

4.1 Introduction

It is essential, as with all types of cancer, to detect the presence of brain cancer early in order to ensure the survival of patients. The brain tumor is caused by the uncontrolled proliferation of certain cells in the brain or around it. Magnetic Resonance Imaging (MRI) is one of the most widely utilized and favored electronic modalities for the diagnosis of brain tumors. It provides an evaluation of the lesion by taking high-resolution and contrast images of the

DOI: 10.1201/9781003461906-4

brain. Tumor detection studies are focused on determining the exact location, size, shape, and type (benign or malignant) of the tumor in the brain [1].

Due to the intricate nature of the brain, the identification of brain tumors through MRI is challenging. Even a qualified radiologist can come to erroneous conclusions in the tumor grading. Image segmentation plays a vital role in medical image processing as it enables the extraction of necessary features for anomaly detection in the scanned image. The analysis of the images with precise image processing techniques is essential for professionals to comprehend the images within a short duration and make rapid decisions. Image processing techniques included in clinical decision support systems will help to increase the diagnostic efficiency of physicians and reduce the possibility of misdiagnosis [1]. The favorable outcomes to be obtained in these systems are important in terms of determining the most appropriate treatment for brain tumors. Given the aforementioned reasons, it appears imperative to implement automated segmentation techniques for MRI images. The objective of this section in the book is to present a thorough examination of the diverse image-processing approaches employed in the segmentation of brain tumors.

4.2 Magnetic Resonance Imaging (MRI)

MRI is one of the commonly used methods to obtain anatomical information from the brain. MRI provides visualization of general morphological features of brain tissues. It is used to detect physical abnormalities, lesions, and damages in the brain.

During the acquisition of an MRI image, the patient is first placed in a large tunnel-shaped device that has a large magnet and a strong magnetic field. The protons in the patient's body are stimulated with radio frequency waves. Protons that receive energy deviate from their positions according to the amount of energy they receive. When the radio frequency energy is cut off, the protons return to their previous positions and emit the energy they received as a signal. MRI images are created using these signals [2].

An MRI procedure poses no risk of radiation exposure as it does not utilize ionizing radiation. Nevertheless, the utilization of a powerful magnet in MRI renders it infeasible to acquire images from patients with pacemakers, aneurysm clips, cochlear implants, or vascular stents [3].

4.2.1 Axial, Coronal, and Sagittal Plane

The locations of structures in the human anatomy are described using hypothetical planes called anatomical planes. During brain imaging, the brain is displayed as two-dimensional (2D) slices. The three planes most commonly used to describe the locations of structures in the brain anatomy are shown in

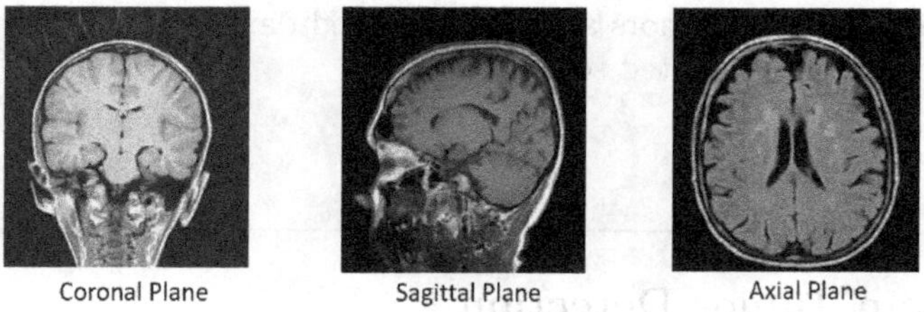

FIGURE 4.1
Anatomical planes. The MRI dataset that was made available as open source on Kaggle was used to create this figure [5].

Figure 4.1. The brain is partitioned into anterior (front) and posterior (back) sections in the coronal plane, and into right and left sections in the sagittal plane. In the horizontal plane, also referred to as the axial plane, the brain is divided into superior (upper) and inferior (lower) sections [4].

4.2.2 T1-weighted MRI and T2-weighted MRI

After figuring out the scan's view, the following step is to determine the image's weight. Two different scan types—T1-weighted and T2-weighted—can be created by adjusting the magnetic fields the scanner produces. Time to echo (TE) and repetition time (TR) are two fundamental time parameters in image acquisition. These serve as key parameters in creating image contrast. TR is the time interval between consecutive radio frequency (RF) pulse sequences applied to the same slice [6]. TE interval occurs between sending out the RF pulse and receiving the echo signal [6]. A short TE and TR are used to construct a T1-weighted MRI and long TE and TR are used to construct a T2-weighted MRI.

T1-weighted scan provides a high anatomical definition in images, whereas T2-weighted scan is effective in detecting pathology [7]. Cerebro-spinal fluid is usually examined to distinguish between T1- and T2-weighted scans. It appears dark on T1-weighted scans and bright on T2-weighted scans [6, 8]. On T1-weighted and T2-weighted scans, tissues containing fat and water can be easily differentiated [9]. Tissues carrying water and fluid appear darker on T1-weighted scans whereas they appear brighter on T2-weighted scans [10]. Conversely, tissues containing fat exhibit the opposite behavior, appearing brighter on T1-weighted scans and darker on T2-weighted scans [10]. On the T1-weighted scan, white and gray matter appear as they do in anatomy. However, on the T2-weighted scan, the white matter appears darker gray than the gray matter, which is contrary to the anatomy [6]. The detection of brain tumors heavily relies on imaging. Tumors are observed to have a darker appearance than brain tissue on T1-weighted scans and a brighter appearance than brain tissue on T2-weighted scans [11]. Inflammations have similar imaging properties as tumors and are displayed darker on T1-weighted scans and brighter on T2-weighted scans [6, 8].

4.3 Brain Tumor Detection

The overall flow of brain tumor detection consists of three phases. The pre-processing phase eliminates noise and undesirable artifacts in the MRI scan, the skull stripping phase eliminates the skull and any surrounding areas from the brain, the segmentation phase partitions the MRI scan into separate regions and detects the tumor. The sections that follow will provide a full introduction to these phases.

4.3.1 Pre-processing and Enhancement

The primary objective of the image pre-processing step is to prevent erroneous results that may occur during the segmentation process. The presence of noise and other undesirable artifacts in the MRI scan can reduce the success of the segmentation process. To tackle this issue, techniques such as image enhancements and noise reduction methods are implemented to improve the image's quality.

4.3.1.1 Histogram Equalization

A histogram is a distribution that shows the frequency of occurrence of each intensity value in the image. It serves as a visual tool to depict the contrast (the highest and lowest pixel intensities difference) in an image. A histogram solely provides statistical information and does not reveal information about the position of pixels. It is worth noting that multiple images can have identical histograms. The clustering of intensity values in particular areas in an image affects the quality of the image. In these cases, histogram equalization is utilized to improve the image's quality.

In histogram equalization, the goal is to achieve a homogeneous distribution of the image's intensity. The definition of histogram equalization in mathematics can be stated as follows [12]:

$$s_k = T(r_k) = (L-1)\sum_{j=0}^{k} p_r(r_j) = (L-1)\sum_{j=0}^{k} \frac{n_j}{n} \quad where\ k = 0, 1, \cdots, L-1 \tag{4.1}$$

In Equation 4.1, r_k and s_k indicate the input and processed kth pixel intensity values respectively. Term L is the maximum intensity value (L=2^n for n bit image), n is the total number of pixels, n_j is the frequency of jth intensity value and $p_r(r_j)$ is the probability of frequency of intensity r_j.

4.3.1.2 Mean Filter

Mean filtering is the process of reducing the intensity difference between one pixel and another pixel in an image. It is commonly used to reduce image noise. The mean filter replaces each pixel with the average of the pixel values in its neighborhood (including itself). The neighborhood is determined by placing the filtered pixel in the center of the sampling window. Let R_{xy} presents a subimage window of dimension mxn and the filtered pixel is centered at the point (x, y). Mean filter can be expressed as Equation 4.2 [13]:

$$J(x,y) = \frac{1}{M * N} \sum_{u,v \in R_{x,y}} K(u,v) \tag{4.2}$$

The filter takes the gray level of the pixel (x, y) in K and replaces it with the surrounding pixel detail $J(x, y)$.

4.3.1.3 Median Filter

The median filter is a commonly employed non-linear filter to remove noise from images. It proves particularly efficient in eliminating salt and pepper-type noise, which refers to random occurrences of black and white pixels. The median filter examines neighboring pixels to determine the value of each pixel. The filter moves through the image one pixel at a time. It arranges all pixel values within the window in ascending order, replacing the current pixel with the median value. The median filter can be expressed as Equation 4.3 [13]:

$$J(x,y) = \underset{(u,v) \in R_{xy}}{median} \{K(u,v)\} \tag{4.3}$$

where R_{xy} is defined as the set of coordinates of window with center at (x, y). The filter takes the gray level of the pixel in K and replaces it with the median value $(J(x, y))$ of the surrounding gray levels. It performs better compared to the mean filter [14].

4.3.1.4 Gaussian Filter

Gaussian filter is a non-uniform low pass filter employed for the purpose of eliminating noise and detail [15]. Its effectiveness lies in its ability to effectively smooth images. Two-dimensional Gaussian functions can be defined as Equation 4.4:

$$g(x,y,\sigma) = \frac{1}{2\pi\sigma^2} e^{-\frac{x^2+y^2}{2\sigma^2}} \tag{4.4}$$

In the equation x and y refer to the plane coordinates, and σ refers to the standard deviation. The mean of the distribution is assumed to be zero. The values of the Gaussian mask are determined by the window size and standard deviation. In this filter, the resulting value obtained by the product of the kernel matrix and the selected region is replaced with the value of the noisy pixel.

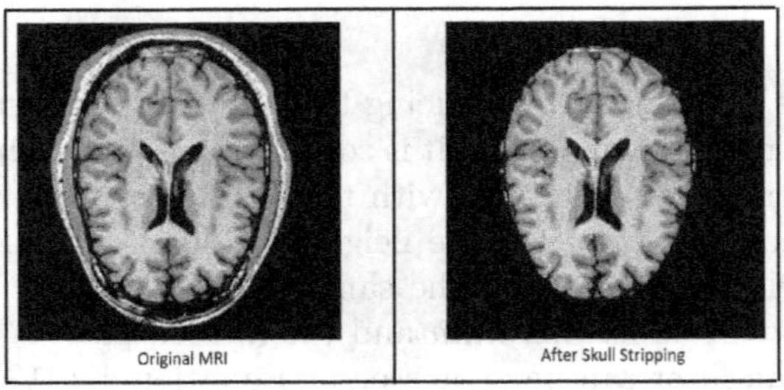

FIGURE 4.2
Original and skull stripped MRI images. The original MRI image featured in this figure was selected from the dataset available as open source on Kaggle [5].

In the literature, different researchers have used various filter types in the pre-processing phase of brain tumor detection. Dandıl proposed a computer-aided approach for the detection of brain tumors [9]. In the pre-processing stage of this approach, the arithmetic median filter was employed to improve the quality of the MRI image, followed by the Laplacian filter to sharpen the tumor boundaries, and finally, the histogram equalization filter was applied to minimize contrast differences. Malathi and Kamal [16] utilized median and Gaussian filters to remove the noise and sharpen MRI images respectively in the pre-processing stage of their study where they detected brain tumors using the k-means clustering technique. Dhage et al. [17] employed bilateral and median filters to eliminate noise from the pre-processing module of the system they suggested for the detection of brain tumors. Based on the results of the performance comparison, the median filter demonstrated better performance. Reddy et al. [18] and Zotin et al. [19] utilized a median filter to reduce the noise and filter out unwanted pixels in MRI during brain tumor detection studies. Aslıyan and Atbakan [20] utilized Gaussian and Wiener filters to improve the quality of the MRI image in their automatic brain tumor segmentation study.

4.3.2 Skull Stripping

Identifying the area that has to be processed and cleaning the other portions are prerequisites before working on images. A skull stripping operation is a procedure used to remove the skull and any surrounding areas from MRI scans of the brain. To ensure the successful completion of subsequent stages, it is essential to define the correct and accurate boundaries of the brain area. An example of a skull-stripping operation is illustrated in Figure 4.2. The figure displays the original MRI image on the left side, while the right side illustrates the appearance of the original MRI image after the skull separation procedure.

A study emphasizing the importance of skull stripping in the detection of brain tumors was carried out by Aslıyan and Atbakan [20]. The success of different brain segmentation techniques was examined with and without the skull stripping step. The finding of the study was that segmentation techniques are significantly more effective when the skull was removed from a brain MRI image.

In the literature there are publicly available and widely used algorithms for brain extraction like Brain Extraction Tool (BET) [21], Brain Surface Extractor (BSE) [22], 3dSkullStrip [23], BridgeBurner (BB) [24], ROBEX (Robust Brain Extraction) [25], and Graph Cuts (GCUT) [26]. Brief descriptions of these methods are presented below.

The BET algorithm [21], uses a deformable model that evolves to adapt to the brain surface. It estimates the intensity threshold between the brain and non-brain regions. Based on the center of gravity of the head, BET first defines an initial sphere. Then, it enlarges the sphere until it achieves the brain border. In the BSE algorithm [22], the process starts with anisotropic diffusion filtering and then edge detection is performed with the 3D Marr Hildret operator. A series of morphological operations are applied to adjust the surface relative to the brain. 3dSkullStrip [23] is a component of the Analysis of Functional NeuroImages (AFNI) package [27]. It modifies the BET by preventing leakage into the skull and the inclusion of the ventricles and eyes. The BB [24] employs a strategy known as thresholding with morphology. BB first locates a small cubic region in the white matter of the brain, and then it calculates a window using its mean intensity, which can be utilized to produce a coarse brain segmentation. A boundary set is created by combining the output of an edge detector with the surface of the preliminary mask. Then, all connections between the brain and non-brain tissue are eliminated through morphological procedures. The ROBEX method [25] accomplishes the final results by combining the discriminative and generative models. The discriminative model is a random forest classifier, employed to detect the brain boundary and the generative model is a point distribution model that guarantees that the outcome is conceivable. The GCUT method [26] compromises of intensity thresholding, graph cuts and post-processing stages. The first step is to find an appropriate threshold value which falls between the gray matter and cerebro-spinal fluid intensities and use it to obtain a preliminary mask. Mask will group the brain and skull, as well as some small interconnections between them. Graph cuts which is a type of graph theoretic image segmentation technique is utilized to eliminate the narrow connections. In post-processing stage, results are improved with morphological closing operation.

Besides the above-mentioned algorithms, semi-automatic or fully automatic brain extraction techniques have been introduced in recent years in order to overcome the drawbacks of manual segmentation. Ilhan and Ilhan [28] used an opening operation with the structure element disk and a series of pixel subtraction operators to remove the skull from the brain image. Unintentionally, some of the pixels from the tumor with the skull were also removed after the opening operation. In order to remove the skull from the brain image more effectively, pixel subtraction was utilized. The image of the brain without the skull is the outcome of the pixel subtraction processes. Dandıl [9] proposed a skull stripping algorithm that includes morphological operations like erosion, dilation and filling. In addition, the study conducted a comparative analysis with Otsu's method to showcase the efficacy of the suggested skull-stripping method. Roy and Maji [29] presented a novel intensity-based algorithm for skull stripping. The steps of the algorithm include adaptively calculating the threshold value and using morphological operations such as opening and closing. The authors compared the results of the algorithm to those of other widely used skull-stripping tools, such as BET, BSE, and ROBEX. The results of the experiment demonstrated that the proposed method can be utilized for synthetic as well as real images. Reddy et al. [18] distinguished and removed the skull regions of the brain based on opening and closing morphological operations. Duarte et al. [30] suggested a paradigm for brain extraction, consisting of data collection, preprocessing, and extraction of the largest connected component, in which they utilized digital image processing approaches at each stage. The purpose of the preprocessing stage was to improve contrast and remove any potential noise from the T1-weighted MRI. The process of extracting the largest connected component—the brain—from an image realized by identifying its largest element and then using mathematical morphological operators to take it out.

In a review study on skull extraction methods, Kalavathi and Prasath [31] stated that although numerous approaches to skull stripping have been put forth, the issue is still not thought to be fully resolved. Numerous systems in the literature perform well on some datasets (T1-weighted images), but when the study populations or acquisition settings are altered, they are unable to yield results that are acceptable. Hence, studies that provide applicable solutions to all the problems presented by skull stripping methods are one of the demanding research areas in the field of brain tumor detection [31].

4.3.3 Segmentation

Image segmentation infers partitioning an image into separate regions according to the characteristics of the pixels in order to reduce the complexity of the image and make its analysis simpler. In this way, pixels with the same characteristics on the image will be grouped together and the image will be divided into subgroups or regions of the same type. Segmentation is utilized in the simplest cases to distinguish objects from the background, therefore the segmented image becomes a binary image containing only the foreground and background [32].

Image segmentation criteria can be stated with the following mathematical expressions [33]. The image R can be partitioned into n regions $R_1, R_2, ..., R_n$ such that:

1. $\bigcup_{i=1}^{n} R_i = R$
2. R_i *is a connected set*, $i = 1, 2, ..., n$

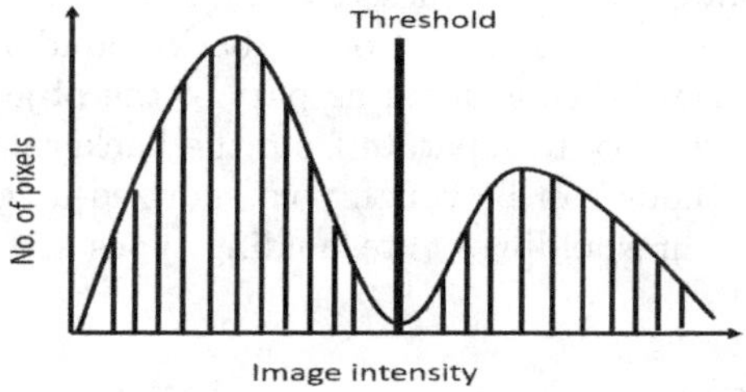

FIGURE 4.3
Histogram of an image.

3. $R_i \cap R_j = , \ i \neq j$
4. $P(R_i) = TRUE \, for \, i = 1, 2, ..., n$
5. $P(R_i \cup R_j) = FALSE, \ i \neq j, \ R_i \, adjacent \, R_j.$

In the expressions ∩ and ∪ symbols denote intersection and union, respectively. The first condition stands for each pixel should belong to a specific region. Second condition specifies that regions are composed of contiguous pixels [34]. Third condition implies that the regions don't intersect each other. Fourth condition determines that each region satisfies the homogeneity predicate P. Last condition implies that two adjacent regions can not be combined into a single region [35].

Various categories exist for brain tumor segmentation techniques, including thresholding, region growing, edge based, clustering, and watershed techniques. The following sections will give an overview of these image segmentation techniques.

4.3.3.1 Thresholding Techniques

The purpose of thresholding techniques is to separate objects in the image from the background by using an appropriate threshold value. For any pixel (x, y) in the source image; if $src(x, y)$ is greater than the threshold value T, it will be a pixel belonging to the object (value 1), otherwise it will be a pixel belonging to the background (value 0).

$$dst(x, y) = \begin{cases} 1, & if \ src(x, y) > T \\ 0, & if \ src(x, y) \leq T \end{cases} \tag{4.5}$$

The histogram, which shows the distributions of gray levels in the image, is widely utilized in determining the threshold value. A suitable threshold can be chosen if the histogram characteristics specified are narrow, tall, symmetrical, and separated by deep valleys [36]. Assuming that we have an image with a histogram shown in Figure 4.3 expressed by the $src(x, y)$ function. The figure displays gray values on the x-axis and the corresponding total number of pixels on the y-axis. A threshold value of T can be determined between the intersection of the lower points of these two valleys [37]. All pixels below the threshold value can be deemed as part of the background and all pixels above the threshold value can be considered as part of the object. In brain tumor detection, the object we try to separate from the background is the tumor.

Thresholding methods can be roughly categorized as global thresholding and local (adaptive) thresholding. Thresholding types are detailed in the following paragraphs.

Global Thresholding

In Global Thresholding, a single value is considered to be a threshold for an entire image. It inputs a source image (src) and a threshold value (T) and outputs an image (dst) based on the comparison of the pixel intensity at the source pixel location (x, y) with the threshold value. Global Thresholding is a widely used and easy-to-implement technique. The following paragraphs discuss the various types of global thresholding methods.

Binary Thresholding is the most basic type of global thresholding. Pixels with an intensity value higher than the threshold will be set to $maxVal$ (white), while those lower than will be set to zero (black) (Equation 4.6) [38].

$$dst(x,y) = \begin{cases} maxVal & if\ src(x,y) > T \\ 0 & otherwise \end{cases} \tag{4.6}$$

The opposite form of binary thresholding is Inverse-Binary Thresholding, in which the pixels whose intensity values are greater than the threshold will be zero (black) and the pixels whose intensity values are lower than the threshold will be $maxVal$ (white) (Equation 4.7) [38].

$$dst(x,y) = \begin{cases} 0 & if\ src(x,y) > T \\ maxVal & otherwise \end{cases} \tag{4.7}$$

In Truncate Thresholding, while pixel values above the threshold are adjusted to the threshold value, other pixels remain same (Equation 4.8) [38].

$$dst(x,y) = \begin{cases} T & if\ src(x,y) > T \\ src(x,y) & otherwise \end{cases} \tag{4.8}$$

The threshold-to-Zero technique will assign a value of zero to the source pixels whose intensity values are lower than the threshold and will not modify the values of the other pixels (Equation 4.9) [38].

$$dst(x,y) = \begin{cases} src(x,y) & if\ src(x,y) > T \\ 0 & otherwise \end{cases} \tag{4.9}$$

The inverted Threshold to Zero technique will do the opposite of the previous method and only change pixels whose intensity values are greater than the threshold (Equation 4.10) [38].

$$dst(x,y) = \begin{cases} 0 & if\ src(x,y) > T \\ src(x,y) & otherwise \end{cases} \tag{4.10}$$

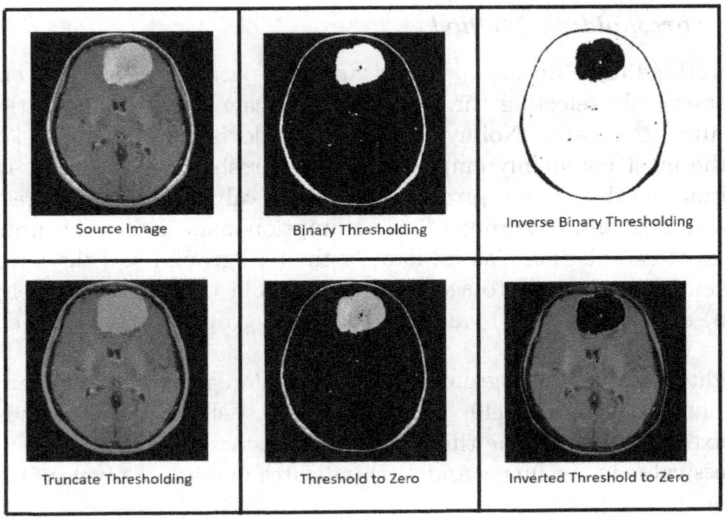

FIGURE 4.4
Various thresholding techniques were applied on same brain MRI images. The source image featured in this figure was selected from the dataset available as open source on Kaggle [5].

Figure 4.4 illustrates the changes that occur in the source image as a result of applying different threshold techniques described above to an example brain MRI image. During these processes, the threshold value (T) and the maximum value ($maxVal$) were determined as 127 and 255, respectively.

While the user can set the threshold T manually, there are also many cases where the user would like to have the threshold to be set automatically by an algorithm. The steps of the iterative algorithm that can automatically estimate the threshold value of each image are given below [33].

Algorithm 1 : Basic Global Thresholding Algorithm

1: Choose an initial threshold value T
2: Segment the image using the selected threshold value T. This will result in the formation of two groups G_1 and G_2
   G_1: contains pixels with intensity values $> T$
   G_2: contains pixels with intensity values $<= T$
3: Calculate the mean intensity values μ_1 and μ_2 for the groups G_1 and G_2
4: Compute a new threshold value $T = \frac{1}{2}(\mu_1 + \mu_2)$
5: Continue to perform steps 2 through 4 until the difference in T between consecutive iterations is less than a predefined parameter ΔT

Otsu's Thresholding Method

Otsu thresholding is an unsupervised and non-parametric method employed for automatically selecting thresholds in grayscale image segmentation. It is named after its creator, Nobuyuki Otsu, who devised this method [39]. It is one of the most commonly employed global thresholding methods. It allows for determining the most appropriate threshold value to be used in reducing a gray-level image into two groups. The assumption made is that the input image comprises of two distinct classes, namely the background and the foreground. Subsequently, it proceeds to ascertain a threshold value (t). The weight (w), mean (μ) and variance (σ_2) values of these two groups are determined for all threshold values.

Weight values for background ($w_b(t)$) and foreground ($w_f(t)$) are calculated as in Equation 4.11 [40]. In the equation, i shows the brightness value of the pixel, t represents the threshold value, I stands for the maximum pixel brightness value in the image and $P(i)$ indicates number of pixels with brightness value i.

$$w_b(t) = \frac{\sum_{i=0}^{t} P(i)}{\sum_{i=0}^{I} P(i)} \quad and \quad w_f(t) = \frac{\sum_{i=t+1}^{I} P(i)}{\sum_{i=0}^{I} P(i)} \tag{4.11}$$

In Equation 4.12, $q_b(t)$ and $q_f(t)$ indicate the total number of pixels in the background and foreground according to the threshold value t, respectively [40].

$$q_b(t) = \sum_{i=0}^{t} P(i) \quad and \quad q_f(t) = \sum_{i=t+1}^{I} P(i) \tag{4.12}$$

Background and foreground mean values are calculated as in Equation 4.13 [40]:

$$\mu_b(t) = \sum_{i=0}^{t} \frac{iP(i)}{q_b(t)} \quad and \quad \mu_f(t) = \sum_{i=t+1}^{I} \frac{iP(i)}{q_b(t)} \tag{4.13}$$

The individual class variances are given in Equation 4.14 [40]:

$$\sigma_b^2(t) = \sum_{i=0}^{t} [i - \mu_b(t)]^2 \frac{P(i)}{q_b(t)} \quad and \quad \sigma_f^2(t) = \sum_{i=t+1}^{I} [i - \mu_f(t)]^2 \frac{P(i)}{q_f(t)} \tag{4.14}$$

The within-class variance is calculated as in Equation 4.15 [40]:

$$\sigma_w^2(t) = w_b(t)\sigma_b^2(t) + w_f(t)\sigma_f^2(t) \tag{4.15}$$

The between class variance is computed using Equation 4.16 [40]:

$$\sigma_B^2(t) = w_b(t)w_f(t)(\mu_b(t) - \mu_f(t))^2 \tag{4.16}$$

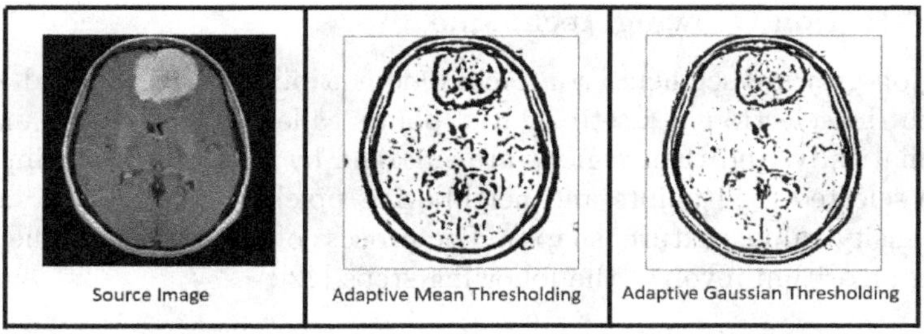

FIGURE 4.5
Adaptive thresholding techniques were applied on same brain MRI images. The source image featured in this figure was selected from the dataset available as open source on Kaggle [5].

In the next step, the most appropriate threshold value is determined. Otsu's method aims to identify the threshold that minimizes the weighted within-class variance, essentially equivalent to maximizing the between-class variance. The threshold value that meets this condition is the optimal threshold value used in image segmentation. Otsu algorithm includes the following steps [41]:

Algorithm 2 : Otsu Algorithm

1: Grayscale image is taken
2: The histogram of the grayscale image is calculated
3: The pixel density probabilities of the image are found
4: Initial values are assigned for $w_b(0)$, $w_f(0)$, $\mu_b(0)$, and $\mu_f(0)$.
5: The following steps are applied for all threshold values from t=0 to the highest pixel intensity value
6: $w_b(t)$, $w_f(t)$, $\mu_b(t)$, and $\mu_f(t)$ values are updated
7: The between class variance $\sigma_B^2(t)$ is calculated
8: The threshold value of t at which $\sigma_B^2(t)$ is maximum is determined

Adaptive Thresholding Method

The adaptive thresholding method divides an image into smaller regions and computes the threshold value for each region. Thus, every region will have different threshold values. For each region, the threshold can be computed either using arithmetic mean or Gaussian mean of the pixel intensities. In the arithmetic mean, each pixel in the neighboring region contributes the same amount to the threshold calculation. In the Gaussian mean, the pixel positions play a significant part in the threshold calculation. Pixels that are further away from the center of the region are less likely to contribute to the calculation. Figure 4.5 demonstrates the resulting output images after applying adaptive thresholding techniques.

4.3.3.2 Region Growing Technique

The region-growing segmentation technique is a pixel-based method and begins with the selection of a set of initial points called as seed points manually or automatically, and then regions are enlarged by looking at the similarities of these selected seed points and neighboring pixels according to a criterion (like intensity value, texture, shape). The process of implementing the Region Growing algorithm involves the following steps [42]:

Algorithm 3 : Region Growing Algorithm

1: The seed pixels, denoted as $s_1, s_2, ..., s_n$, are chosen as the n number of initial points. Additionally, the regions corresponding to these seed pixels are identified as $C_1, C_2, ..., C_n$
2: Determine the similarity between the seed point s_i and the pixel value of neighbouring points. If the similarity measure is less than the specified threshold value, neighboring point can be considered as element of C_i region
3: Recompute the border of C_i and the mean values of all pixels in C_i region are recalculated as new $s_i(s)$ respectively
4: Continue to perform Steps 2 and 3 until all pixels in the image are allocated to a specific region

---

The main difficulties associated with region growing include selecting suitable seeds, determining the similarity criterion, and managing the size and shape of the region.

4.3.3.3 Edge Based Techniques

An edge in an image is a notable local variation in image intensity that is typically connected to a discontinuity in the image intensity or the image intensity's first derivative [35]. Edge detection is a fundamental technique employed in image analysis and holds significant importance in identifying the contours of brain tumors.

Various techniques are available for detecting edges, with most falling under the categories of Gradient and Laplacian. The Gradient method identifies edges by locating the maximum and minimum values in the image's first derivative, while the Laplacian method detects zero crossings in the second derivative to identify edges [43]. This section offers an overview of commonly used edge detection methods, such as Gradient-based, Canny edge detection, and Laplacian-based techniques.

Gradient Based Operator

The gradient operator, represented by the symbol $\bigtriangledown$ and specified as a vector, is the standard tool for determining the magnitude and direction of intensity changes of an image f. The gradient for a two-dimensional image $f(x, y)$ can be defined as a vector as in Equation 4.17 [44]:

$$\nabla f = \begin{bmatrix} G_x \\ G_y \end{bmatrix} = \begin{bmatrix} \frac{\partial f}{\partial x} \\ \frac{\partial f}{\partial y} \end{bmatrix} \tag{4.17}$$

Mathematically, the gradient magnitude is calculated as follows [44]:

$$G\left|f(x,y)\right| = \sqrt{G_x^2 + G_y^2} \tag{4.18}$$

The approximate magnitude is calculated using the Equation 4.19 [44]:

$$G\left|f(x,y)\right| = |G_x| + |G_y| \tag{4.19}$$

The gradient direction $\theta(x, y)$ is calculated using the Equation 4.20 [44]:

$$\theta(x,y) = arctan\left(\frac{G_y}{G_x}\right) \tag{4.20}$$

The partial derivatives $\partial f/\partial x$ and $\partial f/\partial y$ must be calculated at each pixel in the image in order to determine the gradient. Numerical approximations of these derivatives are calculated in the neighborhood of each point while working with digital images [45]. The following paragraphs provide general information about the most commonly used gradient-based edge detectors, Roberts operator, Sobel operator and Prewitt operator; their primary distinction is in the way they carry out this computation.

■ *Roberts Edge Detection*

Roberts edge detector, introduced by Roberts [46], is one of the earliest edge detectors, and is also referred to as the cross gradient operator. It is based on the idea of cross diagonal differences, and is limited to the diagonal elements. It does not take into account horizontal or vertical neighbors. The mask pair for the Roberts edge detector can be found in Equation 4.21:

$$G_x = \begin{bmatrix} 1 & 0 \\ 0 & -1 \end{bmatrix} \quad G_y = \begin{bmatrix} 0 & 1 \\ -1 & 0 \end{bmatrix} \tag{4.21}$$

The computation of the gradient value pair for the $I(x, y)$ pixel on an I image using the Roberts method is as follows [47]:

$$G_x = I(x,y) - I(x+1, y+1) \tag{4.22}$$

$$G_y = I(x+1, y) - I(x, y+1) \tag{4.23}$$

Sobel Edge Detection

Sobel edge detector is proposed by Sobel [48] and used to reveal edge regions in the image. It uses a 3x3 pair of convolution masks to calculate the slope in both x-direction and y-direction. Convolution template of Sobel detector is given in Equation 4.24 where G_x and G_y are used to calculate gradient magnitude in the x-direction and y-direction, respectively.

$$G_x = \begin{bmatrix} -1 & 0 & 1 \\ -2 & 0 & 2 \\ -1 & 0 & 1 \end{bmatrix} \qquad G_y = \begin{bmatrix} 1 & 2 & 1 \\ 0 & 0 & 0 \\ -1 & -2 & -1 \end{bmatrix} \tag{4.24}$$

Equation 4.25 represents the $I(x, y)$ pixel and its neighboring pixels in the image I [47].

$I(x-1, y-1)$	$I(x, y-1)$	$I(x+1, y-1)$
$I(x-1, y)$	$I(x, y)$	$I(x+1, y)$
$I(x-1, y+1)$	$I(x, y+1)$	$I(x+1, y+1)$

(4.25)

The calculation of the gradient value pair for the $I(x, y)$ pixel on an I image using the Sobel method is as follows [47]:

$$\begin{aligned} G_x &= \{I(x+1, y-1) + 2I(x+1, y) + I(x+1, y+1)\} \\ &- \{I(x-1, y-1) + 2I(x-1, y) + I(x-1, y+1)\} \end{aligned} \tag{4.26}$$

$$\begin{aligned} G_y &= \{I(x-1, y-1) + 2I(x, y-1) + I(x+1, y-1)\} \\ &- \{I(x-1, y+1) + 2I(x, y+1) + I(x+1, y+1)\} \end{aligned} \tag{4.27}$$

Prewitt Edge Detection

Prewitt edge detection algorithm is introduced by Prewitt [49]. Prewitt operator utilizes identical equations to those of the Sobel operator. However, it does not give neighbors close to the center of the filter any extra weight. Mask forms are expressed as in Equation 4.28.

$$G_x = \begin{bmatrix} -1 & 0 & 1 \\ -1 & 0 & 1 \\ -1 & 0 & 1 \end{bmatrix} \qquad G_y = \begin{bmatrix} 1 & 1 & 1 \\ 0 & 0 & 0 \\ -1 & -1 & -1 \end{bmatrix} \tag{4.28}$$

The computation of the gradient value pair for the $I(x, y)$ pixel on an I image using the Prewitt method is as follows [47]:

$$\begin{aligned} G_x &= \{I(x+1, y-1) + I(x+1, y) + I(x+1, y+1)\} \\ &- \{I(x-1, y-1) + I(x-1, y) + I(x-1, y+1)\} \end{aligned} \tag{4.29}$$

$$\begin{aligned} G_y &= \{I(x-1, y-1) + I(x, y-1) + I(x+1, y-1)\} \\ &- \{I(x-1, y+1) + I(x, y+1) + I(x+1, y+1)\} \end{aligned} \tag{4.30}$$

Canny Edge Detection

Canny edge detection algorithm is a widely-used method for detecting edges which was proposed in 1986 by John F Canny [50]. It attempts to determine the difference between objects as closely as feasible to reality. The following are the stated steps of the edge detection algorithm.

Algorithm 4 : Canny Edge Detector Algorithm

1: The image is smoothed with a Gaussian filter
2: Gradient magnitude and direction are calculated using Sobel, Prewitt, or Roberts operator.
3: Nonmaxima Suppression is applied to gradient magnitude to find edge points. An edge point is a point whose intensity is locally maximal in the gradient vector's direction.
4: Hysteresis Thresholding: A double thresholding (T_{low} and T_{high}) algorithm is used to detect strong and weak edge pixels
5: **if** $pixelValue > T_{high}$ **then**
6: it is a strong edge pixel
7: **else if** $pixelValue \geq T_{low}$ and $pixelValue \leq T_{high}$ **then**
8: it is a weak edge pixel
9: **else**
10: it is not an edge pixel
11: The detection of edges is completed by suppressing all other edges that are not connected to the weak and strong edges.

Laplacian Based Operator

The Laplacian operator looks for zero crossings and detects edges based on the image's second derivative. The partial second order derivatives in x and y directions are expressed as in Equation 4.31:

$$\begin{aligned} \frac{\partial^2 f(x,y)}{\partial x^2} &= f(x+1,y) + f(x-1,y) - 2f(x,y) \\ \frac{\partial^2 f(x,y)}{\partial y^2} &= f(x,y+1) + f(x,y-1) - 2f(x,y) \end{aligned} \tag{4.31}$$

The Laplace for the two-variable function $f(x, y)$ is computed by the summation of partial derivatives and represented as in Equation 4.32:

$$\nabla^2 f(x,y) = \frac{\partial^2 f(x,y)}{\partial x^2} + \frac{\partial^2 f(x,y)}{\partial y^2}$$

$$\nabla^2 f(x,y) = f(x+1,y) + f(x-1,y) + f(x,y+1) + f(x,y-1) - 4f(x,y) \tag{4.32}$$

Due to the Laplacian's high sensitivity to noise, the image is first smoothed using a Gaussian filter before the zero crossings are found using Laplacian.

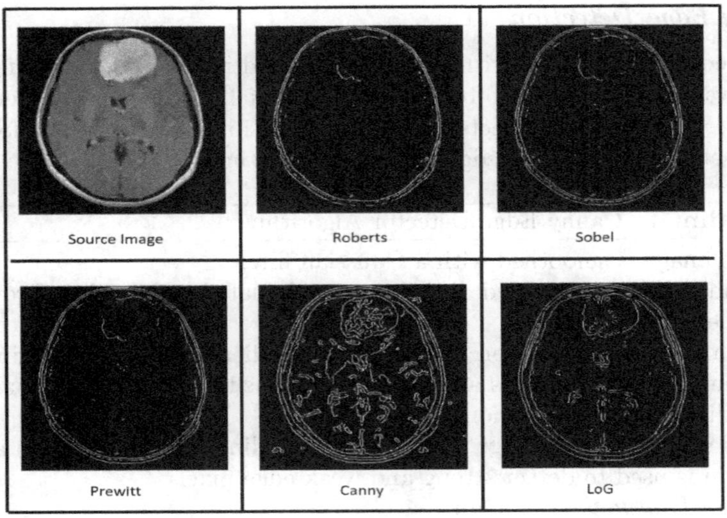

FIGURE 4.6
Edge-based techniques were applied on same brain MRI images. The source image featured in this figure was selected from the dataset available as open source on Kaggle [5].

This is known as the Laplacian of Gaussian (LoG) operation, and it realized in Equation 4.33:

$$LoG(x, y) = -\frac{1}{\pi\sigma^4}\left[1 - \frac{x^2 + y^2}{2\sigma^2}\right] e^{-\frac{x^2 + y^2}{2\sigma^2}} \tag{4.33}$$

Figure 4.6 depicts the resultant images obtained by employing various edge detection methods mentioned above on a sample brain MRI image.

4.3.3.4 Clustering Techniques

Clustering technique is a type of unsupervised learning method and assigns data without label information to classes according to certain attributes. In clustering techniques, k-means and Fuzzy C-means algorithms are frequently used in brain tumor segmentation tasks. These algorithms are mentioned in the following sections.

k-means Clustering Algorithm

The k-means algorithm is an iterative method that assigns each data point to exactly one cluster. Prior to the implementation of the clustering method, the k-value must be determined. Each cluster has a centroid (center point) which is initialized randomly. Distances (like Euclidean distance) between the data points and the cluster centroids are computed using Equation 4.34 [51]:

$$J = \sum_{j=1}^{k} \sum_{i=1}^{n} \left\| x_i^{(j)} - c_{(j)} \right\|^2 \tag{4.34}$$

In the equation k stands for the number of clusters, n stands for a number of data points and c_j stands for the centroid for cluster j. The distance of each data point (x_i) to the centroid of each cluster (c_j) is calculated. Data point is assigned to the nearest cluster. After the placement of all data points is completed, the new cluster centroids are computed for each cluster. Data points are reassigned according to these new cluster centroids. These steps are repeated until the centroids of the clusters are fixed or until the number of iterations is reached. Thus, the image is segmented into regions, in our case the brain is divided into parts.

Fuzzy C-means Clustering Algorithm

In fuzzy clustering, unlike classical clustering, data may belong to more than one cluster, in other words, there are partial memberships of the data. In this method, membership degrees between [0,1] are assigned to the data to indicate the degree to which the data belongs to different clusters. In this case, the membership degree will be the highest for the cluster nearest to the data. This algorithm is designed to minimize the objective function given in Equation 4.35 [51]:

$$J_m = \sum_{i=1}^{N} \sum_{j=1}^{c} u_{ij}^m \left\| x_i - v_j \right\|^2 \ , 1 \leq m < \infty \tag{4.35}$$

In the equation, N represents the total number of data points, c denotes the number of clusters, u_{ij} signifies the membership degree of data point x_i in cluster j, x_i stands for the ith data point, v_j indicates the center of cluster j, and m is the exponent of the partition matrix [51].

The algorithm first assigns a number of clusters and randomly initializes the cluster centers. In the next step, the distances between the data points and the center vectors are calculated and membership degrees are updated using Equation 4.36 [52]:

$$u_{ij} = \frac{1}{\sum_{k=1}^{c} \left(\frac{\|x_i - v_j\|}{\|x_i - v_k\|} \right)^{\frac{2}{m-1}}} \tag{4.36}$$

Then cluster centers are computed using Equation 4.37 [52]:

$$v_j = \frac{\sum_{i=1}^{N} u_{ij}^m . x_i}{\sum_{i=1}^{N} u_{ij}^m} \tag{4.37}$$

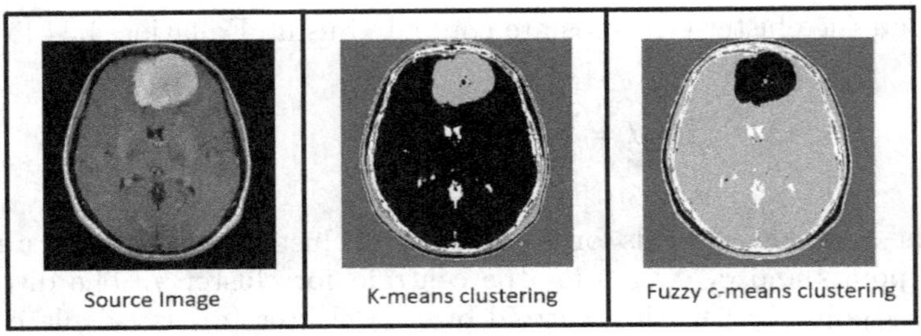

FIGURE 4.7
Clustering based techniques were applied on same brain MRI images. The source image featured in this figure was selected from the dataset available as open source on Kaggle [5].

The algorithm will terminate if $max_{ij}\left\{\left|u_{ij}^{(k+1)} - u_{ij}^{(k)}\right|\right\} < \epsilon$ where ϵ and k stand for the termination and iteration values, respectively [52].

Figure 4.7 depicts the resultant images obtained by employing k-means and Fuzzy c-means clustering methods mentioned above on a sample brain MRI image. For both methods, the number of clusters was taken as four.

4.3.3.5 Watershed Technique

A watershed is essentially the area of land that lies between two rivers. In the realm of image processing, an image can be interpreted as a topographic surface based on its gray levels [53]. Watershed lines are formed if these surfaces are subsequently filled with water from their minimum points while being kept apart from water originating from other sources [54].

Soille and Vincent [55] presented an adaptable algorithm for calculating watersheds in digital images. Let I be a grayscale image and h_{min} and h_{max} are the smallest and largest values of I, respectively. The term $T_h(I)$ represents the threshold of I at level h. A recursion is defined with the gray level h varying from h_{min} to h_{max}. At the beginning of the recursion, the basin set X_h is taken to be equal to the set of points $(T_{h_{min}})$ with the value h_{min}. In Equation 4.38, $T_{h_{min}}$ represents the set of points that water reaches first and $X_{h_{min}}$ denotes the set of points that belong to the minima of the lowest altitude [55].

$$X_{h_{min}} = T_{h_{min}}(I) \tag{4.38}$$

Then, the domain $(IZ_{T_{h+1}(I)}(X_h))$ of the basin cluster X_h within the threshold cluster T_{h+1} is expanded sequentially [56]:

$$X_{h+1} = min_{h+1} \cup IZ_{T_{h+1}(I)}(X_h), \ \ \forall h \in [h_{min}, h_{max} - 1] \tag{4.39}$$

In Equation 4.39, min_h stands for the set of points belonging to the minimum at height h. $X_{h_{max}}$ obtained from this recursion process is the set of basins of the image I. Watershed transformation is expressed as the complement of the $X_{h_{max}}$ basins set within the I image [56].

4.4 Related Work

Several studies have investigated the segmentation of MRI brain images to detect and extract tumor areas. A review of selected literature on brain tumor segmentation techniques and their applications is presented in this section.

In their study, Madhukumar and Santhiyakumari [57] evaluated the capabilities of Fuzzy C-means and k-means segmentation methods to classify tissues (gray matter, white matter, cerebro-spinal fluid, necrotic focus, vasogenic edema and background) in brain MRI images. In the course of the experiments, Fuzzy C-means classified three tissue classes and generated empty clusters, whereas k-means classified six classes. k-means demonstrated better ability to identify vasogenic edema, white matter, gray matter and necrotic focus than Fuzzy C-means.

Dhage et al. [17] accomplished brain tumor segmentation by using the Watershed algorithm and determined the position and shape of the tumor in the MRI image through the use of connected component labeling.

Kaur and Sharma [58] investigated the existing methods for brain tumor detection and segmentation in brain MRI images and reached the following findings. Although the intensity-based thresholding techniques yield good results, they are not effective for images with significant intensity differences. While region-based segmentation techniques work well for images with high contrast, they are ineffective for images with low contrast. Edge-based and clustering-based segmentation techniques obtain better results but fail for noisy images.

A technique for identifying and localizing brain tumors from MRI scans was presented by Hazra et al [59]. During the pre-processing stage, filtering and image enhancement techniques were applied to the image converted to grayscale. The edge detection stage was performed using Sobel, Prewitt, and Canny algorithms. In the last stage, thresholding-based segmentation and k-means clustering techniques were used to detect tumor-affected areas in the MRI.

Mittal et al. [60] proposed an effective algorithm consisting of preprocessing, segmentation and output stages to segment tumor from MRI images. In the first stage, they converted the input image into gray scale, and applied a high pass filter to remove noises and a median pass filter to enhance the quality of image. In the second stage, they utilized the Otsu thresholding method together with the Watershed technique to realize the image segmentation. In the last stage, they carried out morphological operations to segmented the image and detected the tumor on the image.

A new threshold approach to segment brain tumors was proposed by Ilhan and Ilhan [28]. There are three stages to the suggested approach. The first stage is pre-processing, where the image was improved and made ready for analysis using morphological and pixel subtraction operations. The second stage is segmentation, where a novel thresholding technique was suggested to distinguish the tumor region from the enhanced image. In the proposed threshold method, average gray value, which was used to transform a grayscale image into a binary image, was computed by dividing the sum of unique pixel values—excluding zeros—to the count of unique pixel values. In the last stage, they applied a median filter to remove the noise from the segmented image.

A study analyzing the performance of different edge detection techniques on brain MRI images was carried out by Yıldız and Yıldız [61]. The study revealed that the Roberts, Prewitt, and Sobel methods, when used with a threshold value of 0.03, produced better results in comparison to other methods.

Pooja et al. [62] conducted a research on brain tumor detection, where they examined the performance of a variety of segmentation techniques. The techniques analyzed in their study encompassed threshold-based, edge detection, region growing, watershed, and k-means segmentation. The proposed system encompassed the following stages of skull stripping; preprocessing; segmentation; and comparative analysis. The results of the study indicated that region growing and k-means segmentation techniques were more effective than the other segmentation techniques.

Zotin et al. [19] suggested a methodology to determine the location of tumor borders in MRI brain images. They utilized Fuzzy C-means clustering method to segment the images and Canny edge detector to identify fine edges. The performance of the suggested techniques was evaluated against Classic Canny, Prewitt, Roberts, Sobel, and LoG methods. The proposed approach obtained an average of 3–7% more accuracy.

Aslıyan and Atbakan [20] utilized a variety of methods like k-means, Fuzzy C-means, Self Organizing Maps, Otsu, and hybrid k-means+Otsu methods to identify the regions of tumors in brain MRI images. They proposed an algorithm to identify and remove the skull from the image. The success of the different segmentation systems were examined with and without the skull stripping step. Hybrid k-means+Otsu method was reported as the most successful with an accuracy rate of 94% in the skull-removed images and 84% in the non-removed images.

Mahdi et al. [63] applied Sobel, Prewitt, Roberts and Canny edge detection methods to brain, bone, and liver MRI images. Among the edge detection methods, it has been stated that the Canny and Sobel edge detectors perform better than the other techniques.

Traditional edge detection techniques and eight-direction Sobel edge detection algorithm are compared by As and Gopalan [64] in their work and identified that 8-Sobel is the most appropriate method to analyze the MRI images of brain tumors.

In their data analysis study, Sangeeta and Nagendra [65] compared the accuracy and processing times of k-means and Fuzzy C-means clustering techniques in brain tumor detection. In terms of accuracy both of them obtained the same results and achieved 80% accuracy. However, in terms of processing time the situation is different. Since Fuzzy C-means requires more segmentation than k-means, it has longer processing time. Thus, the k-means clustering stands out with its performance in this study.

Nyo et al. [66] employed Otsu's thresholding technique to develop an automated system for segmenting tumors in brain MRI scans. The initial step involves converting the RGB image to grayscale and resizing it. Next, the noise removal stage utilizes a median filter to eliminate any unwanted noise. The segmentation stage employs Otsu's thresholding method to distinguish between tumor and non-tumor regions. Finally, a morphological operation is applied to accurately identify the tumor regions. The system was evaluated using the 2015 BRATS dataset and achieved an accuracy of 68.7%.

4.5 Conclusion

The growth of brain cells that is an abnormal and uncontrolled manner is referred to as a brain tumor. This condition can occur in different anatomical regions within the brain. MRI images are highly effective in detecting even the smallest irregularities in the body, and they are used to visualize the brain and identify any abnormalities, particularly tumors. The research on tumor imaging aims to accurately determine the location, size, shape and type of the tumor.

The identification of brain tumors is a crucial task in the field of medical image processing. The segmentation of medical images is a complex and challenging stage in the study of tumor detection, and various approaches have been proposed in this area. The use of brain tumor segmentation techniques has already demonstrated promise in the detection and analysis of tumors in clinical images. In order to enhance the accuracy of segmentation, it can be considered to employ a combination of segmentation techniques or make modifications in future studies.

Bibliography

[1] R. K. Garg and A. Kulshreshtha, "A review of automated mri image processing techniques employing segmentation & classification," *International Journal of Computer Science Trends and Technology (IJCST)*, vol. 5, no. 2, pp. 117–120, 2017.

[2] E. Çoban Budak and M. R. Bozkurt, "Vertebra lomber disklerde meydana gelen bozulmaların manyetik rezonans görüntüleme mrg ile analizi," *AJIT-e: Academic Journal of Information Technology*, vol. 4, no. 11, pp. 125–144, 2013.

[3] Stanford Medicine, "Risks of magnetic resonance imaging (mri)." https://stanfordhealthcare.org/medical-tests/m/mri/risk-factors.html#:~:text=Because%20radiation%20is%20not%20used,Intracranial%20aneurysm%20clips. Accessed: 2024-02-07.

[4] TeachMeAnatomy, "Anatomical planes." https://teachmeanatomy.info/the-basics/anatomical-terminology/planes/. Accessed: 2024-01-13.

[5] M. Nickparvar, "Brain tumor mri dataset." https://www.kaggle.com/dsv/2645886, 2021. Accessed: 2024-01-30.

[6] D. C. Preston, "Magnetic resonance imaging (mri) of the brain and spine: Basics." https://case.edu/med/neurology/NR/MRI%20Basics.htm#:~:text=Repetition%20Time%20(TR)%20is%20the,receipt%20of%20the%20echo%20signal. Accessed: 2024-01-13.

[7] K. Najarian and R. Splinter, *Biomedical Signal and Image Processing*. CRC Press, 2012.

[8] N. Kumari and S. Saxena, "Review of brain tumor segmentation and classification," in *2018 International conference on current trends towards converging technologies (ICCTCT)*, pp. 1–6, IEEE, 2018.

[9] E. Dandıl, *MR Görüntüleri ve MR Spektroskopi Verileri ile Yapay Öğrenme Tabanlı Beyin Tümörü Tespit Yöntemi ve Uygulaması*. PhD thesis, Sakarya Üniversitesi, 2015.

[10] M. Mafraji, "Magnetic resonance imaging." https://www.msdmanuals.com/professional/special-subjects/principles-of-radiologic-imaging/magnetic-resonance-imaging#:~:text=For%20example%2C%20fat%20appears%20bright,bright%20on%20T2%2Dweighted%20images. Accessed: 2024-01-13.

[11] R. Rulaningtyas and K. Ain, "Edge detection for brain tumor pattern recognition," *Instrumentation, Communications, Information Technology, and Biomedical Engineering (ICICI-BME)*, vol. 3, 11 2009.

[12] TheAILearner, "Histogram equalization." https://theailearner.com/2019/04/01/histogram-equalization. Accessed: 2024-01-08.

[13] C. Maheshan and H. Prasanna Kumar, "Performance of image preprocessing filters for noise removal in transformer oil images at different temperatures," *SN Applied Sciences*, vol. 2, pp. 1–7, 2020.

[14] C. Küpeli and F. Bulut, "Görüntüdeki tuz biber ve gauss gürültülerine karşı filtrelerin performans analizleri," *Haliç Üniversitesi Fen Bilimleri Dergisi*, vol. 3, no. 2, pp. 211–239, 2020.

[15] A. Ravishankar, S. Anusha, H. K. Akshatha, *et al.*, "A survey on noise reduction techniques in medical images," in *2017 International conference of Electronics, Communication and Aerospace Technology (ICECA)*, vol. 1, pp. 385–389, 2017.

[16] R. Malathi and D. N. B. Kamal, "Brain tumor detection and identification using k-means clustering technique," in *Proceedings of the UGC sponsored national conference on advanced networking and applications*, pp. 14–18, 2015.

[17] P. Dhage, M. R. Phegade, and S. K. Shah, "Watershed segmentation brain tumor detection," in *2015 International Conference on Pervasive Computing (ICPC)*, pp. 1–5, 2015.

[18] D. Reddy, Dheeraj, Kiran, *et al.*, "Brain tumor detection using image segmentation techniques," in *2018 International Conference on Communication and Signal Processing (ICCSP)*, pp. 0018–0022, 2018.

[19] A. Zotin, K. Simonov, M. Kurako, *et al.*, "Edge detection in mri brain tumor images based on fuzzy c-means clustering," *Procedia Computer Science*, vol. 126, pp. 1261–1270, 2018.

[20] R. Aslıyan and I. Atbakan, "Automatic brain tumor segmentation with k-means, fuzzy c-means, self-organizing map and otsu methods," *Selçuk-Technical Journal*, vol. 19, no. 4, pp. 267–281, 2020.

[21] S. M. Smith, "Fast robust automated brain extraction," *Human brain mapping*, vol. 17, no. 3, pp. 143–155, 2002.

[22] D. W. Shattuck and R. M. Leahy, "Brainsuite: An automated cortical surface identification tool," *Medical Image Analysis*, vol. 6, no. 2, pp. 129–142, 2002.

[23] AFNI, "Analysis of functional neuroimages." `http://afni.nimh.nih.gov`. Accessed: 2024-01-14.

[24] A. Mikheev, G. Nevsky, S. Govindan, *et al.*, "Fully automatic segmentation of the brain from t1-weighted mri using bridge burner algorithm," *Journal of Magnetic Resonance Imaging*, vol. 27, no. 6, pp. 1235–1241, 2008.

[25] J. E. Iglesias, C.-Y. Liu, P. M. Thompson, *et al.*, "Robust brain extraction across datasets and comparison with publicly available methods," *IEEE Transactions on Medical Imaging*, vol. 30, no. 9, pp. 1617–1634, 2011.

[26] S. A. Sadananthan, W. Zheng, M. W. Chee, *et al.*, "Skull stripping using graph cuts," *NeuroImage*, vol. 49, no. 1, pp. 225–239, 2010.

[27] R. W. Cox, "Afni: Software for analysis and visualization of functional magnetic resonance neuroimages," *Computers and Biomedical Research*, vol. 29, no. 3, pp. 162–173, 1996.

[28] U. Ilhan and A. Ilhan, "Brain tumor segmentation based on a new threshold approach," *Procedia computer science*, vol. 120, pp. 580–587, 2017.

[29] S. Roy and P. Maji, "A simple skull stripping algorithm for brain mri," in *2015 Eighth International Conference on Advances in Pattern Recognition (ICAPR)*, pp. 1–6, 2015.

[30] K. T. N. Duarte, M. A. N. Moura, P. S. Martins, *et al.*, "Brain extraction in multiple t1-weighted magnetic resonance imaging slices using digital image processing techniques," *IEEE Latin America Transactions*, vol. 20, no. 5, pp. 831–838, 2022.

[31] P. Kalavathi and V. S. Prasath, "Methods on skull stripping of mri head scan images—a review," *Journal of digital imaging*, vol. 29, pp. 365–379, 2016.

[32] G. Dougherty, *Digital Image Processing for Medical Applications.* Cambridge University Press, 2009.

[33] R. C. Gonzalez and R. E. Woods, *Digital Image Processing.* Prentice Hall, 2002.

[34] X. M. Pujol, *Image Segmentation Integrating Colour, Texture and Boundary Information.* PhD thesis, University of Girona, 2002.

[35] R. C. Jain, R. Kasturi, and B. G. Schunck, *Machine vision.* McGraw-Hill, 1995.

[36] B. Kim, R. O. Serfa Juan, D.-E. Lee, *et al.*, "Importance of image enhancement and cdf for fault assessment of photovoltaic module using ir thermal image," *Applied Sciences*, vol. 11, no. 18, 2021.

[37] A. Aslantaş, *Kemik Metastazlarının Görüntü Işleme ve Yapay Sinir Ağları Yöntemleri ile Tespiti.* PhD thesis, Sakarya University, 2015.

[38] G. Bradski and A. Kaehler, *Learning OpenCV: Computer Vision with the OpenCV Library.* O'Reilly Media, 2008.

[39] N. Otsu, "A threshold selection method from gray-level histograms," *IEEE transactions on systems, man, and cybernetics*, vol. 9, no. 1, pp. 62–66, 1979.

[40] E. Yücer, *Gece Görüntüleri Kullanılarak Kentsel Alanların Belirlenmesi ve Gelişmişlikle Ilişkisinin Incelenmesi.* PhD thesis, Kocaeli University, 2018.

[41] R. Aşlıyan, "Otsu ve rocchio metotlarıyla beyin tümörü tespiti," *Avrupa Bilim ve Teknoloji Dergisi*, no. 43, p. 69–74, 2022.

[42] B. S. A. Jama and D. N. Baykan, "Modified region growing method for image segmentation using ant lion optimization algorithm," *Avrupa Bilim ve Teknoloji Dergisi*, pp. 404–411, 2020.

[43] O. R. Vincent and O. Folorunso, "A descriptive algorithm for sobel image edge detection," in *Proceedings of informing science & IT education conference (InSITE)*, vol. 40, pp. 97–107, 2009.

[44] E. Arslan, *Hücresel Sinir Ağı Sistemleri Kullanarak Hareketli Nesnelerin Görüntü İşleme Uygulamaları.* PhD thesis, İstanbul University, 2011.

[45] H. Spontón and J. Cardelino, "A Review of Classic Edge Detectors," *Image Processing On Line*, vol. 5, pp. 90–123, 2015.

[46] L. Roberts, "Machine perception of three-dimensional solids," in *Optical and Electro-Optical Information Processing*, pp. 157–197, J. Tippet et al. Eds. Cambridge, MA: MIT Press, 1965.

[47] Y. E. Önal, *Gürültüye Karşı Dayanıklı Bir Kenar Tespit Algoritması Geliştirilmesi.* PhD thesis, Hacettepe University, 2018.

[48] I. E. Sobel, *Camera Models and Perception.* PhD thesis, Stanford University, 1970.

[49] J. M. Prewitt, "Object enhancement and extraction," *Picture processing and Psychopictorics*, vol. 10, no. 1, pp. 15–19, 1970.

[50] J. Canny, "A computational approach to edge detection," *IEEE Transactions on pattern analysis and machine intelligence*, no. 6, pp. 679–698, 1986.

[51] A. Saxena, M. Prasad, A. Gupta, *et al.*, "A review of clustering techniques and developments," *Neurocomputing*, vol. 267, pp. 664–681, 2017.

[52] B. Karun, T. A. Prasath, M. P. Rajasekaran, *et al.*, "Glioma detection using eho based flame clustering in mr brain images," *International Journal of Imaging Systems and Technology*, vol. 34, no. 1, p. e22937, 2024.

[53] N. Dincer, "Beyin tümörlerinin görüntü işleme teknikleri kullanılarak bilgisayar destekli tespiti," master's thesis, Istanbul University-Cerrahpasa, December 2018.

[54] A. Yüksel, "X-ışını el görüntülerinde kemik dokusunun bölütlenmesi," master's thesis, Istanbul Technical University, June 2008.

[55] P. Soille and L. M. Vincent, "Determining watersheds in digital pictures via flooding simulations," in *Visual Communications and Image Processing'90: Fifth in a Series*, vol. 1360, pp. 240–250, SPIE, 1990.

[56] M. Topaloğlu and A. Gangal, "Watershed dönüşümü kullanılarak corpus callosumun bölütlenmesi," *Union Radio-Scientifique Internationale (URSI) (URSI)*, vol. 2, pp. 607–609, 2006.

[57] S. Madhukumar and N. Santhiyakumari, "Evaluation of k-means and fuzzy c-means segmentation on mr images of brain," *The Egyptian Journal of Radiology and Nuclear Medicine*, vol. 46, no. 2, pp. 475–479, 2015.

[58] H. Kaur and D. R. Sharma, "A survey on techniques for brain tumor segmentation from mri," *IOSR Journal of Electronics and Communication Engineering*, vol. 11, no. 05, pp. 01–05, 2016.

[59] A. Hazra, A. Dey, S. K. Gupta, *et al.*, "Brain tumor detection based on segmentation using matlab," in *2017 International Conference on Energy, Communication, Data Analytics and Soft Computing (ICECDS)*, pp. 425–430, 2017.

[60] K. Mittal, A. Shekhar, P. Singh, *et al.*, "Brain tumour extraction using otsu based threshold segmentation," *International Journal of Advanced Research in Computer Science and Software Engineering*, vol. 7, pp. 159–163, 04 2017.

[61] G. Yıldız and D. Yıldız, "Bazı kenar algılama yöntemlerinin manyetik rezonans görüntüleri üzerindeki performans analizi," *International Journal of Multidisciplinary Studies and Innovative Technologies*, vol. 2, no. 2, pp. 13–17, 2018.

[62] V. Pooja, M. K. Kumar, and K. Kamalesh, "Comparative analysis of segmentation techniques on mri brain tumor images," *Materials Today: Proceedings*, vol. 47, pp. 109–114, 2021. NCRABE.

[63] W. H. Mahdi, S. K. Ahmed, Z. H. N. AL-Azzawi, *et al.*, "A comparative study of edge detection technique with mri (magnetic resonance imaging) images," *Webology (ISSN: 1735-188X)*, vol. 19, no. 1, 2022.

[64] R.A.S. Ajai and S. Gopalan, "Comparative analysis of eight direction sobel edge detection algorithm for brain tumor mri images," *Procedia Computer Science*, vol. 201, pp. 487–494, 2022.

[65] S. Sangeeta and H. Nagendra, "Brain tumor detection and classification using clustering and comparison with fcm," in *2022 International Conference on Innovative Computing, Intelligent Communication and Smart Electrical Systems (ICSES)*, pp. 1–6, 2022.

[66] M. T. Nyo, F. Mebarek-Oudina, S. S. Hlaing, *et al.*, "Otsu's thresholding technique for mri image brain tumor segmentation," *Multimedia tools and applications*, vol. 81, no. 30, pp. 43837–43849, 2022.

5

Tumor Growth Simulation

Ihab Elaff

Uskudar University, Istanbul, Türkiye

One of the main causes of death in the world today is thought to be cancer [1, 2]. A World Health Organization information sheet states that 13% of deaths are related to cancer. Brain tumor development simulator modeling can predict a patient's life expectancy, project the impact of brain damage on perception and attitude in the future, and assess the effectiveness of current treatments. The behavior of tumor growth utilizing various factors and models is the main topic of this chapter.

5.1 Brain Tumor

A tumor is characterized as an atypical mass of tissue that arises from an atypical proliferation or division of cells [3]. The most widely used techniques for identifying cancers are CT scans and magnetic resonance imaging (MRI). Based on statistical data, metastatic tumors are more common than original tumors [4], and the ratio of malignant to benign tumors is higher [5]. Glioma is the most prevalent primary central nervous system (CNS)'s tumor, accounting for around 80% of all malignant brain tumors [6]. Based on the pace of tumor growth, two types of glioma can be distinguished: High-Grade Glioma (HGG) and Low-Grade Glioma (LGG). The most prevalent kind of primary brain tumor is the HGG. Chemotherapy, radiation therapy, and surgery are the usual treatments for HGG [5, 7].

DOI: 10.1201/9781003461906-5

5.2 Reaction Diffusion Equations (RDE) for Modeling Brain Tumors

In the literature, spatiotemporal models of tumor growth have been extensively employed to simulate the growth of brain gliomas [5–24]. Based on the Reaction–Diffusion Equation (RDE), these models explain how the pathology progresses through the tumor cells' time of proliferation and the space where they infiltrate into the surrounding tissue. Equation 5.1 and the second Fick's law of Kolmogorov-Petrovsky-Piskounov can be used to create the most basic RDE. Equation 5.2 represents the isotropic version of the formula.

Anisotropic:

$$\frac{dc}{dt} = \nabla.\left(D(x)\nabla\ c\right) + R(c) \tag{5.1}$$

Isotropic:

$$\frac{dc}{dt} = D(x)\nabla^2 c + R\left(c\right) \tag{5.2}$$

Where D(x) is the spatially resolved diffusion tensor that describes cell diffusion rate at certain point x in time t, c is the Glioma cell concentration of the same point x and at the same time t. The function R(c) represents the proliferation component where it is the temporal evolution pattern of the growth. Some research [8, 9, 14, 16, 17] tends to include treatment therapy function T(c) to the equation which makes Equation 5.1 takes the form:

$$\frac{dc}{dt} = \nabla.\left(D(x)\nabla\ c\right) + R\left(c\right) - T(c) \tag{5.3}$$

RDE is bounded by some condition where for each point x:

$$x \in B \tag{5.4}$$

where B is the brain tissue domain

$$t \geq 0 \tag{5.5}$$

$$c\left(x, 0\right) = c_0 \tag{5.6}$$

where, c_0 is initial distribution of tumor cells

$$n.\nabla c = 0\ on \partial B \tag{5.7}$$

5.3 Reaction Models

There are numerous ways to express the reaction part, some of them are as follows [8, 10, 13–18, 20, 21]:

Reaction Method 1 (R1) Exponential Proliferation:

$$R(c) = \rho c \tag{5.8}$$

Reaction Method 2 (R2) Verhulst or logistic function:

$$R(c) = \rho c \, \frac{c_m - c}{c_m} \tag{5.9}$$

Reaction Method 3 (R3) Gompertz equation:

$$R(c) = \rho c \, ln\left(\frac{c_m}{c}\right) \tag{5.10}$$

Where ρ denotes the proliferation rate of cells (also called geometrical rate) and it represent the relative increase of cell concentration per time unit, c_m is the maximum tumor cell concentration parameter. In normalized scale, $c_m = 1$ which makes Verhulst or logistic function becomes Fisher's equation [11, 13, 16, 18, 22]:

$$R(c) = \rho c \,(1 - c) \tag{5.11}$$

and Gompertz equation will take the form:

$$R(c) = \rho c \, ln\left(\frac{1}{c}\right) \tag{5.12}$$

For the HGG, the regularly used value for the proliferation rate is $\rho = 0.012$ per day, however, the LGG employs much lower value such as $\rho = 0.0012$ per day.

5.4 Diffusion Models

The diffusion tensor D(x) has been represented in the literature with different forms and parameters values. The general form can be represented by the following equation:

$$D(x) = D_{WGC}(x)\, W(x) \tag{5.13}$$

where $D_W GC$(x) is the inhomogeneous diffusion coefficient, and W(x) is the diffusion tensor. Inhomogeneous diffusion coefficient $D_W GC$(x) can be determined using:

$$D_{WGC}(x) = \begin{cases} D_{WM} & if\ x \in WM \\ D_{GM} & if\ x \in GM \\ D_{CSF} & if\ x \in CFS \end{cases} \tag{5.14}$$

Such that, D_WM, D_GM, and D_CSF are diffusion coefficients for White Matter (WM), Gray Matter (GM) and Cerebrospinal fluid (CSF) respectively. Different values have been assigned to these for both High-Grade Glioma (HGG) and Low Grade Glioma (LGG); however, the most preferred values in normalized scale are 1, 0.2, and 0 for D_WM, D_GM, and D_CSF respectively where this will keep five-fold difference between the WM and the GM. In this way, the diffusion coefficients for white matter (WM), gray matter (GM), and cerebrospinal fluid (CSF) are, respectively, DWM, DGM, and DCSF. Both High Grade Glioma (HGG) and Low-Grade Glioma (LGG) have been given different values for these; however, the most favored values in a normalized scale are 1, 0.2, and 0 for DWM, DGM, and DCSF, respectively, where this will maintain a five-fold difference between the WM and the GM. The weighted diffusion tensor W(x) has represented using different models such as:

Model 1 (M1) [12, 13, 23]:

$$W(x) = I = \begin{bmatrix} 1 & 0 & 0 \\ 0 & 1 & 0 \\ 0 & 0 & 1 \end{bmatrix} \tag{5.15}$$

Model 2 (M2) [18, 22]:

$$W(x) = \begin{cases} \begin{bmatrix} \lambda_1 & 0 & 0 \\ 0 & \lambda_2 & 0 \\ 0 & 0 & \lambda_3 \end{bmatrix} & x \in WM \\ I & x \in GM \end{cases} \tag{5.16}$$

Model 3 (M3) [21]:

$$W(x) = E \begin{bmatrix} 1+\gamma(x)(\overline{\lambda}-1) & 0 & 0 \\ 0 & 1 & 0 \\ 0 & 0 & 1 \end{bmatrix} E^T \tag{5.17}$$

Model 4 (M4) [10]:

$$W(x) = E \begin{bmatrix} r\lambda_1 & 0 & 0 \\ 0 & \lambda_2 & 0 \\ 0 & 0 & \lambda_3 \end{bmatrix} E^T \tag{5.18}$$

Model 5 (M5) [10]:

$$W(x) = E \begin{bmatrix} \lambda_1(rC_l + rC_p + C_s) & 0 & 0 \\ 0 & \lambda_2(C_l + rC_p + C_s) & 0 \\ 0 & 0 & \lambda_3(C_l + C_p + C_s) \end{bmatrix} E^T \tag{5.19}$$

5.5 Brain Modeling

The first stage in modeling brain tumor simulator is to model the brain itself from medical imaging techniques. Among different medical imaging modality, Diffusion Tensor MRI (DTI) is widely used in that process as it will provide sufficient data to model the 3 main components of the brain namely WM, GM and CSF.

5.5.1 Diffusion Tensor Imaging (DTI)

A magnetic resonance imaging method called diffusion tensor imaging (DTI) makes it possible to assess the limited diffusion of water in tissue [25–30]. The generalized diffusion tensor in three dimensions is given by a symmetric, positive definite, second-order 3×3 matrix D. D's three eigenvectors, or major coordinate directions, e1, e2, and e3, are orthogonal since it is symmetric and positive definite. Accordingly, $\lambda 1$, $\lambda 2$, and $\lambda 3$ are the appropriate eigenvalues (diffusion coefficients) for these vectors, such that $\lambda 1 > \lambda 2 >= \lambda 3$. The two remaining eigenvectors point in the cross-fiber direction, whereas the first eigenvector, e1, indicates the major diffusion direction, which is the fiber direction.

$$D = E\Lambda E^T = \ [\boldsymbol{e_1}|\ \boldsymbol{e_2}|\ \boldsymbol{e_3}] \begin{bmatrix} \lambda_1 & 0 & 0 \\ 0 & \lambda_2 & 0 \\ 0 & 0 & \lambda_3 \end{bmatrix} \begin{bmatrix} \boldsymbol{e_1} \\ \boldsymbol{e_2} \\ \boldsymbol{e_3} \end{bmatrix} \tag{5.20}$$

DTI data can be described using rotational invariant quantities (Table 5.1, Figure 5.1) such as Mean Diffusivity (MD), Fractional Anisotropy (FA), Rational Anisotropy (RA), Linear Anisotropy(Cl), Spherical Anisotropy(Cs), Volume Ratio (VR), Angular Anisotropy (AA), and Diffusion Volume (DV), Aitchison Anisotropy (Aita), Matusita Anisotropy (MA), and Kullback-Leibler Anisotropy (KLA).

5.5.2 Brain Model Segmentation

A thorough understanding of the intricate structure of the brain's constituent parts as well as the DTI scanner's operation principle would enable more accurate selection of the appropriate scalar index to best characterize the targeted tissue in light of its biological properties [31, 32]. These features lead to the conclusion that WM and GM contain the least water, while CSF contains the most. Additionally, the way that the water is contained in each of these components varies: the water in WM is ordered in axon cells, whereas the water in CSF is entirely free (isotropic) (extremely limited or highly anisotropic). Unlike WM and CSF, the organization of GM's water contents is not as severely constrained. Based on these facts, rational quantities like the FA, RA, or

TABLE 5.1
DTI Scalar Indices

Scalar Index Name	Equation
Fractional Anisotropy (FA)	$FA = \frac{\sqrt{3((\lambda_1-\overline{\lambda})^2+(\lambda_2-\overline{\lambda})^2+(\lambda_3-\overline{\lambda})^2)}}{\sqrt{2(\lambda_1{}^2+\lambda_2{}^2+\lambda_3{}^2)}}$
Rational Anisotropy (RA)	$RA = \frac{\sqrt{(\lambda_1-\overline{\lambda})^2+(\lambda_2-\overline{\lambda})^2+(\lambda_3-\overline{\lambda})^2}}{\sqrt{3\overline{\lambda}}}$
Mean Diffusivity (MD)	$MD = (\lambda_1 + \lambda_2 + \lambda_3)/3$
Linear Anisotropy(c_l)	$c_l = \frac{\lambda_1-\lambda_2}{\lambda_1+\lambda_2+\lambda_3}$
spherical Anisotropy(c_s)	$c_s = \frac{3\lambda_3}{\lambda_1+\lambda_2+\lambda_3}$
Volume ratio (VR)	$VR = \frac{\lambda_1\lambda_2\lambda_3}{[\overline{\lambda}]^3}$
Angular Anisotropy (AA)	$AA = arccos\left(\sum_{i=1}^{3}\frac{\lambda_i}{\sqrt{\sum_{j=1}^{3}\lambda_j{}^2}}\frac{\overline{\lambda}}{\sqrt{\sum_{j=1}^{3}\overline{\lambda}^2}}\right)$
Diffusion Volume (DV)	$DV = \frac{4}{3}\pi\lambda_1\lambda_2\lambda_3$
Aitchison Anisotropy(Aita)	$AitA = \sqrt{\sum_{i=1}^{3}(\ln(\lambda_i) - \frac{1}{3}\sum_{j=1}^{3}\ln(\lambda_j))}$
Matusita Anisotropy (MA)	$MA = \frac{\sqrt{\sum_{i=1}^{3}\left(\sqrt{\lambda_i}-\sqrt{\overline{\lambda}}\right)}}{\sqrt{\sum_{i=1}^{3}\lambda_i}}$
Kullback-Leibler Anisotropy (KLA)	$KLA = \sqrt{\frac{2}{3}}\sqrt{ln(\left(\frac{1}{3}\sum_{i=1}^{3}\frac{\lambda_i}{\overline{\lambda}}\right)\left(\frac{1}{3}\sum_{i=1}^{3}ln(\frac{\lambda_i}{\overline{\lambda}})\right))}$

VR might be used to distinguish between WM and non-WM regions, while eigenvalues or MD could be used to categorize CSF and non-CSF regions. K-Means [33], is used for segmenting brain to WM/non-WM from FA images (Figure 5.2) and to CSF/non-CSF from MD images (Figure 5.3).

The John Hopkins Medical Institute's Laboratory of Brain Anatomical MRI website provided the datasets utilized in this study. These files provide large amounts of DTI brain data. There are 50 slices of 256 × 256 voxels in each brain DTI volume. To calculate tensor data, each dataset has a file with 35 gradient orientations. The voxel width and height in each slice are 0.9375 mm

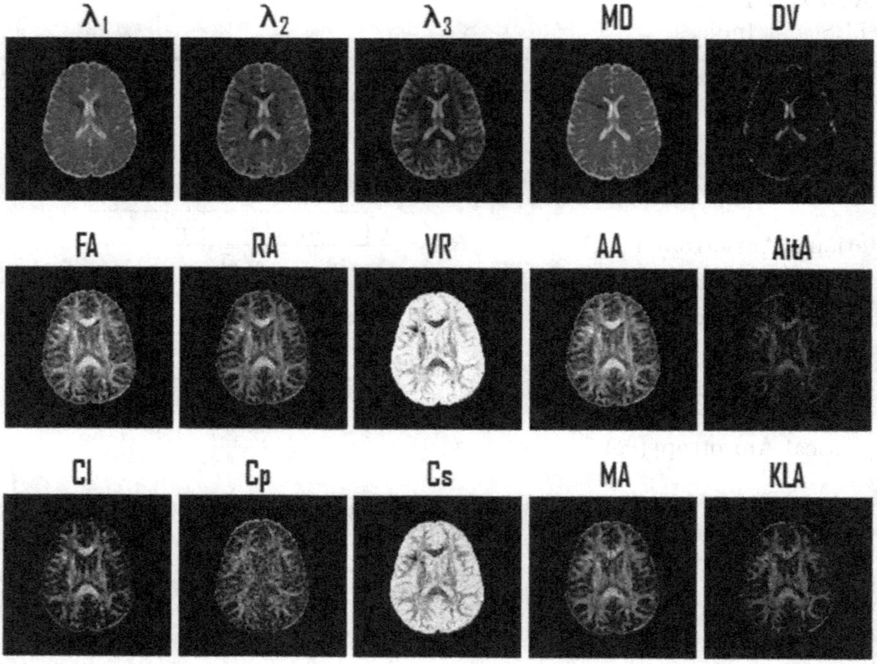

FIGURE 5.1
Illustration of some Scalar Indices at an axial slice.

and 2.5 mm, respectively, as is the distance between two consecutive slices. FA and MD are used to classify brain scan model to WM, GM and CSF.

5.5.3 Finite Element Modeling RDE

The solution to Equation 5.1 can be written in discrete form as follows:

$$c^{t+1} = c^t + dt[\nabla.(D\nabla c^t)] + dtR(c) \tag{5.21}$$

where dt is the time step and c^{t+1} and c^t represents the next and the current values of the variable respectively. The initial value of R(c) is taken to be equal zero. The diffusion term can be written as:

$$\nabla.(D\nabla c) = \begin{bmatrix} d_{11}\frac{\partial^2 c}{\partial x^2} + d_{22}\frac{\partial^2 c}{\partial y^2} + d_{33}\frac{\partial^2 c}{\partial z^2} + \\ 2d_{12}\frac{\partial^2 c}{\partial x \partial y} + 2d_{23}\frac{\partial^2 c}{\partial y \partial z} + 2d_{13}\frac{\partial^2 c}{\partial x \partial z} + \\ \frac{\partial c}{\partial x}\left[\frac{\partial d_{11}}{\partial x} + \frac{\partial d_{21}}{\partial y} + \frac{\partial d_{31}}{\partial z}\right] + \\ \frac{\partial c}{\partial y}\left[\frac{\partial d_{12}}{\partial x} + \frac{\partial d_{22}}{\partial y} + \frac{\partial d_{32}}{\partial z}\right] + \\ \frac{\partial c}{\partial z}\left[\frac{\partial d_{13}}{\partial x} + \frac{\partial d_{23}}{\partial y} + \frac{\partial d_{33}}{\partial z}\right] \end{bmatrix} \tag{5.22}$$

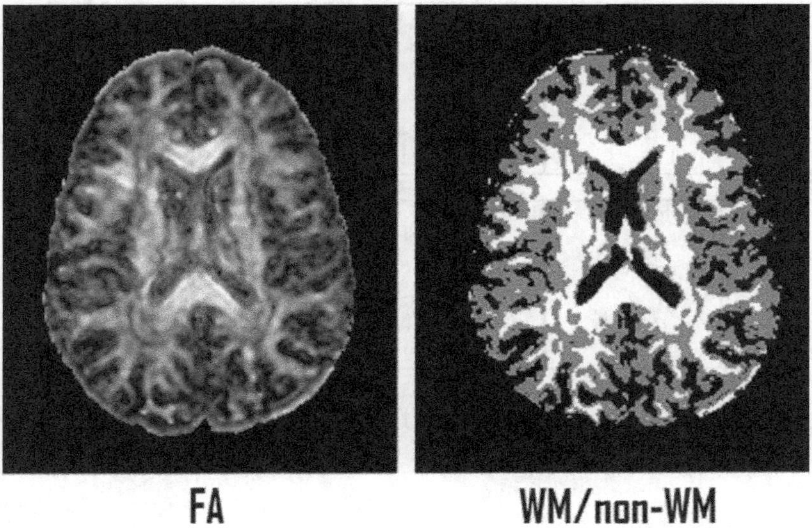

FIGURE 5.2
WM/none-WM classifications of brain tissues using k-means.

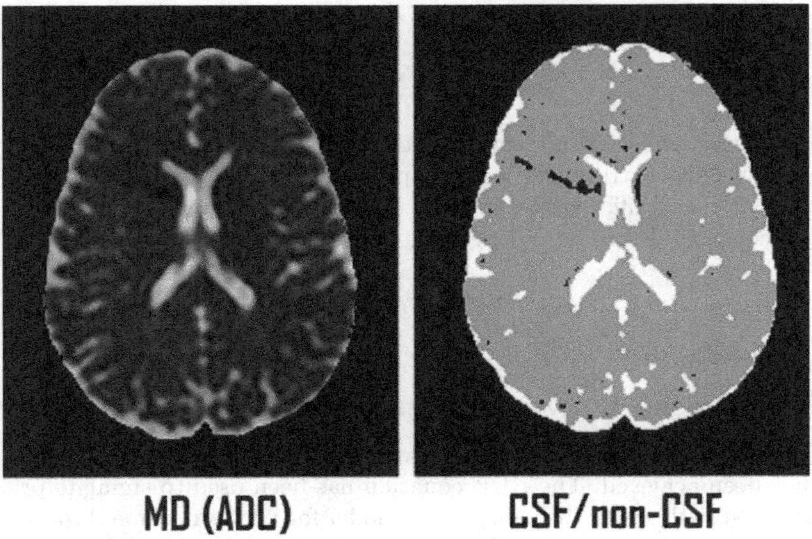

FIGURE 5.3
CSF/none-CSF classifications of brain tissues using k-means.

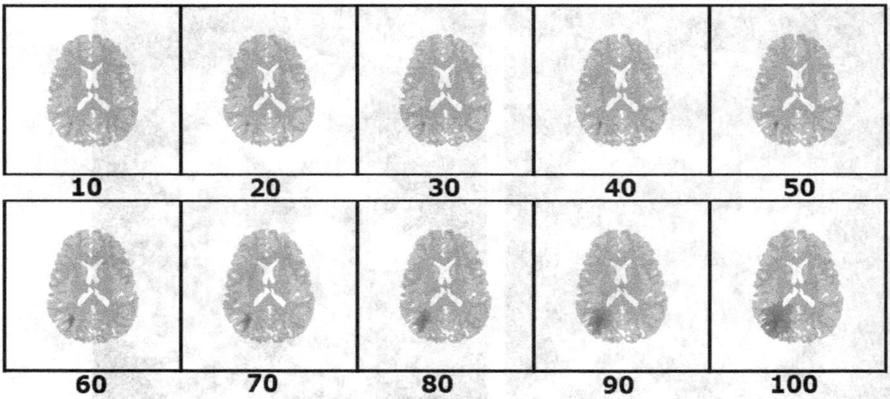

FIGURE 5.4
Sample simulation of primary Glioma growth.

By applying Taylor's expansion series such that

$$\frac{\partial c}{\partial x} = \frac{c_{x+1,y,z} - c_{x-1,y,z}}{2h_x} = \frac{(c_{x+1,y,z} - c_{x,y,z}) + (c_{x,y,z} - c_{x-1,y,z})}{2h_x} \tag{5.23}$$

$$\frac{\partial^2 c}{\partial x^2} = \frac{c_{x+1,y,z} - 2c_{x,y,z} + c_{x-1,y,z}}{h_x^2} = \frac{(c_{x+1,y,z} - c_{x,y,z}) - (c_{x,y,z} - c_{x-1,y,z})}{h_x^2} \tag{5.24}$$

$$\frac{\partial^2 c}{\partial x \partial y} = \frac{c_{x+1,y+1,z} - c_{x-1,y+1,z} - c_{x+1,y-1,z} + c_{x-1,y-1,z}}{4h_x h_y} \tag{5.25}$$

where h's are the displacements between nodes in each direction. Deriving the first derivative as a central difference will provide less solution error than the forward or backward difference. The term *dtR(c)* is set to 1 when the desired location is considered tumor starting point.

5.6 Comparison between Different Model Combinations

Using a C++ finite element model, spatiotemporal simulation of glioma growth has been achieved. The RDE equation has been used to simulate primary glioma growth using the same brain model for the same time duration of 10000 time units (where one keyframe is saved after every 100 times unites) and from the same starting point where the WM, GM, and CSF of the brain model have been segmented for applying inhomogeneous diffusion coefficients (Figure 5.4). The five diffusion methods (M1 to M5) in addition to the three reaction equations (R1 to R3) have been used in the RDE equation. As a guide, the homogenous-isotropic (M0-Iso) scenario is used.

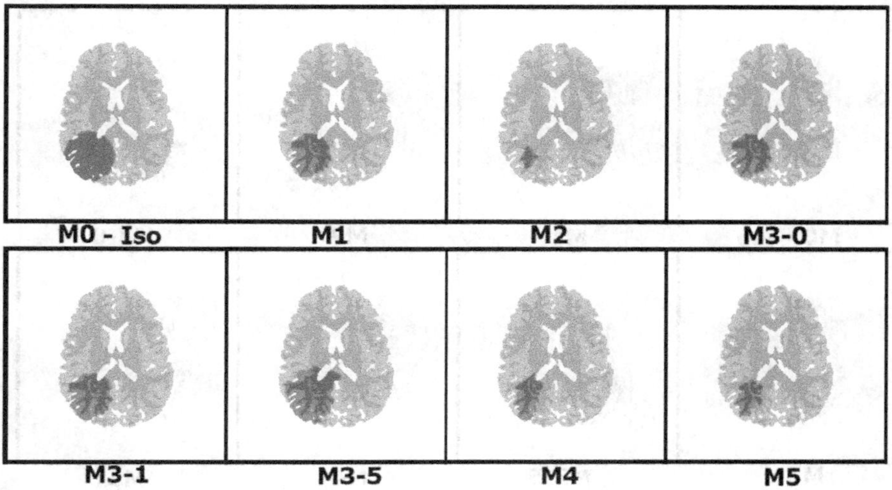

FIGURE 5.5
Tumor growth simulation using R1 with different diffusion methods.

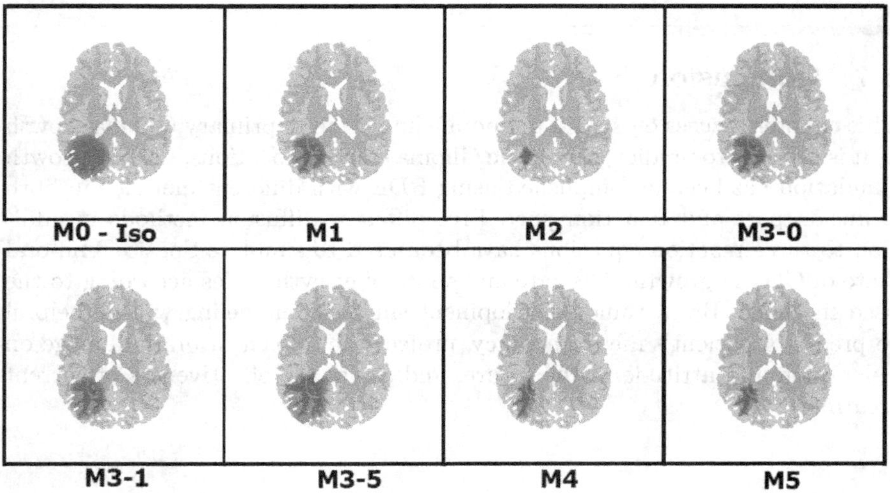

FIGURE 5.6
Tumor growth simulation using R2 with different diffusion methods.

For evaluating the effect of different diffusion methods and different reaction methods, all possible combinations between them have been tested where different shapes and sizes of tumors have been produced as shown in Figures 5.5, 5.6, and 5.7.

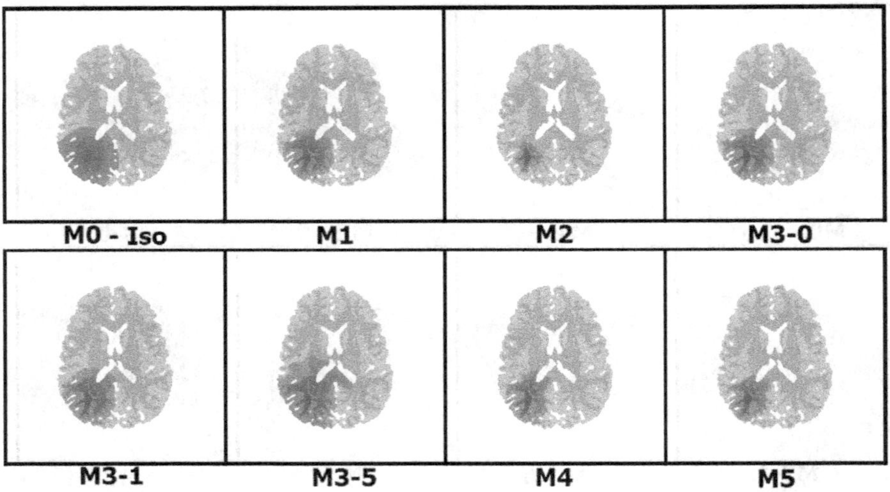

FIGURE 5.7
Tumor growth simulation using R3 with different diffusion methods.

5.7 Conclusion

This chapter focuses on spatio-temporal simulation of primary Glioma growth as it is difficult to predict metastatic Glioma starting locations. Glioma growth simulation has been accomplished using RDE with different methods in both Diffusion part and Reaction part. Five different diffusion methods in addition to three reaction equations have been used to simulate Spatio-Temporal state of Glioma growth. The rate and space of growth varies according to the used methods. Brain tumor development simulator modeling will be helpful to predict a patient's life expectancy, project the impact of brain damage on perception and attitude in the future, and assess the effectiveness of current treatments.

Bibliography

[1] A. Parent, *Carpenter's Human Neuroanatomy.* 1996.

[2] S. Standring, *Gray's Anatomy: The Anatomical Basis of Clinical Practice.* 2015.

[3] M. Kemp, "Style and non-style in anatomical illustration: From renaissance humanism to henry gray," *Journal of Anatomy*, vol. 216, 2010.

[4] N. E. Gilhus, *Barnes MP, Brainin M. European Handbook of Neurological Management: Volume 1.* 2011.

[5] R. T. Merrell, E. C. Quant, and P. Y. Wen, "Advances in treatment options for high-grade glioma - current status and future perspectives," *European neurological review*, vol. 06, p. 49, 2010.

[6] M. L. Goodenberger and R. B. Jenkins, "Genetics of adult glioma," *Cancer genetics*, vol. 205 12, pp. 613–21, 2012.

[7] S. S. Talibi, S. S. Talibi, B. Aweid, *et al.*, "Prospective therapies for high-grade glial tumours: A literature review," *Annals of Medicine and Surgery*, vol. 3, pp. 55–59, 2014.

[8] O. Clatz, M. Sermesant, P.-Y. Bondiau, *et al.*, "Realistic simulation of the 3-d growth of brain tumors in mr images coupling diffusion with biomechanical deformation," *IEEE Transactions on Medical Imaging*, vol. 24, pp. 1334–1346, 2005.

[9] P. Tracqui, "From passive diffusion to active cellular migration in mathematical models of tumour invasion," *Acta Biotheoretica*, vol. 43, pp. 443–464, 1995.

[10] S. Jbabdi, E. Mandonnet, H. Duffau, *et al.*, "Simulation of anisotropic growth of low-grade gliomas using diffusion tensor imaging," *Magnetic Resonance in Medicine*, vol. 54, 2005.

[11] E. Konukoglu, O. Clatz, B. H. Menze, *et al.*, "Image guided personalization of reaction-diffusion type tumor growth models using modified anisotropic eikonal equations," *IEEE Transactions on Medical Imaging*, vol. 29, pp. 77–95, 2010.

[12] E. Stretton, E. Geremia, B. Menze, *et al.*, "Importance of patient dti's to accurately model glioma growth using the reaction diffusion equation," 2013.

[13] A. Roniotis, K. Marias, V. Sakkalis, and M. Zervakis, 'Diffusive modelling of glioma evolution: a review,' *Journal of Biomedical Science and Engineering*, 3, 501-508, 2010. doi: 10.4236/jbise.2010.35070.

[14] A. Roniotis, K. Marias, V. Sakkalis, and M. Zervakis, 'Diffusive modelling of glioma evolution: a review,' Journal of Biomedical Science and Engineering, 3, 501-508, 2010. doi: 10.4236/jbise.2010.35070.

[15] A. Roniotis, G. C. Manikis, V. Sakkalis, *et al.*, "High-grade glioma diffusive modeling using statistical tissue information and diffusion tensors extracted from atlases," *IEEE Transactions on Information Technology in Biomedicine*, vol. 16, pp. 255–263, 2012.

[16] H. Enderling and M. A. J. Chaplain, “Mathematical modeling of tumor growth and treatment,” *Current pharmaceutical design*, vol. 20 30, pp. 4934–40, 2014.

[17] K. R. Swanson, C. A. Bridge, J. D. Murray, *et al.*, “Virtual and real brain tumors: using mathematical modeling to quantify glioma growth and invasion,” *Journal of the Neurological Sciences*, vol. 216, pp. 1–10, 2003.

[18] E. Konukoglu, O. Clatz, P.-Y. Bondiau, *et al.*, “Extrapolating tumor invasion margins for physiologically determined radiotherapy regions,” *Medical image computing and computer-assisted intervention : MICCAI ... International Conference on Medical Image Computing and Computer-Assisted Intervention*, vol. 9 Pt 1, pp. 338–46, 2006.

[19] E. Konukoglu, O. Clatz, P.-Y. Bondiau, *et al.*, “Extrapolating glioma invasion margin in brain magnetic resonance images: Suggesting new irradiation margins,” *Medical image analysis*, vol. 14 2, pp. 111–25, 2010.

[20] H. L. Harpold, E. C. Alvord, and K. R. Swanson, “The evolution of mathematical modeling of glioma proliferation and invasion,” *Journal of Neuropathology and Experimental Neurology*, vol. 66, pp. 1–9, 2007.

[21] F. Dittmann, B. Menze, E. Konukoglu, J. Unkelbach, ‘Use of Diffusion Tensor Images in Glioma Growth Modeling for Radiotherapy Target Delineation’ In: Shen, L., Liu, T., Yap, PT., Huang, H., Shen, D., Westin, CF. (eds) Multimodal Brain Image Analysis. MBIA 2013. Lecture Notes in Computer Science, vol 8159. Springer, Cham. 2013.

[22] A. Gholami, A. Mang, and G. Biros, “An inverse problem formulation for parameter estimation of a reaction–diffusion model of low grade gliomas,” *Journal of Mathematical Biology*, vol. 72, pp. 409–433, 2015.

[23] J. Unkelbach, Bjoern H. Menze, A. Motamedi, F. Dittmann, Ender Konukoglu, et al.. Glioblastoma growth modeling for radiotherapy target delineation. Image-Guidance and Multimodal Dose Planning in Radiation Therapy, INRIA, Nice, France. pp. 9–16, 2012.

[24] I. Elaff, M. Aqraa, O.M. Badawy, 'Spatio-temporal models for brain tumor grow simulation,' 4th International Conference on Electronics, Biomedical Engineering and its Applications (ICEBEA'2014) Jan. 28-29, 2014 Bangkok.

[25] S. Mori, “Introduction to diffusion tensor imaging,” 2007.

[26] P. Hagmann, L. Jonasson, P. Maeder, J-P Thiran, V.J. Wedeen, R. Meuli, ‘Understanding Diffusion MR Imaging Techniques: From Scalar Diffusion-weighted Imaging to Diffusion Tensor Imaging and Beyond, RadioGraphics, Vol. 26, No. suppl_1, 2006.

[27] M. Zarei, H. J. Berg, and P. M. Matthews, "Diffusion tensor imaging and tractography in clinical neurosciences," *Iranian Journal of Radiology*, vol. 1, pp. 45–52, 2003.

[28] P. J. Basser, J. Mattiello, and D. LeBihan, "Mr diffusion tensor spectroscopy and imaging," *Biophysical Journal*, vol. 66 1, pp. 259–67, 1994.

[29] P. J. Basser and C. Pierpaoli, "Microstructural and physiological features of tissues elucidated by quantitative-diffusion-tensor mri. 1996," *Journal of Magnetic Resonance*, vol. 213 2, pp. 560–70, 1996.

[30] A. Vilanova, S. Zhang, G. L. Kindlmann, *et al.*, "An introduction to visualization of diffusion tensor imaging and its applications," in *Visualization and Processing of Tensor Fields*, 2006.

[31] B. Mortamet, D. Zeng, G. Gerig, *et al.*, "Effects of healthy aging measured by intracranial compartment volumes using a designed mr brain database," *Medical image computing and computer-assisted intervention: MICCAI ... International Conference on Medical Image Computing and Computer-Assisted Intervention*, vol. 8 Pt 1, pp. 383–91, 2005.

[32] R. C. Gur, F. M. Gunning-Dixon, *et al.*, "Sex differences in temporolimbic and frontal brain volumes of healthy adults," *Cerebral Cortex*, vol. 12 9, pp. 998–1003, 2002.

[33] K. Wagsta, C. Cardie, S. Rogers, *et al.*, "Constrained k-means clustering with background knowledge," 2001.

6

Mathematical Modeling for Brain Tumors Including Fractional Operator

Arife Aysun Karaaslan

Üsküdar University, İstanbul, Türkiye

Mathematical modeling is a way of representing real-life problems. Firstly, a problem is defined and according to the problem, a system can be constructed using variables. Systems can be solved using different methods. Outcomes give us a cycle between real life and mathematical life. This cycle is a formulation and the formulation can be graphs, equations, sometimes inequations etc. Differential equations may be included in some models while they may not be in others. They may include statistical terms and regression analysis. But our models include mathematical structures and ordinary differential equations or partial differential equations. There are various solution methods but in this chapter, we will give information about fractional operators. Fractional operator studies with non-integer order of derivatives and effects of fractional calculus over brain tumor growth will be examined.

6.1 Introduction

Uncontrolled cell growth and proliferation is referred to as a tumor. Benign and malignant are the terms used to describe the resulting formation. Benign tumors do not spread to other areas; they are confined to the area in which they originate. Tumors that are malignant can grow and spread to other tissues. Malignant growths are referred to as cancer. One or more cell mutations are the source of cancerous tumors, which typically develop quickly and uncontrollably. We'll talk about the unchecked growth and dissemination of brain tumors. Three stages are present in brain tumors. Gliomas in their fourth and worst stage are the most deadly tumors. Following a tumor diagnosis, treatment is crucial, and "The problem of how gliomas spread" is one of

DOI: 10.1201/9781003461906-6

the main issues that arises. This means that the tumor is not the only thing being imaged. It is the spread of the cell, which may not be observed by imaging techniques. As a result, researchers concentrated on understanding how gliomas grow. Growth of tumor models, a developing study in glioma research, became a field. Researchers study mathematical models to better understand the glioma growth process. Mathematical models are utilized to comprehend complex structures while studying processes and diseases. Theoretical models mainly focus on the total amount of cells in a tumor and assume exponential growth, Gompertzian, or logistic.

6.2 Obtaining the Models

A mathematical model is a language for describing a system. This description may be made, among other things, by mathematical formalism and abstraction, which may allow for extrapolation beyond situations that were initially examined, quantitative predictions, and/or inference of mechanisms [1]. Three basic steps make up the procedure of mathematical modeling: first, a problem set from the actual world is formulated as a mathematical issue; this, along with any presumptions made, is the mathematical model. After the mathematical difficulty is resolved and the answer is eventually applied to the original situation, the outcomes that the model assessed may be deciphered and applied to assist in resolving the original issue [2]. The behavior of developing gliomas under scientific investigation can possibly be described mathematically in the case of gliomas. Murray's diffusion model is the first glioma development model [3–5].

6.3 Some Solution Methods for Mathematical Models

There are different solution methods for solving mathematical models. All have some advantages and disadvantages compared to each other. In this section, we give some information about basic solution methods; finite element, finite difference, and finite volume.

6.3.1 Finite Element Method

A numerical analytical method for approximating solutions to a wide range of engineering issues is the finite element method (FEM) [6]. The governing equations of a problem can be approximated piecewise using a finite element model. The basic concept behind the FEM is that a solution area may be discretized—that is, replaced with an assembly of discrete elements—in order to be mathematically modeled or approximated. These pieces may be utilized to represent extremely complex forms because of the number of ways in which they can be assembled. The concepts of finite element analysis go far further back, even though the term "finite element method" was originally used in 1960 to tackle planar elasticity problems. The first usage of piecewise continuous functions defined over triangular domains in practical mathematics literature dates back to 1943. The concept of minimizing a functional by linear approximation over sub-regions is established, in which values are supplied at discrete places which fundamentally act as the node points of an element mesh [6].

The problem becomes simpler by the finite element separation process, that breaks a continuum into elements that can be a body of matter such as a solid, liquid, gas, or just a patch of space. The unknown field variable is then expressed in terms of presumptive approximation functions inside each element [7]. The values that occur of the field's variables at designated places identified as nodes or nodal points are used to create the approximation functions, which are additionally often referred to as interpolation functions. Nodes often sit on the edges of elements when neighboring components are joined. An element may have a few internal nodes in addition to its perimeter nodes. The behavior of the field variable inside the elements is fully defined by the nodal values of the field variable and the interpolation functions for the elements. Finite element method can be written with respect to dimensions as shown in the following subsections [8].

6.3.1.1 One Dimensional Finite Elements

The one-dimensional ones are the initial and most basic kind. Throughout its length, the area cross-section may change even while their area remains constant. This is the issue with one-dimensional objects.

6.3.1.2 Two Dimensional Finite Elements

The two-dimensional area model uses two broad groups of components. These forms are quadrilaterals and triangles. Higher order elements, including quadratic and cubic, have either linear, curvilinear, or both types of edges. Linear components in each family have linear edges. The first finite element to be suggested for continuous problems was the triangle finite element. These elements can be represented in xy plane [8].

6.3.1.3 Three Dimensional Finite Elements

The most commons are variations of two-dimensional elements such as tetrahedrons and parallelepipeds. One can examine it using a xyz coordinate plane.

6.3.2 Finite Difference Method

The finite difference approach is one of the "grid-point" approaches. The grid-point techniques use a space-time grid to cover a computational domain, with each function's values represented at grid points. Although the grid points' space-time distribution is essentially random, it has a big impact on how accurate the approximation is. Generally, the values located within the grid points are not assumed. The function values at a predetermined set of grid points are used in the so-called finite-difference formula, which approximates a derivative of a function. Even if the finite-difference approach is not used to solve the differential equation, it is still useful to understand its fundamentals. This is due to the fact that finite-difference formula and other numerical approaches often estimate the temporal dependence of the functions [9]. The following actions play a role in applying the approach to a specific differential problem:

a. *Building the problem's discrete finite-difference model:*

- Coverage of the computational domain by a space-time grid,
- Estimates for functions, derivatives, and/or beginning and/or boundary conditions
- Creation of a finite-difference system, all at the grid points (i.e., algebraic) equations

b. *Analyzing the model with finite differences:*

- The order and consistency of the approximation
- Stability
- Convergence

c. *Numerical computations*

6.3.3 Finite Volume Method

Similar to FEM, the finite volume technique (FVM) also relies on an unstructured mesh, such as a triangle. It is hence appropriate for complicated and irregular geometry. For issues involving fluid mechanics, FVM is superior to FEM in a different manner. The numerical techniques we have so far shown are based on PDEs. As opposed to this, FVM is predicated on the conservation laws' integral form as compared with their differential form. Generally, FVM is more applicable to fluid mechanic problems when it is compared with other methods [10].

6.4 Fractional Operators

The commonly used expression "fractional calculus," which relates to the calculus of non-integer order, is as ancient as the calculus of integer order, that was established individually by Newton and Leibniz [11]. Only in 1974 was fractional calculus designated as a distinct field of mathematics, in contrast to calculus of integer order. Fractional calculus began to get interest from scholars in the 1980s, and explicit applications started to show up in a number of domains. One reason fractional calculus has gained popularity is that its applications are more practical. In mathematics, fractional calculus may be regarded as a frontier field as its applications have been studied just as thoroughly as those of calculus of integer order. First, the notion of the fractional integral in the Liouville sense—a specific instance of the Riemann-Liouville sense—will be discussed. This may be thought of as an extension of the integral of integer order. We will then talk about the concepts of derivatives proposed by Riemann-Liouville and Caputo [11].

6.4.1 Caputo Derivative

The Cauchy-Riemann integral may be produced as an extension of the fractional integral of Riemann-Liouville, which is an integral that generalizes the idea of an integral in the classical sense. First, the definition of the Riemann-Liouville fractional integral was established. This was followed by a description of the fractional derivative of Riemann-Liouville and the fractional integral in the sense of Riemann-Liouville. Mathematicians, in particular, utilize this term the most when solving problems where beginning conditions are not involved [11]. The differential operator of non-integer order in the Riemann-Liouville sense and the differential operator of non-integer order in the Caputo sense are comparable. The key distinction is that, in the Riemann-Liouville sense, the derivatives operate on the integral, meaning that we compute the derivative after evaluating the integral, but in the Caputo view, the derivative acts first on the function. When compared to the Riemann-Liouville derivative, the Caputo derivative is more restrictive. We also see that the Riemann-Liouvile fractional integral is used to define both derivatives. The significance of this derivative lies in the fact that it may be applied in the Caputo sense, for instance, when dealing with fractional differential equations that have well-established beginning conditions, like integral order calculus. There are multiple studies relevant to this [12–21].

6.4.2 Fractional Equations

Applications where a particle cloud expands faster than expected by a classical equation could profit by the use of fractional diffusion equations [22].

6.4.2.1 Fractional Diffusion Equations

In several branches of science and engineering, reaction-diffusion equations are important tools. Applications of population biology are well studied; the diffusion term takes into account migration, while the response term simulates growth. The physics model serves as the source of the classical diffusion term [23–33]. In accordance with recent studies, the typical diffusion equation is unable to accurately describe a wide range of real-world situations in which a particle plume spreads more quickly than the classical model predicts and may show notable asymmetry. These circumstances are known as anomalous diffusion. The fractional diffusion equation, which substitutes a fractional derivative of order $0 < \alpha < 2$ for the typical second derivative in space, is a well-liked model for anomalous diffusion. The fractional diffusion equation's solutions may show asymmetries and spread more quickly than those of the conventional diffusion equation. Still, these equations' fundamental solutions have useful scaling characteristics that draw applications to them. The classical diffusion equation $\frac{\partial u}{\partial t} = D\frac{\partial^2 u}{\partial x^2}$ is strongly related to statistics' central limit theorem, which asserts that when the number of summands goes to infinity, the probability distribution of a normalized sum of independently distributed random variables converges to a normal distribution. The fractional diffusion equation $\frac{\partial u}{\partial t} = D\frac{\partial^\alpha u}{\partial x^\alpha}$ relates to another central limit theorem. According to the usual discovering, individual random leap has a limited standard deviation [22].

6.4.2.2 Fractional Reaction Equations

The common reaction-diffusion equation in one dimension

$$\frac{\partial u(x,t)}{\partial t} = D\frac{\partial^2 u(x,t)}{\partial x^2} + \tilde{f}(u(x,t)), u(x,0) = u_0(x) \tag{6.1}$$

acts as a model for the spread of invasive species in population biology. Here $u(x,t)$ is the population density at location $x \in \mathbf{R}$ and time $t > 0$ [22]. The diffusion component, which is the first term on the right, models migration. The reaction term, which simulates growth in population, is the second term; a typical choice is the Kolmogorov-Fisher equation $\tilde{f}(u(x,t)) = ru(x,t)(1 - u(x,t)/K)$ where r is a species' intrinsic growth rate and K is the carrying capacity of the ecosystem, or the highest sustainable population density [22]. A fractional reaction-diffusion equation with more generality is:

$$\frac{\partial u(x,t)}{\partial t} = D\frac{\partial^\alpha u(x,t)}{\partial x^\alpha} + \tilde{f}(u(x,t)), u(x,0) = u_0(x) \tag{6.2}$$

with $0 < \alpha \leq 2$.

6.5 Impact of Fractional Calculus on Tumor Growth Models

Complex in nature, cancer is a significant public health issue [1]. Because cancer is a chronic disease and current therapies include side effects, it places a significant load on health care systems. Personalized adaptive radiation treatment has the potential to benefit from the incorporation of mathematical models into radiation oncology by considering either fractionation or dose adaptation to patients based on their unique clinical responses. By using numerical simulations that utilize tumor growth models and person's gene expression, predictive oncology may be able to assist in the personalization of radiation dosages. Research efforts have been focused on applying mathematics and physics to cancer genesis and early growth, as well as tumor and intercellular interactions, because thorough modeling may possibly improve the development and implementation of innovative cancer treatments [34]. In fact, the subject of mathematical oncology is founded on the ideas that biology presents novel mathematical problems that require the development of improved mathematical tools, and that mathematics may be employed to advance biological knowledge about the disease. From the investigation of tumor growth to the implementation of tailored treatment plans, mathematical oncology encompasses the development and use of models for phenomena relevant to cancer. It's a growing field for research that obtains from the data produced by the present bioinformatics boom. Given its significance, mathematical oncology makes the case for comprehensive theoretical models to comprehend, organize, or utilize clinical data with an eye toward oncology decision-making, for example. All solid cancers originate from the formation of a primary tumor, despite being an extremely complex collection of diseases. By concentrating on this shared location, we may be able to better understand key aspects of early tumor development. While the pathways and signals leading to the emergence of malignant cells have become increasingly clear due to the sequencing of genes and molecular biology, it is as crucial to comprehend the phenomenological principles driving the proliferation of tumor population cells. In terms of general vascular tumor growth, approaches based on ecological models and explained via ordinary differential equations (ODE) have the prospect of expanding notions and insights [34].

Numerous ODE models have been created to characterize dynamic tumor development by including special adjustments to account for biological particularities and experimental data. Most of them are based on a sigmoidal rule that relies on the population's carrying capacity and growth rate. The several phases that a primary tumor goes through in relation to the resources at hand, and like tumor surface area and small heterogeneity, justify this behavior. Even though ODE-based approaches are not as complex as cancer models that include partial differential equations (PDEs), their continued use is motivated by their ease. Their relative simplicity makes it possible to derive analytical solutions, which may be used to analytically characterize the evolution of events.

Additionally, the flexibility of ODE-based models and the ability to fine-tune their free parameters versus experimental data to represent various tumor phases make them a good choice for supporting therapeutic recommendations. Nevertheless, there is disagreement about whether ODE-based model is best suited for particular types of cancer. An inappropriate model selection may end up in significant variations in cancer predictions, indicating the need for more study. Thus, ODE models for tumor development may be expanded so that complexity is contained in simplicity, while maintaining their deductive-reductionist features to better suit experimental data. Fractional calculus examines integral calculus and non-integer order differential among other mathematical options. The ability to handle unique behavior according to an arbitrary degree of differentiation (or integration) is a characteristic shared by fractional models, which broadens the application scope. Even in comparatively smaller models, this is a crucial feature of non-integer order calculus that makes it a fascinating instrument for reductionist methods. Additionally, the fundamental attributes of fractional calculus, such as its capacity to indicate complex procedures like long-term memory and/or geographic heterogeneity, may enhance ODE-based tumor models. Fractional models have gained popularity and been effectively used in a variety of fields, including signal processing, thermoacoustics, economics, robotics, viscoelasticity, chemical kinetics, electromagnetism, agricultural computing, and traffic control, attributed to their many outstanding advantages [35–38]. As a matter of fact, there is already what could be called "fractional mathematical oncology"—a number of recent studies have used non-integer calculus to deal with various aspects of cancer, such as the dynamics of chemotherapy, radiotherapy, and immunotherapy, as well as numerical solutions and control for invasion structures, bioengineering, and tumor growth [39–42]. As more research is conducted in this field, fractional calculus may be supported as an alternative reductionist phenomenological modeling (method) to study early avascular general tumor growth controlled by ODEs [43–50]. The general form of tumor development models driven by ODE equations are usually the following:

$$\frac{dV(t)}{dt} = af(V(t)) - bg(V(t)), \tag{6.3}$$

where $V(t)$ is tumor volume at a given time and $t, \frac{dV(t)}{dt}$ represents tumor growth rate. Tumor growth is determined by a parameter called a, whereas tumor size is constrained by a parameter called b. Functions $f(V(t))$ and $g(V(t))$ define whether or not the model is logistic, exponential, or in some other form.

For certain ordinary differential equations, models, differential equations, maximum size, and growth conditions are provided, respectively in [51]:

- *Exponential* model is represented with differential equation $\frac{dV(t)}{dt} = aV(t)$, max.size ∞ and growth condition is $a > 0$,

- *Logistic* model is represented with differential equation $\frac{dV(t)}{dt} = aV(t)(1 - \frac{V(t)}{V_\infty})$, max.size $V_\infty = a/b$ and growth condition is $a > 0$,

- *Gompertz* model is represented with differential equation $\frac{dV(t)}{dt} = bV(t)ln(\frac{V_\infty}{V(t)})$, max.size $V_\infty = ln^{-1}(a/b)$ and growth condition is $b > 0$,

- *Bertalanffy* model is represented with differential equation $\frac{dV(t)}{dt} = aV(t)^{2/3} - bV(t)$, max.size is $V_\infty = (a/b)^3$ and growth condition is $a > b$,

- *Guiot − West* model is represented with differential equation $\frac{dV(t)}{dt} = aV(t)^{3/4} - bV(t)$, max.size is $V_\infty = (a/b)^4$ and growth condition is $a > b$.

The study's findings indicate that each model's fractional version outperforms its integer order equivalents in terms of indicators. Numerical findings imply that fractional models can be important to tumor prediction.

It may be worthwhile to investigate the details and characteristics of fractional calculus in connection to the measurement of tumor development. A potential explanation for the better prediction accuracy of fractional models might be the memory effect, which is a natural consequence of the non-integer order derivative specification. Considering that cells in tumors have accumulated several mutations and alterations throughout their development, fractional models may be able to account for these non-local (past) occurrences. Another intriguing pattern is that larger, rapidly growing tumors appear to be best demonstrated using fractional orders. The previously stated models have to be taken into consideration in order to support therapeutic advice. Even though the initial findings and potential characteristics are very promising, further research has to be done, especially to find out how versatile arbitrary order α is and to compare these models to other experimental sets of data and advice [34].

6.6 Mathematical Modeling of Brain Tumors Using Fractional Operator

Fractional differential equations, fractional integro-differential equations, fractional partial differential equations, and so on are variant classes of fractional equations that have been applied recently in the areas of control, mechanics, chemistry, physics, biology, signal processing, and economics to model various real phenomena like viscoelasticity and damping, diffusion and wave propagation, control systems, and signal processing [34]. As a consequence, a great deal of research has been done by several scientists in the domains of biology, engineering, physics, and other sciences to illustrate many significant phenomena in these subjects via the FC. These can be seen in [52–59]. For instance, the authors have provided a fractional operator model for the co-infection of HIV and HSV-2. Furthermore, a Covid-19 mathematical model is worked out. A COVID-19 fractional model was utilized in Galicia, Spain, and Portugal. Study was done on a fractional model of the tumor-immune system using fractional derivative and a mathematical model of Parkinson's disease in the basal ganglia. A fractional operator is used to describe the growth of brain tumors (glioblastomas) during medical therapy [51]. The model was initially built to resemble a case of chemotherapy-treated recurrent anaplastic astrocytoma. Later, it was adjusted to enable assessment of the impacts of surgical resection extent as well as growth and diffusion changes to cover the complete spectrum of glioma behavior. Although this glioma can develop at any age, individuals over 45 are more likely to get glioma. They can occur in the cerebellum as well as the cerebral hemispheres, where they typically occur. A number of researchers have examined the mathematical equation of tumor growth and have provided explanations of the basic two-dimensional tumor model.

In mathematical words, rate of change of tumor cell density = diffusion of tumor cells + growth of tumor cells,

$$\partial_\tau B(x,\tau) = D\nabla^2 B(x,\tau) + \rho B(x,\tau) \tag{6.4}$$

The two major processes in the development of an invading brain tumor are taken into account in these models, cell proliferation (ρ) and diffusion (D), and combines them to create an equation for reaction and diffusion:

$$\partial_\tau B(x,\tau) = D\frac{1}{x^2}\partial_x(x^2\partial_x B(x,\tau)) + \rho B(x,\tau) \tag{6.5}$$

The tumor cells in these models are considered to grow at a constant pace, exponentially. Owing to the significance of these models, it can sometimes be difficult to obtain the results. As a consequence, there is a great deal of focus on developing methods for estimating solutions associated with these models. A number of researchers analyzed a patient's final year of CT images to create a mathematical model of glioma development and diffusion. The patient had recurrent anaplastic astrocytoma. By using the quantitative measures of proliferation and diffusion, the model described the development of the glioma cell population.

In mathematical words, rate of change of tumor cell density = diffusion of tumor cells + growth of tumor cells,

$$\partial_\tau B(x,\tau) = D\frac{1}{x^2}\partial_x(x^2\partial_x B(x,\tau)) + \rho B(x,\tau) \tag{6.6}$$

The model above was created to add a lethal term to equation (6.6) as follows:

In mathematical words, rate of change of tumor cell density = diffusion of tumor cells + growth of tumor cells-killing rate of tumor cells,

$$\partial_\tau B(x,\tau) = D\frac{1}{x^2}\partial_x(x^2\partial_x B(x,\tau)) + \rho B(x,\tau) - k_\tau B(x,\tau) \tag{6.7}$$

This model is expressed as follows:

$$\partial_\tau B(x,\tau) = D(\partial_{xx} B(x,\tau) + \frac{2}{x}\partial_x B(x,\tau)) + (\rho - k_\tau)B(x,\tau) \tag{6.8}$$

This problem was solved by Ganji and friends as a fractional Burgess equation [51]. The most prevalent primary brain tumor in adults, glioblastoma, usually results in early death. Radiation therapy, chemotherapy, and surgery are the usual treatments for brain tumors. In recent years, brain tumors that have been treated and those that have not, have been investigated by applying mathematical models. The Burgess equation is used to simulate glioblastomas (brain tumors) and includes the two main variables controlling tumor growth: the rate of cell proliferation and the diffusion of cancer cells. This model aims to improve on previous studies. The fractional Burgess equation is taken to be considered in terms of Caputo in their study. Owing to the model being studied, a method to solve this model is suggested.

6.7 Conclusions

Expressing real-world problems by mathematical modeling has shown to be very effective. Following the creation of the modeling, solution approaches are looked at, contrasted, and the best approach is found. Fractional operators and equations have improved the effectiveness of events that had been expressed using ordinary differential equations. It has completed the missing parts of ordinary differential equations. Fractional derivatives offered by fractional equations allow for a better description of occurrences. Fractional calculus, like in many other aspects of life, has proven to be useful in the study of brain tumors, including their pathogenesis and the identification of the best course of therapy. In the future, mathematical models are expected to be more successful in handling the simulation of actual events. Additionally, because mathematical modeling provides the ability to formulate problems, develop solutions, derive both numerical and non-numerical results, analyze collected data, and make ideas a reality, it may be included in glioma studies.

Bibliography

[1] L. C. Vieira, R. S. Costa, and D. Valério, "An overview of mathematical modelling in cancer research: Fractional calculus as modelling tool," *Fractal and Fractional*, 2023.

[2] J. Berry and K. Housten, *Mathematical modelling.* Modular Mathematics Series, 2004.

[3] J. D. Murray, *Mathematical Biology II: spatial models and biomedical applications.* Springer, 2003.

[4] A. Roniotis, K. Marias, V. Sakkalis, *et al.*, "Diffusive modelling of glioma evolution: a review," *Biomedical Science and Engineering*, pp. 501–508, 2010.

[5] K. R. Swanson, E. C. Alvord, and J. D. Murray, "Virtual brain tumours (gliomas) enhance the reality of medical imaging and highlight inadequacies of current therapy," *British Journal of Cancer*, vol. 86, pp. 14–18, 2002.

[6] V. Jagota, A. S. Sethi, and K. Kumar, "Finite element method: An overview," 2013.

[7] O. C. Zienkiewicz, "The finite element method in engineering science," 1971.

[8] G. Nikishkov, "Introduction to the finite element method," *Finite Element Analysis*, 2021.

[9] P. Moczo, J. Kristek, and L. Halada, "The finite-difference method for seismologists ; an introduction," 2004.

[10] B. E. Rapp, "Chapter 31 – finite volume method," 2017.

[11] E. C. Grigoletto and E. C. D. Oliveira, "Fractional versions of the fundamental theorem of calculus," *Applied Mathematics-a Journal of Chinese Universities Series B*, vol. 2013, pp. 23–33, 2013.

[12] K. S. Miller and B. Ross, "An introduction to the fractional calculus and fractional differential equations," 1993.

[13] K. B. Oldham and J. Spanier, "The fractional calculus: Theory and applications of differentiation and integration to arbitrary order," 1974.

[14] R. L. Bagley and P. J. Torvik, "A theoretical basis for the application of fractional calculus to viscoelasticity," *Journal of Rheology*, vol. 27, pp. 201–210, 1983.

[15] T. Machado, V. S. Kiryakova, and F. Mainardi, "A poster about the recent history of fractional calculus," *Fractional Calculus and Applied Analysis*, vol. 13, pp. 329–334, 2010.

[16] J. T. Machado, V. S. Kiryakova, and F. Mainardi, "Recent history of fractional calculus," *Communications in Nonlinear Science and Numerical Simulation*, vol. 16, pp. 1140–1153, 2011.

[17] K. Diethelm, "The analysis of fractional differential equations: An application-oriented exposition using differential operators of caputo type," 2010.

[18] R. Hilfer, "Applications of fractional calculus in physics," 2000.

[19] A. A. Kilbas, H. M. Srivastava, and J. J. Trujillo, "Theory and applications of fractional differential equations," 2006.

[20] I. Podlubny, "Fractional differential equations," 1998.

[21] S. G. Samko, A. A. Kilbas, and O. I. Marichev, "Fractional integrals and derivatives: Theory and applications," 1993.

[22] B. Baeumer, M. Kovács, and M. M. Meerschaert, "Numerical solutions for fractional reaction-diffusion equations," *Computers & Mathematics with Applications*, vol. 55, pp. 2212–2226, 2008.

[23] N. F. Britton, "Reaction-diffusion equations and their applications to biology," 1989.

[24] R. S. Cantrell and C. Cosner, "Spatial ecology via reaction-diffusion equations," 2003.

[25] P. M. Grindrod, "The theory and applications of reaction diffusion equations: Patterns and waves," 1996.

[26] F. Rothe, "Global solutions of reaction-diffusion systems," 1984.

[27] L. b. Bachelier, "Theorie de la speculation, doctor thesis, annales scientifiques ecole normale sperieure iii -17,"

[28] A. Einstein, *Investigations on the theory of the Brownian movement.* Dover Publications Inc., 1956.

[29] I. M. Sokolov and J. Klafter, "From diffusion to anomalous diffusion: a century after einstein's brownian motion," *Chaos*, vol. 15 2, p. 26103, 2004.

[30] R. Metzler and J. Klafter, "The random walk's guide to anomalous diffusion: a fractional dynamics approach," *Physics Reports*, vol. 339, pp. 1–77, 2000.

[31] M. M. Meerschaert, D. A. Benson, and B. Bäumer, "Multidimensional advection and fractional dispersion," *Physical Review. E, Statistical Physics, Plasmas, Fluids, and Related Interdisciplinary Topics*, vol. 59 5 Pt A, pp. 5026–8, 1999.

[32] M. M. Meerschaert, D. A. Benson, and B. Baeumer, "Operator lévy motion and multiscaling anomalous diffusion," *Physical Review. E, Statistical, Nonlinear, and Soft Matter Physics*, vol. 63 2 Pt 1, p. 021112, 2001.

[33] R. Schumer, D. A. Benson, M. M. Meerschaert, *et al.*, "Multiscaling fractional advection-dispersion equations and their solutions," *Water Resources Research*, vol. 39, 2003.

[34] C. A. Valentim, N. A. Oliveira, J. A. Rabi, *et al.*, "Can fractional calculus help improve tumor growth models?," *Journal of Computational and Applied Mathematics*, vol. 379, p. 112964, 2020.

[35] N. Miljković, N. Popovic, O. Djordjevic, *et al.*, "Ecg artifact cancellation in surface emg signals by fractional order calculus application," *Computer Methods and Programs in Biomedicine*, vol. 140, pp. 259–264, 2017.

[36] C. A. Valentim, F. D. C. Bannwart, and S. A. David, "Fractional calculus applied to linear thermoacoustics: A generalization of rott's model," 2018.

[37] S. A. David, J. A. T. Machado, D. D. Quintino, *et al.*, "Partial chaos suppression in a fractional order macroeconomic model," *Mathematics and Computers in Simulation*, vol. 122, pp. 55–68, 2016.

[38] K. Leyden and B. Goodwine, "Using fractional-order differential equations for health monitoring of a system of cooperating robots," *2016 IEEE International Conference on Robotics and Automation (ICRA)*, pp. 366–371, 2016.

[39] H. Enderling, J. C. L. Alfonso, E. G. Moros, *et al.*, "Integrating mathematical modeling into the roadmap for personalized adaptive radiation therapy," *Trends in Cancer*, vol. 5 8, pp. 467–474, 2019.

[40] A. d'Onofrio and A. Gandolfi, "Mathematical oncology 2013," 2014.

[41] A. Chauviere, H. Hatzikirou, J. S. Lowengrub, *et al.*, "Mathematical oncology: How are the mathematical and physical sciences contributing to the war on breast cancer?," *Current Breast Cancer Reports*, vol. 2, pp. 121 –129, 2010.

[42] T. L. Jackson, N. L. Komarova, and K. R. Swanson, "Mathematical oncology: Using mathematics to enable cancer discoveries," *The American Mathematical Monthly*, vol. 121, pp. 840–856, 2014.

[43] V. Cristini, E. J. Koay, and Z. Wang, "An introduction to physical oncology: How mechanistic mathematical modeling can improve cancer therapy outcomes," 2017.

[44] R. A. Gatenby and P. K. Maini, "Mathematical oncology: Cancer summed up," *Nature*, vol. 421, pp. 321–321, 2003.

[45] E. A. Sarapata and L. de Pillis, "A comparison and catalog of intrinsic tumor growth models," *Bulletin of Mathematical Biology*, vol. 76, pp. 2010 – 2024, 2014.

[46] E. Uçar, N. Özdemir, and E. Altun, "Fractional order model of immune cells influenced by cancer cells," *Mathematical Modelling of Natural Phenomena*, 2019.

[47] C. M. Ionescu, A. M. Lopes, D. Copot, *et al.*, "The role of fractional calculus in modeling biological phenomena: A review," *Communications in Nonlinear Science and Numerical Simulation*, vol. 51, pp. 141–159, 2017.

[48] P. T. Sowndarrajan, J. Manimaran, A. Debbouche, *et al.*, "Distributed optimal control of a tumor growth treatment model with cross-diffusion effect," *The European Physical Journal Plus*, vol. 134, pp. 1–21, 2019.

[49] J. E. Solís-Pérez, J. F. Gómez-Aguilar, and A. Atangana, "A fractional mathematical model of breast cancer competition model," *Chaos, Solitons & Fractals*, 2019.

[50] F. M. Atici, M. Atici, W. J. M. Hrushesky, *et al.*, "Modeling tumor volume with basic functions of fractional calculus," 2015.

[51] R. M. Ganji, H. Jafari, N. Nkomo, *et al.*, "A mathematical model and numerical solution for brain tumor derived using fractional operator," *Results in Physics*, vol. 28, p. 104671, 2021.

[52] D. Baleanu, A. Jajarmi, H. Mohammadi, *et al.*, "A new study on the mathematical modelling of human liver with caputo–fabrizio fractional derivative," *Chaos Solitons & Fractals*, vol. 134, p. 109705, 2020.

[53] A. A. Alderremy, J. F. Gómez-Aguilar, *et al.*, "A fuzzy fractional model of coronavirus (covid-19) and its study with legendre spectral method," *Results in Physics*, vol. 21, pp. 103773–103773, 2020.

[54] P. Pandey, Y. Chu, J. F. Gómez-Aguilar, *et al.*, "A novel fractional mathematical model of covid-19 epidemic considering quarantine and latent time," *Results in Physics*, vol. 26, pp. 104286–104286, 2021.

[55] N. H. Tuan, H. Mohammadi, and S. Rezapour, "A mathematical model for covid-19 transmission by using the caputo fractional derivative," *Chaos, Solitons, and Fractals*, vol. 140, pp. 110107–110107, 2020.

[56] J. Danane, Z. Hammouch, K. Allali, *et al.*, "A fractional-order model of coronavirus disease 2019 (covid-19) with governmental action and individual reaction," *Mathematical Methods in the Applied Sciences*, 2021.

[57] H. Singh, H. M. Srivastava, Z. Hammouch, and other, "Numerical simulation and stability analysis for the fractional-order dynamics of covid-19," *Results in Physics*, vol. 20, pp. 103722–103722, 2020.

[58] G. C. Cruywagen, D. E. Woodward, P. Tracqui, and other, "The modelling of diffusive tumours," *Journal of Biological Systems*, vol. 03, pp. 937–945, 1995.

[59] P. K. Burgess, P. M. Kulesa, J. D. Murray, *et al.*, "The interaction of growth rates and diffusion coefficients in a three-dimensional mathematical model of gliomas," *Journal of Neuropathology and Experimental Neurology*, vol. 56 6, pp. 704–13, 1997.

7

EEG-based BCI Systems in Neuropsychiatric Diseases

Emine Elif Tülay

Muğla Sıtkı Koçman University, Muğla, Türkiye

Due to the rapid and substantial advancements in technology over the past decades, intelligent systems have become an indispensable part of our lives. Therefore, Brain-Computer Interface (BCI) applications have become effective in a wide variety of fields, starting with the motivation to control computer systems and external devices directly with their thoughts. Moreover, BCI systems hold significant promise in advancing our understanding and management of neuropsychiatric diseases including Alzheimer's Disease, Parkinson's Disease, and various mood and mental disorders. The chapter begins by elucidating the fundamental principles of electroencephalography (EEG) and its relevance in capturing real-time brain activity. Subsequently, it delves into the multifaceted landscape of neuropsychiatric diseases, emphasizing the potential of EEG-based BCIs in enhancing diagnosis, treatment, and rehabilitation strategies.

7.1 Introduction

The communication between a human and a machine, more simply computers, has always been an attractive topic for scientists since the invention of computing systems. However, especially in the last decade, intelligent systems have become an indispensable part of our lives, and new technologies have started to be used to interact with these systems. Brain-computer interface (BCI) technology is one of the current technologies that provide a control ability on machines via human brain functions without needing physical contact. In recent years, BCI has expanded its applications beyond the previously mentioned purposes to include the detection of several diseases in medicine. During the development of distinct BCI applications, various neuroimaging modalities

DOI: 10.1201/9781003461906-7

(e.g., functional resonance imaging (fMRI), electroencephalography (EEG)), acquisition techniques, feature extraction methods, and decoding algorithms (Machine Learning (ML), Deep Learning (DL) techniques) are utilized. The main aim of this chapter is to provide an overview of EEG-based BCI applications to detect neuropsychiatric diseases, including Alzheimer's Disease (AD), Parkinson's Disease (PD), Mood Disorders, Schizophrenia (SCZ) Spectrum, and other psychotic disorders. In the meanwhile, the fundamental technologies for acquiring, encoding, and decoding phases of BCI are briefly described.

This chapter is organized as follows: Section 7.2 introduces the background information about EEG-based BCI including its definition, history, categories, and technologies. Section 7.3 presents the application steps of EEG-based BCI, starting with the acquisition of EEG signals followed by pre-processing, feature extraction/selection phases, and application of artificial intelligence techniques. Section 7.4 illustrates current BCI applications. Section 7.5 discusses the challenges and future perspectives of BCI technologies. Section 7.6 concludes the chapter.

7.2 Understanding the Brain-Computer Interface (BCI)

In this section, the background information related to BCI technology is given starting with the definition of BCI and followed by the idea of emergence, the current types and the hardware and software technologies to implement BCI.

7.2.1 What is BCI?

The Brain-Computer Interface (BCI) term, also sometimes called brain-machine interface or Human-Machine Interface in the recent literature, was originally used in the study by Vidal [1] and described as a direct link between man and machine (in particular, a computer) to provide a dialog by utilizing brain signals. However, due to the rapid improvement of technology in the last decades, there has been an exponential growth of BCI applications [2] and various types of BCI systems emerged, such as active BCI, and passive BCI (see Section 7.2.3). Therefore, multiple terms have been started to be used for the description of BCI systems due to the high heterogeneity of devices, protocols, applications, and disciplines. According to Antonietti [3], 34 definitions of the different BCI types have been used in the current literature of various fields, including neuroscience, psychology, clinical neurology, computer science, and engineering.

The common goal of the earliest BCI systems is to provide an alternative way of controlling peripheral movements without using neural pathways, especially for people with motor impairment or paralysis (see the review by Xu [4]). These kinds of systems were accepted as promising tools that translate brain activity into specific commands or messages to control external devices, such as robotic arms and wheelchairs, or to communicate with the outside world via several applications (see Section 7.4.1). On the other hand, the recent motivation for developing BCI technology is detection of the diseases by decoding brain activity, especially for early diagnosis (see Section 7.4.2) as well as emotion and face recognition processes [5]. For all purposes of using BCI, EEG is the most preferred modality to capture neural activations among other neuroimaging techniques (e.g., fMRI) due to attractive characteristics such as being non-invasive, portable, and affordable in cost as well as having excellent temporal resolution.

Various investigations have been carried out with the EEG method over the last decades and BCI systems that use this method are called EEG-based BCI systems. Besides non-invasive EEG, different types of intracranial EEG (iEEG) could be also used to obtain electrical activity of the brain for BCI systems as an invasive method (please see Section 7.2.3). Although they provide high-quality and accurate signals with better spatial resolution and fewer artifacts, these recording techniques require a more expensive setup than EEG, and risky surgery [6].

7.2.2 History of EEG-based BCI

EEG-based BCI studies started almost 60 years ago with a mere idea and reached today's complex implementations by gaining momentum with the fast improvement of technology over the past years. According to most of the literature, the milestone and the most famous study of BCI, where the term BCI was first proposed, was published by Jacques Vidal in 1973 [1] in California (UCLA). However, one of the first documented examples of BCI technology was conducted by Alvin Lucier, an American composer, in 1965 when the term BCI had not yet been coined [7]. In his experiment, he attempted to generate resultant sounds with "Music for Solo Performer" by using enormously amplified brain waves, in particular, alpha waves. After this pioneering study in art, multiple artists have done similar performances over further years [8].

In fact, the history of BCI systems with EEG dates back to Hans Berger, who is a German psychiatrist. Berger developed a system that recorded brain activity including alpha and beta waves from a human brain in 1929 [9] after the animal studies by Richard Caton (1842–1926), Adolf Beck (1863–1939), Pavel Yurevich Kaufman (1877–1951) and Vladimir Vladimirovich Pravdich Neminsky (1879–1952) [6, 10]. After the invention of brain activity by Berger, slow brain waves below alpha, delta, and theta, have been first reported by Walter [11]. After that, Jaspers and Andrews [12] demonstrated a cortical origin of the beta rhythm and introduced the term "gamma rhythms" for the first time.

Throughout the 1950s to the 1970s, several researchers had doubts about the cortical origin of the alpha rhythm, due to challenges in deciphering the fundamental neuronal mechanisms behind brain wave generation persisted.

Therefore, there was an increasing focus on research exploring Event-Related Potentials (ERPs) as a neurological reaction to both external and internal stimuli until the end of the 1980s (see the review by [13]). In the 1990s, EEG was started to be considered as an important signal of the brain with the different oscillatory systems rather than a background noise [14, 15].

Over the past few decades, EEG has been employed for various purposes, including BCI applications, neuro-marketing, gaming, emotion, and face recognition as well as clinical diagnosis (see Section 7.4).

7.2.3 Categories of EEG-based BCI

In the literature, the current BCI systems are classified based on various factors, including the way of recording brain signals, the elicitation way of brain signals, synchronization, and dependability and timing (Please see the comprehensive reviews, [16–18]).

a) *The way of recording brain signals*: EEG-based BCI systems can be divided into three groups including invasive, semi-invasive, and non-invasive based on the recording style of brain signals. In BCI terminology, non-invasive methods, like EEG, are called procedures without penetrating the brain to record the electrical activity, which means that no surgical operation is needed. Therefore, they are accepted as secure methods despite poor signal quality and poor spatial resolution and are preferred by most scientists and researchers. In contrast, the methods with neurosurgical operation, such as iEEG, implant electrodes to obtain brain signals for BCI systems. As a type of iEEG, Electrocorticography (ECoG) is called a semi-invasive method that uses electrodes placed on the exposed surface of the cortex [19] whereas stereotactic electroencephalogaphy (sEEG), called invasive method, uses depth electrodes that are penetrated in deeper structures of the brain [20]. iEEG could not be broadly used since they have a risk for brain damage as well as they are expensive systems.

b) *The elicitation way of brain signals*: EEG-based BCI systems could also be classified into four categories according to the elicitation way of brain signals. One of them is active, also called endogenous, BCIs, which transform the users' self-induced brain activity to commands to use machines, independently of external stimulations. The neural signals used in these systems are generated through a mental task, such as motor imagery (MI) by which the user imagines a movement of a limb to use a BCI system. In contrast, passive BCIs utilize the brain activities that arise without voluntary control upon application of various types of stimuli (e.g., visual, auditory, or emotional), especially cognitive tasks. Although the initial motivation was to develop active BCI systems in this field, passive systems become an emerging trend in recent years. Besides these two types, there is also one more BCI type that uses the brain signals generated as a reaction to stimuli, often tactile, pain, audio, or video. Such systems are called reactive BCI systems. Several studies can also mix two or more different kinds of BCI types in one application and develop hybrid BCI systems to provide more robust control.

c) *Synchronization*: The categorizing of the BCI systems can also be done based on operating approaches which are synchronous or asynchronous protocols. Synchronous (cue-paced) systems direct the user via cognitive tasks at a desired time. Conversely, in asynchronous (self-paced) systems, the users can think freely at any time without any cue from the system.

d) *Dependability*: The other classification type of BCI systems is based on the interaction between the user and the system. If the users need their muscles for system control, then this system is called a dependent BCI system whereas in independent BCI systems, muscle activity is not required to generate the brain signals that the system uses.

e) *Timing*: Another aspect of using BCI systems is related to implementing the system in real-time or offline.

7.2.4 Hardware and Software Technology of EEG-based BCI Systems

According to Nicolas-Alonso and Gomez-Gil [21], BCI is a system where the hardware and software communicate with each other to provide user-machine interaction. The diversity of both software and hardware has increased with the development of technology.

Multiple hardware technologies developed by various companies are used in the current investigations, especially in the EEG signal acquisition phase of BCI. Generally, hardware technologies consist of electrodes, amplifiers, an A/D converter, and a recording device. There are many technologies currently in use and they mostly vary based on the type of transmission (wireless or wired), wearability, sensor type (wet and dry sensors), number of electrodes (from 1 to 280), and sampling frequency property (128, 256, 512 Hz, and so on) [6]. Also, one company could manufacture more than one device with different characteristics (please see the comprehensive review: [22]).

The acquisition unit (e.g., headsets) and the translation unit (e.g., amplifier) could be connected via wired technologies as well as wireless technologies such as Wi-Fi or Bluetooth. Both of them have several advantages and disadvantages [17]. In the EEG signal acquisition, wired and wireless devices use different sensor technology that is used to capture the brain activities of the users [23]. Wired devices use wet sensor technology that requires a conductive gel as an interface between sensors and scalps whereas wireless devices use dry sensor technology without the need for the use of gels. Moreover, EEG devices may contain different numbers of sensors (electrodes) starting from 1 and up to 280, which are placed according to various types of montage with the standard electrode positions [24, 25]. In the literature, the number of electrodes is associated with the sampling frequency. While the devices with a low number of electrodes have a general sampling rate of 500 Hz, the devices with high electrode numbers archive a sampling rate of higher than 1,000 Hz. After the sensors acquire the brain activity, the amplifiers enlarge the amplitude of EEG signals and the A/D converter digitalizes the signal to store it in a recording device.

Most of the companies that produce hardware devices for EEG acquisition also develop software packages to analyze signals, obtain outputs, and provide feedback [26]. The software developed by a company is mostly commercial software (e.g., Brain Products, Emotiv). However, there are open-source software packages (e.g., EEGlab [27], FieldTrip [28]) that can be run, shared, and modified by anyone.

7.3 Phases of EEG-based BCI Systems

EEG-based BCI systems are implemented in several sequential steps, starting with the acquisition of EEG signals followed by pre-processing and feature extraction/selection phases. After these steps, various artificial intelligence (AI) techniques fed by the extracted features can be applied to finalize the BCI system (please see the details of each step in further sub-sections).

7.3.1 Acquisition of EEG Signals

All types of BCI systems require the acquisition of brain signals so this step is mandatory. To capture and record the desired brain activities, various hardware technologies (please see Section 7.2.4) and well-designed paradigms are used during the signal-acquisition phase (please see the following sub-section 7.3.2). A recent comprehensive review by Mridha et al. [29] provides a compilation of datasets that encompass BCI paradigms, including motor imagery, P300-based BCI speller, and cognitive paradigms.

7.3.2 Encoding Paradigms for EEG-based BCI

The paradigms are used during the EEG signal acquisition phase to modulate and encode the neural signals via specially designed mental tasks, thus target brain activities are generated. Since the invention of BCI, multiple paradigms have been designed to elicit different brain activities such as motor-related (e.g., MI), sensory-related (e.g., Steady-state visual evoked potential (SSVEP)), cognitive-related (e.g., Visual and/or Auditory oddball, Go/nogo paradigms) or Hybrid [30] that corresponds to two or more different mental strategies (such as EEG signal upon application of visual attention and motor imagery paradigms). Among various kinds of paradigms, MI, P300 as a component of event-related potentials and SSVEP are the most widely used ones in BCI applications. Regarding active BCI, MI paradigm has a common usage that requires imagining specific movement whereas P300 and SSVEP are the preferred paradigms, regarding reactive BCI. A compressive review by Xu et al. [4] overviewed various encoding paradigms for BCI systems.

7.3.3 Pre-processing of EEG Signals

The pre-processing stage prepares the recorded signals in a suitable form for further steps by removing any unwanted components embedded within the EEG signal and reorganizing the data. Effective pre-processing contributes to an elevation in signal quality, thereby resulting in enhanced feature separability and improved performance in classification [31].

Although EEG allows us to measure brain electrical signals, it does not solely display these signals. Many noises, referred to as artifacts, can occur during EEG recording, and these noises can interfere with the signals obtained from the brain. Some of these noises are related to the individual being recorded (body movement, eye movements and/or blinks, sweating, etc.), while others arise from technical reasons (50/60 Hz artifact, cable movement, improper placement of electrodes, etc.) [32]. Various methods are used to clean EEG data from noise [33, 34].

The most important sources of physiological artifacts in BCI systems are Electrooculography (EOG) and electromyography (EMG) artifacts, including eye and body movements. Especially for eye movements and blinks, Independent Component Analysis (ICA) is the most preferred methodology to exclude blinking patterns from the EEG signals. Although ICA is also used for EMG artifacts, automatic artifact rejection algorithms based on defined criteria or manual rejections by identifying specific regions affected by artifacts are the common ways to eliminate muscle artifacts. However, both ways of cleaning processes are challenging since automatic techniques could cause the loss of valuable data whereas manual rejection is more labor intensive and sometimes subjective evolution [31]. Therefore, it could be more reliable if cleaning processes are done by experts.

Moreover, technical problems could occur during the recording of EEG and destroy the actual brain activity data. One of them is line interference, also called 50/60 Hz noise. These kinds of noise can be eliminated from the data by using Notch Filtering. The second technical problem most often encountered is damaged electrodes which could not record the signal accurately. In that case, instead of losing the data completely, interpolation techniques that fill in missing or rejected data points by estimating values from neighboring electrodes are used.

During the EEG recording, utilizing a physical reference is essential and the signal at each electrode is determined by subtracting the electric potential at its designated location from the electric potential at the location of the reference electrode. In the pre-processing phase, the reference electrode used in recording could be reorganized by applying a re-referencing process to data. Re-referencing is preferred for various purposes, including noise reduction, adjusting for head model variability, and Adaptation to Analysis Techniques.

The most common reference types are average reference, linked mastoids, reference electrode standardization technique (REST), or a specific EEG channel such as Cz, or FCz [35].

Downsampling and segmentation are the other two steps in pre-processing. Downsampling is a technique used in digital signal processing to reduce the sampling rate by an integer factor which causes a decrease in the resolution and file size and speeds up the further analysis. On the other hand, it can lead to the loss of information as well. Segmentation, also called epoching, is the division of the EEG data into blocks, often aligned with specific events or tasks.

7.3.4 Feature Extraction Methods for EEG-based BCI

EEG reflects distinct characteristics of brain signals and feature extraction is a signal processing stage in BCI, which captures the relevant information to explain mental conditions. Various feature extraction approaches could be utilized to develop EEG-based BCI systems.

If we endeavor to gain a more comprehensive understanding, it would be better to start with the properties of EEG. An EEG signal is formed by five crucial different natural frequencies (oscillatory activity), which are traditionally divided into delta (1–3 Hz), theta (4–7 Hz), alpha (8–13 Hz), beta (15–30 Hz), and gamma (above 30 Hz) frequency bands. These fundamental EEG bands are believed to indicate distinct functional processes within the brain. Brain functions are not only associated with oscillatory activities but also with functional connections within the brain [36, 37]. Various parameters can be used to characterize any oscillation and include important information. These are the oscillation's (i) frequency, (ii) amplitude, and (iii) phase [38].

All these parameters of EEG are represented in different domains that help in analyzing and understanding the characteristics of brain activity [37]. One of them is time domain representation which examines the EEG signal over time for understanding the temporal aspects of brain activity. The second representation is the frequency domain that decomposes the signal into various frequency bands, including delta, theta, alpha, beta, and gamma, and provides insights into the dominant frequencies associated with different cognitive states. Furthermore, the other informative representation is called the time-frequency domain which combines both time and frequency information, providing a more comprehensive view of EEG data [32].

In each domain, there exist diverse types of analyses [29]. In the EEG literature, the most popular time domain analysis is the Event-Related Potential (ERP) which is a time-locked average of EEG activity in response to specific stimuli or events. Various sensory, cognitive, or motor stimuli have the potential to elicit ERPs. The second most common analysis of the time domain is the digital filtering of EEG to determine the oscillatory activity in different frequency bands. To gather statistical features, amplitude (magnitude of EEG voltage fluctuations over time) and latency (the time delay between the occurrence of a stimulus and the corresponding neural response) could be evaluated in both analyses. Additionally, Hjorth parameters that include three statistical parameters (activity, mobility, and complexity) [39] are another useful analysis, especially for real-time systems due to low computation cost.

In BCI systems, the other prevailing and standard analyses could be categorized in the frequency domain. Fourier decomposition is the most widely used method to convert the time domain to the frequency domain, resulting in a complex spectrum in which each frequency is represented by power and phase. Wavelet analysis and Hilbert transformation after band-pass filtering are the other common methods for the transformation to the frequency domain. By utilizing the outputs of the analysis, multiple features could be calculated such as mean and/or peak frequencies, mean and/or maximum power in specific frequency bands, etc. Subsequently, frequency domain analyses contain various functional connectivity metrics that are estimated to evaluate neuronal interactions, including coherence, phase synchronization, phase-slope index, and Granger causality [40].

On the other hand, if there is a need to assess changes in amplitude or power spectrum over time, it is recommended to choose the time-frequency domain analysis. This domain can include techniques like event-related spectral perturbations (ERSPs) that could be obtained via different mathematical methods (e.g., wavelet transform) focus on changes in spectral properties over time, and inter-trial phase coherence (ITPC) that represent phase consistency over trials (typically within the range of zero to one) [41]. The percentage of using the time-frequency domain features is higher than the other domains in the EEG MI-BCI systems [42]. In recent motor imagery BCI applications, spatial domain analyses are also employed for the feature extraction step. One of the popular algorithms in this domain is Common Spatial Patterns (CSP) which involves converting EEG signals into a different space through spatial filtering techniques, aiming to optimize the variance of one group while minimizing the variance of the second group [43].

7.3.5 Artificial Intelligence Techniques in EEG-based BCI Systems for Neural Decoding

The mid-20th century saw the birth of Artificial Intelligence (AI) as a field of study, with early applications focusing on problem-solving and symbolic methods. With today's technological advancement in AI, from industries to home appliances, it has become a ubiquitous reality that is integral to our daily experiences.

Once the feature-extraction process has been established in a BCI system, proper neural decoding models should be selected to recognize feature patterns (e.g., ERP features when a paralyzed user's intent to move a cursor using their thoughts or oscillatory activities when an individual with cognitive decline pay attention to external stimuli). To date, various AI techniques, including conventional ML and DL approaches, have been developed and introduced to detect task-specific patterns in the BCI field (please see the comprehensive review [44]).

In the BCI context, conventional decoding techniques have been pioneering the field for understanding how machines and humans can work together, as they require extensive feature extraction and selection mechanisms to decode effectively. This was necessary to identify meaningful patterns within the complex data generated by the brain, facilitating the development of effective BCI systems. Some widely employed ML approaches used in BCI applications are Linear Discriminant Analysis (LDA), Support Vector Machines (SVM), k-nearest neighbors (k-NN), Naive Bayes classifier, Decision Trees (DT), and Random Forests [45]. These techniques have allowed researchers to decode complex brain data, enabling the development of BCIs that can perform various tasks, from translating motor imagery into commands to recognizing P300 signals by attention to stimuli, and even interpreting SSVEPs for control interfaces.

In particular, LDA and SVM are some of the most efficient classification approaches among the conventional ML techniques. However, due to LDA's strict reliance on the linear separability of the data, its performance heavily deteriorates when dealing with multiclass classification tasks or complex data where there is significant overlap among classes [46]. Despite the limitations, SVM is considered a more robust classifier that can work with a limited number of training samples in a high-dimensional setting [47]. In some cases, DT and Artificial Neural Networks, which are algorithms that do not assume linear separability, are capable of modeling overlapping class distributions more effectively [46]. Among the ML approaches, along with DT, LDA, SVM, and k-NN, non-linear approaches have also proven effective in BCIs for classifying more complex tasks and handling multiclass problems, often outperforming other classifiers in accuracy [48].

Additionally, conventional ML approaches have paved the way for more sophisticated DL approaches that are an extension of artificial neural networks (ANN). Over the last decade, the integration of DL with EEG-based BCIs has significantly advanced the field in terms of more intricate and practical applications. The adoption of DL and transfer learning techniques within EEG-based BCI systems has revolutionized the way we decode and interpret brain signals, showing the invaluable insights and necessary groundwork laid by conventional ML approaches. Convolutional Neural Networks (CNN), deep neural networks (DNN), Long Short-Term Memory Networks (LSTMs), and Generative Adversarial Networks (GANs) are some of the popular DL methods in the literature.

CNN has widespread use and the ability to work and extract features across temporal, spatial, and spectral domains, which overall characterizes the nature of EEG data in a broad sense. As mentioned in Section 7.3.4, EEG signal encapsulates a variety of information across its temporal, spatial, and spectral domains, each holding great clues into brain function and cognitive states. CNN architectures, when compared to conventional ML techniques, enable efficient and effective feature extraction that does not require extensive manual feature engineering. In the temporal domain, CNNs can analyze the functions of brain signals over time, capturing dynamic neural responses to stimuli as well as spontaneous brain activity. On the other hand, the spectral quality of EEG signals is complementary to CNN's ability to identify patterns within specific frequency bands, which are crucial for discriminating between different states of brain activities and cognitive tasks [49]. CNNs, although somewhat limited, extend their feature workspace to the spatial domain, where a varied number of EEG electrodes collect data from the different regions of the human brain. The spatial features are essential qualities for locating changes on the scalp that occur during different cognitive processes. Recent research explored the integration of multi-domain strategies for decoding in BCI systems [50, 51]. The use of CNN to combine features from multiple domains has been shown to improve interpretability and decoding accuracy [52, 53].

The other DL method that is Transfer learning has emerged as a key strategy in overcoming the inherent challenges of cross-subject and cross-session variability in EEG-based BCI systems, enabling more adaptability. Early transfer learning efforts in BCI focused on configuring decomposition algorithms to provide easier adaptation across sessions and subjects. Krauledat et al. [54] focused on stable prototype filters to reduce the need for extensive calibration at the start of new sessions, which may cause fatigue on the subject. Similarly, Kang et al. [55] introduced a composite Common Spatial Pattern (CSP) approach with regularized covariance matrices to provide subject-to-subject transfer. Some other studies focused on statistical aspects of the EEG signals. One notable approach is the Stationary Subspace Analysis (SSA) [56], which separates EEG signals into stationary and non-stationary components, focusing analysis on the more consistent stationary components to improve the classification tasks. A more recent study [57], applied a sophisticated cross-subject data augmentation-focused deep learning framework for enhancing the cross-subject capabilities of motor imagery BCI applications. The architecture of the proposed framework incorporates a multi-domain feature extractor based on CSP equipped with a sliding window mechanism, alongside a parallel two-branch CNN.

7.4 Current BCI Systems Applications

This chapter intended to provide a short overview of the application domains of BCI, encompassing systems facilitating the control of external devices and the diagnosis of neuropsychiatric diseases.

7.4.1 Control of Computer Systems and External Devices

With the integration of technology into every aspect of our lives, the diversity of BCI applications has increased, covering various fields. One of the most prominent applications of BCI systems is in the healthcare sector, particularly in neurorehabilitation by allowing its users to control computer systems and external devices (e.g., robotic arms, wheelchairs) directly with their thoughts [58, 59]. The direct translation of neural signals into commands allows users to navigate interfaces, type messages, and execute various tasks solely through their cognitive intentions. The possibility of this significantly enhances accessibility, especially for individuals with motor disabilities, making everyday tasks more manageable and providing greater independence and autonomy. Various studies in the literature attempted to develop robust MI-BCI systems with the implementations of ML and DL models to enable the person to communicate with their surroundings [42]. Besides neurorehabilitation systems, several detection systems have also emerged such as stress detection [60] and disease detection [61] (see also the following section).

Over the past ten years, BCI has become a prominent focus in research on human-computer interaction (HCI) for non-clinical applications. The BCI recognition systems play a crucial role not only in healthcare but also for non-clinical technology including neuro-marketing [62], security and authentication [63], smart home appliances [64], communication [65], emotion recognition [66], novel sound recognition [67], and natural language processing (NLP) [68] to make our daily lives easier.

The gaming and entertainment industry has also embraced BCI systems, introducing immersive experiences where users can control elements of the virtual environment through neural commands [69]. This novel integration enhances user engagement and sets the stage for a new era of interactive entertainment. Moreover, BCI offers a novel avenue for art [70], enabling artists to convey their inner thoughts, and emotions directly through their neural patterns; for creativity [71] to explore how BCI can be utilized to understand and augment creative ideation; for sports [72] to improve the performance of athletics.

7.4.2 Decoding Mental States in Neuropsychiatric Diseases

Over the past decades, neuroimaging has gained prominence, with the advancements in computing technology and enhanced our understanding of the brain mechanisms with various unimodal modalities such as EEG, fMRI, magnetoencephalography (MEG), positron emission tomography (PET), and near-infrared spectroscopy (NIRS), that provides functional insights (such as neural activity and cognitive functions). Additionally, methods like computed tomography (CT), structural MRI (sMRI), and diffusion tensor imaging (DTI) offer structural and anatomical information (e.g., gray matter and white matter tracts). Besides unimodal modalities, the combination of two or more modalities, aka Multimodal Neuroimaging (MN), is another approach that allows to examination of brain structural and functional changes [73]. However, due to practical use and high temporal resolution, EEG is the prominent modality for neural decoding. Neuropsychiatric diseases present substantial public health challenges as they play a major role in the global burden of disease and significantly influence the social and economic welfare of populations. Although the large majority of EEG studies in the literature have been investigated various biomarkers specific to the neuropsychiatric diseases ([74] for bipolar disorder (BD); [75] for SCZ, AD, and BD; [76] for AD, PD), evaluating the results and identification of biomarkers, particularly in the context of distinguishing these diseases, are challenging processes, and requires expertise; therefore, although some challenges (such as sample size) remain, there is a growing interest in the prevalence of EEG studies employing AI techniques as a prognostic or computer-aided diagnostic tool that decodes the brain activities [73].

Decoding is an essential phase that predicts the course of diseases using brain activities as well as the connections among structures. To achieve this, various AI models (see Section 7.3.5) are used to investigate significant distinct EEG patterns associated with numerous illnesses including neurodegenerative diseases (e.g., AD, PD), mood disorders (e.g., BD, Major depressive disorder (MDD)) and different mental disorders such as Schizophrenia (SCZ) spectrum.

AD is a progressive neurodegenerative illness characterized by progressive cognitive decline, memory loss, and impaired daily functioning. AD typically progresses slowly mainly in three stages which are (1) The preclinical phase characterized by the absence of clinical symptoms, although neuropathological changes have initiated. (2) The Mild Cognitive Impairment (MCI) stage where the individuals do not meet the criteria for AD, but there is notable memory impairment, particularly in the area of episodic memory, when compared to individuals without cognitive issues. (3) Dementia stage that is marked by substantial memory loss, along with observable impairments in various cognitive domains, including language [77]. BCI studies have held paramount significance in impeding the advancement of dementia in AD by paving the way for early detection. A large majority of AI models were utilized by novel researches to enhance diagnostic precision, facilitate early detection, subtype recognition, predictive modeling, and personalized treatment planning for the AD continuum [78]. Among different ML techniques, the Support Vector Machine (SVM) with different kernels is the most used model, followed by K-nearest neighbor (KNN) and Linear Discriminant Analysis (LDA). One of the most recent studies that distinguish AD and healthy control (HC) was published by Nour et al. [79]. They employed Deep Ensemble Learning (DEL) without applying any feature extraction after cleaning from noise and artifacts and reached an average accuracy of 97.9%. Another study attempted to differentiate MCI from HC, applying a comparative deep-learning analysis of resting-state EEG time series [80].

PD is the second most common neurodegenerative disorder, following AD. PD is primarily identified by motor symptoms like hypokinesia, resting tremors, and a mask-like face. In addition to motor symptoms, non-motor manifestations of PD encompass cognitive and sensory deficits, including hearing loss, olfactory dysfunction, and sleep problems [81]. The utilization of contemporary AI techniques fed by various EEG characteristics plays a substantial role in improving the sensitivity of clinical diagnosis of PD via cognitive symptoms. This effect is observed even when symptoms are under control with medication [82–85]. In the literature, both EEG in resting state [86] and upon application of cognitive tasks were evaluated by using continuous data or distinct extracted features such as Hjorth features [87] and phase locking factor [88]. Moreover, some studies have aimed not only to distinguish patients from healthy individuals but also to differentiate between different diseases. For example, one of the latest studies [89] used a graph neural network fed by effective brain connectivity to classify AD and PD (97.4% accuracy) as well as PD and HC (94.2% accuracy).

SCZ is a serious mental health disorder characterized by disturbances in thinking, emotions, and behavior, involving positive symptoms like hallucinations and delusions, negative symptoms such as social withdrawal, and cognitive impairments [90]. AI techniques with EEG features have also been employed for diagnosing SCZ. A recent comprehensive review by Jafari et al. [91] summarized EEG-based ML and DL research for the diagnosis of SCZ with various methodological approaches, and reported promising outcomes of the studies, achieving maximum 100% performance.

Mood disorders are broadly divided into BD [92] and depressive disorders, mainly including MDD [93]. While both bipolar disorder and major depressive disorder involve episodes of depression, bipolar disorder is distinguished by the occurrence of manic or hypomanic episodes. In the literature, both ML models [94, 95] and DL models [96] were utilized to predict BD and depression. Also, Yasin et al. [97] conducted a review of studies that adopted neural network and deep learning approaches to detect both mental disorders.

7.5 Challenges and Future Perspectives

Although BCI technology gained momentum among researchers in the last decades and numerous feature extraction and decoding techniques have been implemented, achieving promising outcomes, several challenges in different aspects need to be overcome. These challenges could be methodological as well as technological which consist of reliability, reactivity, and flexibility [17, 98]. In the study of Aggarwal and Chugh [45], multiple problems were categorized based on ideal signal processing and classification methods, BCI functioning, performance assessment, and commercialization. Additionally, from the technological point of view, Donoghue [99] claimed that the foremost difficulty is stable and reliable long-term recording. Furthermore, Maiseli et al. [2] draw attention to possible threats in the application of BCI, including medical safety, privacy, ethics, and security.

In many fields of EEG-based BCI, maybe the major challenge is the individual differences in the EEG signal of the subjects. In general, ML approaches work under the assumption that the feature space of a sample data set should somewhat represent the overall characteristics and variabilities of all potential data. However, with BCI, this assumption often holds only on a subject-specific basis. Thus, a single model would not guarantee the same consistency for all other subjects. This cross-subject variability of brain signals poses a unique challenge for creating subject-independent models that are universally applicable to everyone. Adding to the cross-subject variability, there is also the factor of temporal variability (cross-session variability), where an individual's brain signal patterns may change over time due to factors present such as mood, fatigue, or even the time of day. Many transfer learning and EEG analysis studies approach this problem in a variety of innovative ways [4].

In the development of BCI applications, achieving high signal quality and accuracy in EEG recordings remains a persistent challenge that is also caused by environmental noise, electrode placement variability in addition to individual differences. However, ongoing developments in electrode technology, such as dry and flexible electrodes, can address issues related to comfort, variability, and signal quality.

BCI technology is still in its early stages despite notable advancements in recent years. In the not-too-distant future, new solutions for all kinds of challenges in any application field will be produced by the researchers as computing resources and sensor technologies are enhanced.

7.6 Conclusion

This chapter provides an overview of the current landscape of EEG-based BCI systems in the context of neuropsychiatric diseases. It is evident that EEG-based BCI systems hold promise not only in unraveling the complexities of neural patterns but also in transforming the way we diagnose, treat, and support individuals facing these challenges. The road ahead involves addressing methodological, technological, and ethical considerations to fully harness the capabilities of EEG-based BCIs in clinical settings.

7.7 Acknowledgment

The author would like to thank M.Sc. Muhammed Enes Özelbas (Yıldız Technical University, Istanbul, Türkiye) for his scientific support.

Bibliography

[1] J. Vidal, "Toward direct brain-computer communication," *Annual Review of Biophysics and Bioengineering*, vol. 2, pp. 157–180, 06 1973.

[2] B. Maiseli, A. T. Abdalla, L. V. Massawe, *et al.*, "Brain–computer interface: trend, challenges, and threats," *Brain Informatics*, vol. 10, p. 20, 08 2023.

[3] A. Antonietti, P. Balachandran, A. Hossaini, *et al.*, "The bci glossary: a first proposal for a community review," *Brain-Computer Interfaces*, vol. 8, no. 3, pp. 42–53, 2021.

[4] L. Xu, M. Xu, T.-P. Jung, *et al.*, "Review of brain encoding and decoding mechanisms for eeg-based brain–computer interface," *Cognitive Neurodynamics*, vol. 15, pp. 569–584, 04 2021.

[5] E. H. Houssein, A. Hammad, and A. A. Ali, "Human emotion recognition from eeg-based brain–computer interface using machine learning: a comprehensive review," *Neural Computing and Applications*, vol. 34, p. 12527–12557, 05 2022.

[6] A. Kawala-Sterniuk, N. Browarska, A. Al-Bakri, *et al.*, "Summary of over fifty years with brain-computer interfaces—a review," *Brain Sciences*, vol. 11, p. 43, 01 2021.

[7] V. Straebel and W. Thoben, "Alvin lucier's music for solo performer: Experimental music beyond sonification," *Organised Sound*, vol. 19, pp. 17–29, 02 2014.

[8] A. Wadeson, A. Nijholt, and C. S. Nam, "Artistic brain-computer interfaces: state-of-the-art control mechanisms," *Brain-Computer Interfaces*, vol. 2, pp. 70–75, 04 2015.

[9] H. Berger, "Über das elektrenkephalogramm des menschen," *Archiv für Psychiatrie und Nervenkrankheiten*, vol. 87, pp. 527–570, 12 1929.

[10] M. A. B. brazier, *A History of the Electrical Activity of the Brain: the first half-century.* Pitman, 1961.

[11] W. G. Walter, "The location of cerebral tumours by electro-encephalography," *The Lancet*, vol. 228, p. 305–308, 08 1936.

[12] H. H. Jasper and H. Andrews, "Electroencephalography. iii. normal differentiation of occipital and precentral regions in man.," *Archives of Neurology and Psychiatry*, vol. 39, p. 96, 01 1938.

[13] C. S. Herrmann, D. Strüber, R. F. Helfrich, *et al.*, "Eeg oscillations: From correlation to causality," *International Journal of Psychophysiology*, vol. 103, pp. 12–21, 05 2016.

[14] E. Başar, *Brain Function and Oscillations. I. Brain Oscillations: Principles and Approaches.* Springer, 09 1998.

[15] E. Başar, *Brain Function and Oscillations. Brain Function and Oscillations. II. Integrative Brain Function. Neurophysiology and Cognitive Processes.* Springer, 1999.

[16] D. Yadav, S. Yadav, and K. Veer, "A comprehensive assessment of brain computer interfaces: Recent trends and challenges," *Journal of Neuroscience Methods*, vol. 346, p. 108918, 12 2020.

[17] M. Rashid, N. Sulaiman, A. P. P. Abdul Majeed, *et al.*, "Current status, challenges, and possible solutions of eeg-based brain-computer interface: A comprehensive review," *Frontiers in Neurorobotics*, vol. 14, 06 2020.

[18] A. Bonci, S. Fiori, H. Higashi, *et al.*, "An introductory tutorial on brain–computer interfaces and their applications," *Electronics*, vol. 10, p. 560, 02 2021.

[19] M. P. Branco, S. H. Geukes, E. J. Aarnoutse, *et al.*, "Nine decades of electrocorticography: A comparison between epidural and subdural recordings," *European Journal of Neuroscience*, vol. 57, pp. 1260–1288, 03 2023.

[20] C. Herff, D. J. Krusienski, and P. Kubben, "The potential of stereotactic-eeg for brain-computer interfaces: Current progress and future directions," *Frontiers in Neuroscience*, vol. 14, p. 123, 02 2020.

[21] L. F. Nicolas-Alonso and J. Gomez-Gil, "Brain computer interfaces, a review," *Sensors*, vol. 12, pp. 1211–1279, 01 2012.

[22] M. Soufineyestani, D. Dowling, and A. Khan, "Electroencephalography (eeg) technology applications and available devices," *Applied Sciences*, vol. 10, p. 7453, 10 2020.

[23] X. Gu, Z. Cao, A. Jolfaei, *et al.*, "Eeg-based brain-computer interfaces (bcis): A survey of recent studies on signal sensing technologies and computational intelligence approaches and their applications," *IEEE/ACM Transactions on Computational Biology and Bioinformatics*, vol. 18, pp. 1645 – 1666, 2021.

[24] R. Srinivasan, *Acquiring Brain Signals from Outside the Brain*, pp. 106–122. Brain–Computer Interfaces: Principles and Practice, Oxford University Press eBooks, 01 2012.

[25] J. N. Acharya, A. Hani, J. Cheek, *et al.*, "American clinical neurophysiology society guideline 2," *Journal of Clinical Neurophysiology*, vol. 33, pp. 308–311, 08 2016.

[26] P. Stegman, C. S. Crawford, M. Andujar, *et al.*, "Brain–computer interface software: A review and discussion," *IEEE Transactions on Human-Machine Systems*, vol. 50, pp. 101–115, 04 2020.

[27] A. Delorme and S. Makeig, "Eeglab: an open source toolbox for analysis of single-trial eeg dynamics including independent component analysis," *Journal of Neuroscience Methods*, vol. 134, no. 1, pp. 9–21, 2004.

[28] R. Oostenveld, P. Fries, E. Maris, *et al.*, "Fieldtrip: Open source software for advanced analysis of meg, eeg, and invasive electrophysiological data," *Computational Intelligence and Neuroscience*, vol. 2011, 2011.

[29] M. F. Mridha, S. C. Das, M. M. Kabir, *et al.*, "Brain-computer interface: Advancement and challenges," *Sensors*, vol. 21, p. 5746, 08 2021.

[30] S. Sadeghi and A. Maleki, "Recent advances in hybrid brain-computer interface systems: A technological and quantitative review," *Basic and Clinical Neuroscience*, vol. 9, p. 373–388, 2018.

[31] M. M. Fouad, K. M. Amin, N. El-Bendary, *et al.*, *Brain Computer Interface: A Review*, vol. 74 of *Brain-Computer Interfaces*, pp. 3–30. Springer, Cham, 11 2015.

[32] A. Keil, E. M. Bernat, M. X. Cohen, *et al.*, "Recommendations and publication guidelines for studies using frequency domain and time-frequency domain analyses of neural time series," *Psychophysiology*, vol. 59, p. e14052, 04 2022.

[33] J. A. Urigüen and B. Garcia-Zapirain, "Eeg artifact removal-state-of-the-art and guidelines," *Journal of neural engineering*, vol. 12, p. 031001, 2015.

[34] C. Y. Jung and S. S. Saikiran, "A review on eeg artifacts and its different removal technique," *Asia-pacific Journal of Convergent Research Interchange*, vol. 2, pp. 43–60, 12 2016.

[35] X. Lei and K. Liao, "Understanding the influences of eeg reference: A large-scale brain network perspective," *Frontiers in Neuroscience*, vol. 11, p. 205, 04 2017.

[36] E. Başar, "The theory of the whole-brain-work," *International Journal of Psychophysiology*, vol. 60, pp. 133–138, 05 2006.

[37] E. Başar, B. T. Gölbaşı, E. Tülay, *et al.*, "Best method for analysis of brain oscillations in healthy subjects and neuropsychiatric diseases," *International Journal of Psychophysiology*, vol. 103, pp. 22–42, 05 2016.

[38] P. Sauseng and W. Klimesch, "What does phase information of oscillatory brain activity tell us about cognitive processes?," *Neuroscience and Biobehavioral Reviews*, vol. 32, pp. 1001–1013, 07 2008.

[39] B. Hjorth, "Eeg analysis based on time domain properties," *Electroencephalography and Clinical Neurophysiology*, vol. 29, pp. 306–310, 09 1970.

[40] A. M. Bastos and J.-M. Schoffelen, "A tutorial review of functional connectivity analysis methods and their interpretational pitfalls," *Frontiers in Systems Neuroscience*, vol. 9, 01 2016.

[41] S. Makeig, S. Debener, J. Onton, *et al.*, "Mining event-related brain dynamics," *Trends in Cognitive Sciences*, vol. 8, pp. 204–210, 05 2004.

[42] Pawan and R. Dhiman, "Machine learning techniques for electroencephalogram based brain-computer interface: A systematic literature review," 08 2023.

[43] Z. J. Koles, M. S. Lazar, and S. Z. Zhou, "Spatial patterns underlying population differences in the background eeg," *Brain Topography*, vol. 2, pp. 275–284, 1990.

[44] A. E. Hramov, V. A. Maksimenko, and A. N. Pisarchik, "Physical principles of brain–computer interfaces and their applications for rehabilitation, robotics and control of human brain states," *Physics Reports*, vol. 918, pp. 1–133, 06 2021.

[45] S. Aggarwal and N. Chugh, "Review of machine learning techniques for eeg based brain computer interface," *Archives of Computational Methods in Engineering*, vol. 29, 01 2022.

[46] 9th International Conference on Emerging Technologies (ICET), *Evaluation of ANN, LDA and Decision trees for EEG based Brain Computer Interface*, IEEE, 12 2013.

[47] 30th International Symposium on Computer-Based Medical Systems (CBMS), *A Comparison Study on EEG Signal Processing Techniques Using Motor Imagery EEG Data*, IEEE Xplore, 06 2017.

[48] 2009 International Conference on Information and Automation, *Comparison of different classification methods for EEG-based brain computer interfaces: A case study*, IEEE, 06 2009.

[49] A. M. Roy, "An efficient multi-scale cnn model with intrinsic feature integration for motor imagery eeg subject classification in brain-machine interfaces," *Biomedical Signal Processing and Control*, vol. 74, p. 103496, 04 2022.

[50] Y. Li, L. Guo, Y. Liu, *et al.*, "A temporal-spectral-based squeeze-and-excitation feature fusion network for motor imagery eeg decoding," *IEEE Transactions on Neural Systems and Rehabilitation Engineering*, vol. 29, pp. 1534–1545, 2021.

[51] H. Li, M. Ding, R. Zhang, *et al.*, "Motor imagery eeg classification algorithm based on cnn-lstm feature fusion network," *Biomedical Signal Processing and Control*, vol. 72, p. 103342, 02 2022.

[52] V. J. Lawhern, A. J. Solon, N. R. Waytowich, *et al.*, "Eegnet: a compact convolutional neural network for eeg-based brain–computer interfaces," *Journal of Neural Engineering*, vol. 15, p. 056013, 07 2018.

[53] C. Ieracitano, F. C. Morabito, A. Hussain, *et al.*, "A hybrid-domain deep learning-based bci for discriminating hand motion planning from eeg sources," *International Journal of Neural Systems*, vol. 31, p. 2150038, 08 2021.

[54] M. Krauledat, M. Tangermann, B. Blankertz, *et al.*, "Towards zero training for brain-computer interfacing," *PLoS ONE*, vol. 3, p. e2967, 08 2008.

[55] H. Kang, Y. Nam, and S. Choi, "Composite common spatial pattern for subject-to-subject transfer," *IEEE Signal Processing Letters*, vol. 16, p. 683–686, 08 2009.

[56] P. von Bünau, F. C. Meinecke, F. J. Király, *et al.*, "Finding stationary subspaces in multivariate time series," *Physical Review Letters*, vol. 103, 11 2009.

[57] M. E. Özelbaş, E. E. Tülay, and S. Ozekes, "Improving cross-subject classification performance of motor imagery signals: A data augmentation-focused deep learning framework," *Machine Learning: Science and Technology*, 01 2024.

[58] R. Mane, T. Chouhan, and C. Guan, "Bci for stroke rehabilitation: motor and beyond.," *Journal of neural engineering*, vol. 17, p. 041001, 2020.

[59] M. J. Young, D. J. Lin, and L. R. Hochberg, "Brain–computer interfaces in neurorecovery and neurorehabilitation," *Seminars in Neurology*, vol. 41, pp. 206–216, 03 2021.

[60] R. Katmah, F. Al-Shargie, U. Tariq, *et al.*, "A review on mental stress assessment methods using eeg signals," *Sensors*, vol. 21, p. 5043, 07 2021.

[61] 2021 9th International Winter Conference on Brain-Computer Interface (BCI), *Evaluation and Diagnosis of Brain Diseases based on Non-invasive BCI*, IEEE, 02 2021.

[62] F. S. Rawnaque, K. M. Rahman, S. F. Anwar, *et al.*, "Technological advancements and opportunities in neuromarketing: a systematic review," *Brain Informatics*, vol. 7, 09 2020.

[63] M. P. Orenda, L. Garg, and G. Garg, *Exploring the Feasibility to Authenticate Users of Web and Cloud Services Using a Brain-Computer Interface (BCI)*, vol. 10590 of *Lecture Notes in Computer Science*, pp. 353–363. Springer, Cham, 01 2017.

[64] A. Zakzouk, K. Menzel, and M. Hamdy, *Brain-Computer-Interface (BCI) Based Smart Home Control Using EEG Mental Commands*, pp. 720–732. PROPRO-VE 2023: Collaborative Networks in Digitalization and Society 5.0, Springer, Cham, 01 2023.

[65] S. Garcia and M. Andujar, *Neurochat: Artistic Affective State Facial Filters in Online Video Communication*, pp. 23–32. Augmented Cognition, Springer, Cham, 2021.

[66] X. Si, D. Huang, Y. Sun, *et al.*, "Transformer-based ensemble deep learning model for eeg-based emotion recognition," *Brain Science Advances*, vol. 9, pp. 210–223, 09 2023.

[67] E. E. Tülay, "Detection of orienting response to novel sounds in healthy elderly subjects: A machine learning approach using eeg features," *Acta Infologica*, vol. 7, pp. 71–80, 04 2023.

[68] N. Hollenstein, C. Renggli, B. Glaus, *et al.*, "Decoding eeg brain activity for multi-modal natural language processing," *Frontiers in Human Neuroscience*, vol. 15, 07 2021.

[69] B. Kerous, F. Skola, and F. Liarokapis, "Eeg-based bci and video games: a progress report," *Virtual Reality*, vol. 22, pp. 119–135, 10 2018.

[70] D. Friedman, ""brain art: Brain-computer interfaces for artistic expression"," *Brain-Computer Interfaces*, vol. 7, pp. 36–37, 04 2020.

[71] M. E. Vanutelli, M. Salvadore, and C. Lucchiari, "Bci applications to creativity: Review and future directions, from little-c to c2," *Brain Sciences*, vol. 13, p. 665, 04 2023.

[72] C. Jeunet, D. Hauw, and J. d. R. Millán, "Sport psychology: Technologies ahead," *Frontiers in Sports and Active Living*, vol. 2, 02 2020.

[73] E. E. Tulay, B. Metin, N. Tarhan, *et al.*, "Multimodal neuroimaging: Basic concepts and classification of neuropsychiatric diseases," *Clinical EEG and Neuroscience*, vol. 50, pp. 20–33, 06 2019.

[74] A. Ozerdem, B. Guntekin, M. I. Atagun, *et al.*, "Brain oscillations in bipolar disorder in search of new biomarkers," *Supplements to Clinical neurophysiology*, vol. 62, pp. 207–221, 01 2013.

[75] E. Başar, C. Schmiedt-Fehr, B. Mathes, *et al.*, "What does the broken brain say to the neuroscientist? oscillations and connectivity in schizophrenia, alzheimer's disease, and bipolar disorder," *International Journal of Psychophysiology*, vol. 103, p. 135–148, 05 2016.

[76] B. Güntekin, T. Aktürk, X. Arakaki, *et al.*, "Are there consistent abnormalities in event-related eeg oscillations in patients with alzheimer's disease compared to other diseases belonging to dementia?," *Psychophysiology*, vol. 59, 08 2022.

[77] E. E. Tülay, B. Güntekin, G. Yener, *et al.*, "Evoked and induced eeg oscillations to visual targets reveal a differential pattern of change along the spectrum of cognitive decline in alzheimer's disease," *International Journal of Psychophysiology*, vol. 155, pp. 41–48, 09 2020.

[78] A. Modir, S. Shamekhi, and P. Ghaderyan, "A systematic review and methodological analysis of eeg-based biomarkers of alzheimer's disease," *Measurement*, vol. 220, pp. 113274–113274, 10 2023.

[79] M. Nour, U. Senturk, and K. Polat, "A novel hybrid model in the diagnosis and classification of alzheimer's disease using eeg signals: Deep ensemble learning (del) approach," *Biomedical Signal Processing and Control*, vol. 89, pp. 105751–105751, 03 2024.

[80] M. Şeker and M. S. Özerdem, "Deep insights into mci diagnosis: A comparative deep learning analysis of eeg time series," *Journal of Neuroscience Methods*, vol. 403, pp. 110057–110057, 01 2024.

[81] B. R. Bloem, M. S. Okun, and C. Klein, "Parkinson's disease," *The Lancet*, vol. 397, pp. 2284–2303, 04 2021.

[82] A. M. Maitín, A. J. García-Tejedor, and J. P. R. Muñoz, "Machine learning approaches for detecting parkinson's disease from eeg analysis: A systematic review," *Applied Sciences*, vol. 10, p. 8662, 12 2020.

[83] Q. Wang, L. Meng, J. Pang, *et al.*, "Characterization of eeg data revealing relationships with cognitive and motor symptoms in parkinson's disease: A systematic review," *Frontiers in Aging Neuroscience*, vol. 12, 11 2020.

[84] M. S. Alzubaidi, U. Shah, H. Dhia Zubaydi, *et al.*, "The role of neural network for the detection of parkinson's disease: A scoping review," *Healthcare*, vol. 9, p. 740, 06 2021.

[85] H. W. Loh, W. Hong, C. P. Ooi, *et al.*, "Application of deep learning models for automated identification of parkinson's disease: A review (2011–2021)," *Sensors*, vol. 21, p. 7034, 10 2021.

[86] S. Q. A. Rizvi, G. Wang, A. Khan, *et al.*, "Classifying parkinson's disease using resting state electroencephalogram signals and u^{<i>en</i>}-pdnet," *IEEE Access*, vol. 11, pp. 107703–107724, 01 2023.

[87] B. F. O. Coelho, A. B. R. Massaranduba, C. A. d. S. Souza, *et al.*, "Parkinson's disease effective biomarkers based on hjorth features improved by machine learning," *Expert Systems with Applications*, vol. 212, p. 118772, 02 2023.

[88] E. E. Tülay, E. Yıldırım, T. Aktürk, *et al.*, "Classification of parkinson's disease with dementia using phase locking factor of event-related oscillations to visual and auditory stimuli," *Journal of Neural Engineering*, vol. 20, p. 026025, 03 2023.

[89] J. Cao, L. Yang, P. G. Sarrigiannis, *et al.*, "Dementia classification using a graph neural network on imaging of effective brain connectivity," *Computers in Biology and Medicine*, vol. 168, pp. 107701–107701, 01 2024.

[90] R. A. McCutcheon, T. Reis Marques, and O. D. Howes, "Schizophrenia—an overview," *JAMA Psychiatry*, vol. 77, 10 2019.

[91] M. Jafari, D. Sadeghi, A. Shoeibi, *et al.*, "Empowering precision medicine: Ai-driven schizophrenia diagnosis via eeg signals: A comprehensive review from 2002–2023," *Applied Intelligence*, vol. 54, pp. 35–79, 12 2024.

[92] E. Vieta, M. Berk, T. G. Schulze, *et al.*, "Bipolar disorders," *Nature Reviews Disease Primers*, vol. 4, p. 18008, 03 2018.

[93] C. Otte, S. M. Gold, B. W. Penninx, *et al.*, "Major depressive disorder," *Nature Reviews Disease Primers*, vol. 2, 09 2016.

[94] N. Agnihotri and D. S. K. Prasad, "Review on machine learning techniques to predict bipolar disorder," *www.techrxiv.org*, vol. 13, pp. 195–206, 04 2022.

[95] D. Watts, R. F. Pulice, J. Reilly, *et al.*, "Predicting treatment response using eeg in major depressive disorder: A machine-learning meta-analysis," *Translational Psychiatry*, vol. 12, 08 2022.

[96] A. Safayari and H. Bolhasani, "Depression diagnosis by deep learning using eeg signals: A systematic review," *Medicine in Novel Technology and Devices*, vol. 12, p. 100102, 12 2021.

[97] S. Yasin, S. A. Hassan, S. Aslan, *et al.*, "Eeg based major depressive disorder and bipolar disorder detection using neural networks:a review," *Computer Methods and Programs in Biomedicine*, vol. 202, p. 106007, 04 2021.

[98] S. Saha, K. A. Mamun, K. Ahmed, *et al.*, "Progress in brain computer interface: Challenges and opportunities," *Frontiers in Systems Neuroscience*, vol. 15, 02 2021.

[99] J. P. Donoghue, *Brain–Computer Interfaces: Why Not Better?*, pp. 341–356. Neuromodulation (Second Edition) Comprehensive Textbook of Principles, Technologies, and Therapies, Academic Press, 01 2018.

8

Bioinformatics of Brain Diseases

Tuba Sevimoglu

University of Health Sciences, İstanbul, Türkiye

As the renowned theoretical physicist Michio Kaku says "Sitting on your shoulders is the most complicated object in the known universe". The complexity of the tasks the brain carries also makes it difficult for researchers to comprehend its mechanism in disease and health. For a thorough comprehension of how the brain functions, understanding the molecular basis of the brain's general activity is crucial. The study of how DNA is expressed as proteins and other molecules is known as transcriptomics. Brain transcriptomics technologies help us gather information regarding gene expression. Microarray and RNA-seq technologies have been used in this regard for quite a while. Understanding brain diseases and disorders require the use of bioinformatics which is the acquisition and interpretation of big biological data gathered through the use of these technologies and more.

8.1 Introduction

Researchers had hoped that the majority of human diseases will be fully comprehended and cured after the Human Genome Project was completed. However, they were left with a massive amount of data to be analyzed and interpreted and many more questions to be answered. Bioinformatics, a multidisciplinary field that uses computer approaches to make sense of large amounts of biological data, comes in help here. This field makes use of biology, genetics, medicine, computer science, and engineering [1].

Dayhoff was the first to use computer techniques in biology to analyze protein sequence similarities [2]. She is regarded as a bioinformatics pioneer. In the present day, bioinformatics is concerned with not just sequence similarities but the sequencing of DNA, RNA, and proteins as well as the storing and comparison of data, the analysis of protein interactions, the knowledge

DOI: 10.1201/9781003461906-8

of gene evolution, and the modeling and understanding of protein structure and functions. There are countless databases and tools in this area to help understand the big data which is the result of analysis of numerous characters of hundreds of large molecules in a single run.

To understand the brain however, we need more than genomics and proteomics. Imaging of the brain is also an important aspect of brain research. So, understanding the brain requires combining various data types including as gene expression, atlases of brain anatomy, positron emission tomography (PET), and magnetic resonance imaging (MRI). This field is also called neuroinformatics [3]. This area is an expanded use of analogous technologies crucial for the progress of bioinformatics, however, applied to broader, diverse types of data at various levels of function.

It should be noted that programming languages are at the core of bioinformatics. They are utilized in the development of novel tools for the processing of biological data as well as in every facet of bioinformatics, from data analysis to visualization. Coding is also necessary to address the broad spectrum and intricate nature of challenges that arise in the field of bioinformatics. The most used programming languages in this area are R programming, Python, and Perl [4, 5].

8.2 Analyzing the Brain Transcriptome

One of the basic bioinformatics applications in this area is analyzing the brain transcriptome which is the set of coding and non-coding RNA scripts expressed in the brain. Researchers are interested in the transcriptome since it correlates well with cellular responses. In this chapter, we will focus on two approaches to obtain transcriptomic data: hybridization-based microarrays and RNA-seq (Figure 8.1) [6].

8.2.1 Microarrays

Microarrays were invented by a group of scientists with the leadership of bioenterpreneur Alejandro (Alex) Zaffaroni in the late 1980s [7]. They are traditional hybridization techniques that lets us study a plethora of genes. In this technique a myriad of DNA sequences is deposited on a glass slide called a chip. Each DNA fragment has its own location on the chip. The technique is based on the fact that mRNA will be translated to proteins, thus if we analyze mRNA we will be able to get genetic information or the gene expression. Considering that the degrading of mRNA is quick, it is being converted into a cDNA (complementary DNA) form which is labeled with fluorochrome dyes Cy3 (green) and Cy5 (red). The approach is based on the idea that complementary sequences will bind to one another (Figure 8.1A) [8].

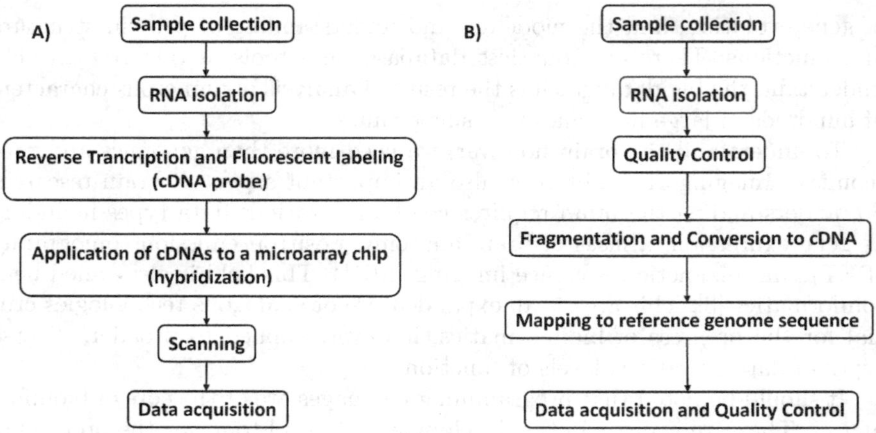

FIGURE 8.1
A simplified **A.** Microarray **B.** RNA-seq workflow.

There are various types of microarrays with DNA microarrays being the most widely used one. The other microarray technologies include protein, peptide, antibody, transfection, cell, and tissue microarrays [9]. Making use of microarray technology, one can investigate the concurrent gene expression patterns of thousands of different genes, determine transcription factor binding sites or genotype single-nucleotide-polymorphism (SNP) [10]. The most important purpose of using this technology is to identify a pattern in the investigated areas. Subsequently, qPCR (quantitative polymerase chain reaction) is used to validate the microarray findings. There are different microarray platforms such as Affymetrix (https://www.thermofisher.com/tr/en/home/brands/applied-biosystems.html), Illumina (https://www.illumina.com) and Agilent (https://www.agilent.com). Various characteristics set these microarray technologies apart. For instance, while Illumina arrays use multiple copies of a single 50-nucleotide probe attached to microbeads to quantify target levels and Agilent uses a single 60-nucleotide probe per gene on the microarray, Affymetrix arrays characterize gene expression using a set of different 25-nucleotide probes synthesized *in situ* [11, 12].

There are quite a few benefits to using microarray technology. Microarrays have well defined protocols for hybridization and the data submission is standardized. They are also low cost compared to RNA-seq. However, since microarrays use hybridization techniques prior knowledge of a sequence is required. There also have been several problems identifying very low and highly expressed genes using this technique. Background noise can be high. Furthermore, microarrays generally do not identify splice variants and they do not give paralogue information. Most commonly used microarray platforms use a single set of manufacturer-designed probes, resulting in an absence of oversight over the collection of analyzed transcripts. Another major drawback of microarrays is the elevated cost for each experiment and the growing number of probe designs that utilize low-specificity sequences [13]. These disadvantages propelled researchers to come up with a sequence-based technique: RNA-seq. Nevertheless, it is wise to use microarrays when there are a large number of samples and cost is an issue or if you wish to directly compare the expression profiles with data from another microarray platform.

8.2.2 RNA-seq Technologies

RNA sequencing (RNA-seq) is a technique that is being used to detect and quantify mRNA molecules in a biological sample consisting of millions of cells [14]. It uses high throughput sequencing to not only quantify gene expression but also to determine alternatively spliced genes and detect allele specific expression and more. RNA-seq may be applied to various types of RNA such as mRNA, total RNA, microRNA, single cell RNA and long noncoding RNA [15]. With RNA-seq, firstly the RNA is isolated and converted to cDNA. Next, a sequencing library is prepared following a PCR amplification. The cDNA is fragmented into short pieces, and finally sequencing is done using an NGS (Next Generation Sequencing) platform (Figure 8.1B). Following the production of sequence reads in FASTQ format, a reference sequence is then used to align the reads [16].

There are several NGS platforms with Illumina (www.illumina.com) being the most popular one. Other major platforms can be listed as Roche 454 (www.424.cm), Pacific Biosciences (www.pacificbiosciences.com), Ion Torrent (www.iontorrent.com), and SOLID (www.invitrogen.com). These platforms differ in terms of sequencing and detection chemistry. Each NGS platform has its own protocol. Selection of a platform may depend on the level of accuracy needed, the number and the length of the reads, whether RNA or DNA is sequenced, amount of sample material, cost of the job, and the amount of time needed to get the job done [17]. RNA-seq is an intricate, interwoven process which involves steps such as PCR amplification, fragmentation, purification, and sequencing. Any error in any of these stages could make the data unreliable. Which is why quality control (QC) is an important aspect of RNA-seq. QC of RNAs is a critical step prior to library preparation. To obtain high quality RNA, it is essential to stabilize the sample after collection, fully lyse it, and eliminate any potential DNA contamination. Furthermore, RNA-seq data of poor quality can dramatically bias the outcomes of analysis and result in false conclusions. Additionally, biases such as GC-content (guanine-cytosine content) and nucleotide composition and complexity of the transcriptome can also cause flawed data [18]. Rigorous QC methods must be applied to the raw data before any downstream analysis [19].

Unlike hybridization-based methods RNA-seq uses sequence-based approaches to determine the transcripts directly. Alternative splicing may be detected if aligned to the genome. Furthermore, SNPs and paralogous genes can be identified with this technology. The background noise is relatively low. These additional application options make it more advantageous over microarrays. The optimization of protocols, the demand for high-power computer facilities, high setup costs, and complex analysis in the case of splice variants or paralogues are some problems that still need to be overcome for this technology [20].

8.3 Repositories

Various types of microarrays and RNA-seq technology were employed in hopes of identifying the genetic mechanism of diseases and disorders in wet lab experiments. These studies are archived in several online repositories.

The National Center for Biotechnology Information's (NCBI) Gene expression omnibus (GEO) is the most widely used public functional genomics data repository that has both array and sequence-based data (https://www.ncbi.nlm.nih.gov/geo/). Here researchers can search for studies done on any disease that comes to mind. There are currently 4348 datasets, 206863 series, 25300 platforms and 6640900 samples in this repository (as of August 2023). All the brain diseases and disorders discussed in the first chapter of this book were searched in the GEO database and a chart was drawn with the number of experiments (number of series) done for each brain disease/disorder (Figure 8.2). Here, we can see that among the three groups of diseases and disorders investigated in this book, major transcriptomic research was done on brain tumors, with gliomas being the leading disease group. The second mostly experimented brain disease group is the neurodegenerative diseases, with Alzheimer's Disease (AD) leading the group. Here, we should also highlight that numerous genes have been linked to autism, despite the fact that there aren't as many studies about this complex condition in GEO database.

ArrayExpress (https://www.ebi.ac.uk/biostudies/arrayexpress) is another public repository that stores data from high-throughput functional genomics experiments such as gene expression, methylation profiling, chromatin immunoprecipitation assays, RNA-seq, and single-cell RNA-seq (scRNA-seq) [21]. There is also The DNA Data Bank of Japan (DDBJ) Center (https://www.ddbj.nig.ac.jp) which has developed the Genomic Expression Archive (GEA) for functional genomics data obtained from microarray and high-throughput sequencing studies [22]. The data can be downloaded from these repositories freely.

8.4 Data Analysis and Visualization Tools

The data obtained from wet lab experiments employing microarray and RNA-seq technology needs to be analyzed to give comprehensible meaning to

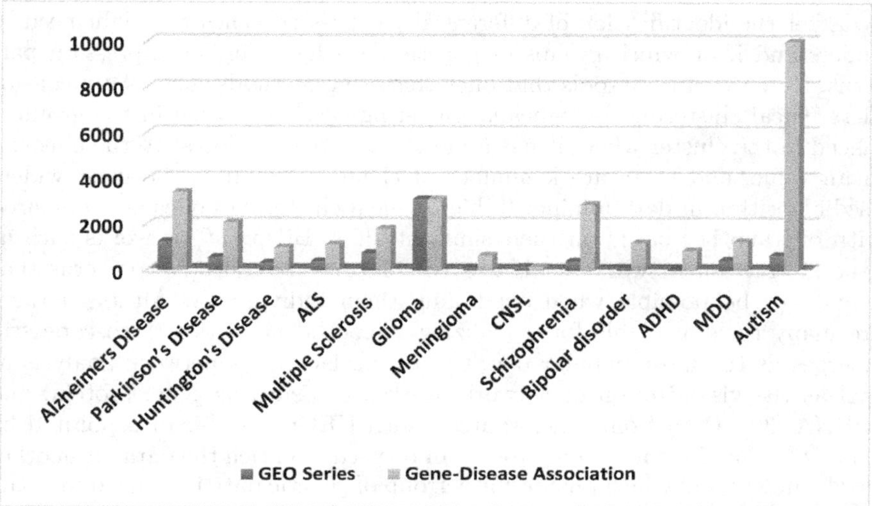

FIGURE 8.2
Total number of experiments in the GEO repository for brain diseases and disorders and total number of genes associated with the studied diseases and disorders from the DisGeNET database (As of August 2023).

biological information. Most manufacturers provide analysis tools along their microarray or RNA-seq products. However, there are also open-source tools that include various methods in analyzing the data.

Bioconductor is an open-source software based on R programming language that helps analyze genomic data (both microarray and RNA-seq) generated by wet lab experiments (https://www.bioconductor.org) [23]. It is essentially a repository of R packages. There are currently 3593 packages in its environment which are mostly software packages (2230) but there are also annotation (912) and experimental data (421) packages as well as workflow packages (30) (as of August 2023). Here, we can find genomic data analysis packages like LIMMA (linear models for microarray data), an algorithm that uses RMA (Robust Multi-array Average) and other normalization techniques to account for data noise before using a linear model to determine the differential expression of genes [24]. In addition to LIMMA, there are other packages in Bioconductor that are used in analyzing RNA-seq and microarray data such as EdgeR and DESeq2 [25]. EdgeR is a package that uses a Poisson model to include both biological and technical variations [26]. Shrinkage estimation for dispersions and fold changes are used in the DESeq2 approach to improve estimate stability and perception [27]. As previously stated, these and other packages implement a variety of statistical methodologies for differential analysis. Once the analysis results are out there, we can identify significant differential expression through the use of several cut offs such as p-value's and fold changes.

After the identification of differentially expressed genes we might need to understand if or which groups of genetic data have similar expression patterns. Here we can use tools that offer clustering methods such as k-means or hierarchical clustering. In k-means clustering each individual in the group is placed in the cluster where it has a mean value that is closest to the cluster's mean value, and there are k number of clusters [28]. It is the most widely used algorithm in data mining. In hierarchical clustering nodes are compared with one another based on their similarity [29]. Biological networks such as gene interaction networks enable us to comprehend collective patterns that would not be possible when examining them individually. Although there are many tools available for visualizing biological networks, Cytoscape still emerges as the most popular one. Cytoscape facilitates network analysis as well as the visualization of network interactions such as gene, protein, and miRNA [30]. Data from other sources, such KEGG, is also incorporated by this tool. Enrichment analysis tools can be used to enrich the data, or in other words understand which phenotype a group of genetic data is associated with. These tools make use of databases such as The Cancer Genome Atlas (TCGA) [31], Kyoto Encyclopedia of Genes and Genomes (KEGG) [32], Gene Ontology, and PANTHER [33]. Here the above-mentioned databases and others are used to identify common biological functions, signaling pathways and interactions networks and more. A widely used enrichment analysis tool is Gene Set Enrichment Analysis: (GSEA) [34]. Another enrichment analysis tool in use is The Database for Annotation, Visualization and Integrated Discovery (DAVID) (https://david.ncifcrf.gov/home.jsp) [35].

There are also databases for storing the discoveries made through techniques mentioned here and/or others. The Genetic Association Database (GAD) is a repository of information from genetic association studies that have been published, in which the data and metadata presented in each study have been structured into a common format [36]. An extensive collection of human genes and genetic features can be found in the OMIM (Online Mendelian Inheritance in Man) database [37]. DisGeNET is a database that compiles data on human gene-disease and variant-disease relationships from numerous sources, including GAD and OMIM [38]. Figure 8.2 also displays the number of genes retrieved from DisGeNET that are connected to the diseases and disorders under study.

8.5 Bioinformatics Studies on Brain Diseases and Disorders

There are numerous experiments accomplished since the emerge of microarray and RNA-seq technologies. Accordingly, only recent studies involving microarray and RNA-seq technologies on the studied diseases will be presented in the following sections.

8.5.1 Microarray Studies

Brain tumors have received the most research attention among the diseases and disorders under study. The prevalence of glioblastoma multiforme (GBM), the most frequent form of glioma, is rising in many nations as a result of advancing age, errors in diagnosis, ionizing radiation, polluted air, and other environmental factors [39]. Mostly tissue microarrays and transcript microarrays are used to analyze the gene expression patterns for these cancer types [40]. For instance, Wang and coworkers performed a comprehensive evaluation of 34 microarray datasets to identify a diagnostic tool for glioblastoma [41]. Here, they discovered that CBX3 silencing reduces the capacity of cells to proliferate by stopping the cell cycle in the G2/M phase. In another study, Zhang and coworkers aimed to identify prognostic markers of the disease through the comparison of GBM microarray datasets, The Cancer Genome Atlas (TCGA), and Chinese Glioma Genome Atlas (CGGA) [42]. They identified PRKCG, PRKCB, and CAMK2A as possible prognostic indicators of GBM.

The most frequent primary intracranial neoplasm is meningioma and only a very small portion of these tumors are malignant (around 1 %). Wedemeyer and colleagues looked at the differences between specific tumors and the neighboring normal dura, which is the top layer of the three meninges that cover and safeguard the brain [43]. They also looked at copy number variations and epigenetic changes. They performed whole-exome sequencing, single-nucleotide polymorphism (SNP) and methylation array and identified dysregulation of FOXC1. In another study Menghi and coworkers identified CKS2 and LEPR as potential biomarkers of the disease performing DNA microarray on tumor tissues and blood samples of individuals with meningioma [44].

Central nervous system lymphoma (CNSL) is a rare and incredibly aggressive disease that appears in the white blood cells of the brain or spinal cord. Villa and coworkers performed tissue microarray for primary CNSL with diffuse large B-cell lymphoma [45]. Their population-based analysis demonstrated that key molecular characteristics of primary CNSL are distinct from those of systemic diffuse large B-cell lymphoma. In another study Takashima and colleagues used total RNA extracted from tumor tissue of patients with primary CNSL to identify distinct expression patterns of miRNAs [46]. Their findings showed that miR-101/548b/554/1202, which are linked to cancer immunity, can serve as an effective predictive marker in PCNSL that may aid in our understanding of the target pathways for PCNSL therapy.

Currently the most extensively studied neurodegenerative condition is Alzheimer's disease (AD). This is due to the unclear pathophysiology of the condition and lack of a currently available treatment. Increases in life expectancy and the diagnosis of AD patients will have a significant negative impact on the economies of countries. There are a multitude of studies involving microarray techniques and many more are to be added till a cure for this complex mind-boggling brain disease is established. In a comprehensive study done by Takei and coworkers, a tissue microarray technique was used to identify diffuse pathological processes in late stages of AD, dementia, and amyotrophic lateral sclerosis (ALS) [47]. In another study Blauwendraat and coworkers identified a diverse spectrum of mutation carriers observed novel genotype-phenotype correlations in AD and Parkinson's Disease (PD) [48].

Given how challenging it is to obtain a premortem brain tissue sample, it is clear from the research that considerable effort has been made to identify blood biomarkers for particular brain diseases and disorders in addition to tissue biomarkers. Collection of blood samples is minimally intrusive, simple to use, and economical. Such studies may involve the use of peripheral blood mononuclear cells (PBMC), whole blood cells, lymphocytes, serum T-cells, or red blood cells. For instance, Sakharkar et al. did a comparison of brain and peripheral blood cell gene expression profiles of PD patients to assess early indicators of the disease [49]. Their analysis results determined that the identified genes do not represent a common biological pathway due to the heterogenic structure of the disease. In another study, Miki and colleagues performed whole transcriptome assay using PBMC from PD patients [50]. According to their findings, PD exhibits considerably elevated upstream autophagy protein levels as well as negative feedback on the mRNA expression of these proteins.

Neurons in the brain gradually degenerate due to Huntington's disease (HD), an uncommon hereditary condition. Zhou and colleagues analyzed postmortem prefrontal cortical tissue using microarrays from patients with HD [51]. Their research revealed that reduced brain derived neurotrophic factor expression is involved in HD pathogenesis and may be regulated by cAMP, MAPK, and Ras signaling pathways. Revealing HD mechanism can be challenging due to the intricacy of the affected regions of the brain and cell types. Thus, it is most likely to come across studies in animal models of this disease. For instance, in a mouse cell line model of HD, Marfil-Marin, and colleagues used microarray technology to discover the circRNAs (circular RNA's) with differential expression and the biochemical pathways regulated through these circRNAs [52]. In a study that is first of its kind they discovered 23 circRNAs with variable expression, and they found that several pathways, like the dopaminergic synapse, MAPK, and long-term depression were notably enriched.

There is a significant genetic predisposing factor for amyotrophic lateral sclerosis (ALS), a fatal neurodegenerative illness which mostly impacts the motor neuron system of humans. A whole blood transcriptome microarray analysis of ALS carried out by Van Rheenen and coworkers discovered 2,943 transcripts that were differently expressed, mostly associated with RNA binding and intracellular trafficking [53]. Swindell and coworkers analyzed microarray data of blood samples derived from ALS patients and their healthy counterparts [54]. They discovered 61 genes that collectively considerably enhance survival prediction.

It is very difficult to diagnose Multiple Sclerosis (MS) early due to its chaotic and complex nature. Li and coworkers attempted to construct a diagnosis model for MS microarray data using peripheral blood RNA [55]. According to their findings, the diagnosis model used in this study had a high specificity (93.93 %), making it effective for differential diagnosis. In another study, Loveless and colleagues employed a tissue microarray methodology using tissue blocks from neocortex and subcortical sites of MS patients (Loveless et al., 2018). Their research demonstrated complement dysregulation in MS grey matter lesions, incorporating a relationship between tissue lesions and the numerical density of C1q+ cells.

Depression is on the rise as a result of genetic susceptibility, growing daily stress, and global difficulties. Lind and Tsai have compiled microarray studies regarding major depression disorder (MDD) in hopes of identifying the current understanding and limits of this disorder [56]. They have also determined the limitations of these studies. The key drawback in MDD studies was the small cohort size, which may have resulted in insufficient statistical data for the identification of important biomarkers. In a more current investigation, Yu and colleagues used the analysis of microarray data in identifying Arc and Homer1 involved in both epilepsy and depression [57]. They also identified mutual pathways such as regulation of angiogenesis and cellular response to interleukin-1. Feng and coworkers performed bioinformatics analysis on MDD data from GEO database where they identified several deregulated genes in connection with the disorder [58].

Although genetics play a significant part in its onset, the exact cause of schizophrenia (SCZ) is still unknown. Therefore, determining the origins of SCZ is essential to enhancing the effectiveness of treatments and the prognosis of those who suffer from the condition. Wagh and associates performed a systematic assessment of peripheral blood microarray studies using SCZ patients' and healthy controls' blood. They investigated 61 studies on gene expression, of which 17 used microarrays and two used RNA sequencing [59]. Microarray study outcomes compared between drug-naive and drug-treated SCZ patients revealed discrepancies. They concluded that cohort studies including a variety of groups, the application of high-throughput sequencing technologies, and the use of computational analysis based on artificial intelligence (AI) will considerably advance our comprehension and diagnostic capacities for this complicated condition. Long non-coding RNAs (lncRNAs) were the subject of an investigation by Wang et al. using a microarray dataset to examine how they altered the molecular mechanisms and pathways underlying SCZ pathophysiology [60]. Their findings suggested the pathophysiology of the disease involved a competing endogenous RNAs subnetwork that may be employed as possible diagnostic biomarkers. In another study, three microarray datasets were used in a meta-analysis carried out by Piras et al. to look for peripheral SCZ indicators [61]. Their findings indicated abnormalities in ATL3 peripheral expression in SCZ.

Extreme mood fluctuations, including mania and depression, are symptoms of bipolar disorder (BD), a heritable mental health illness. Choi and coworkers evaluated microarray data with postmortem tissue samples from patients with bipolar disorder (BD) and healthy controls. They also raised issues with this disease's research limitations, such as the inability of many studies to converge and the consequent difficulty in drawing general conclusions from individual findings [62]. To this end, they integrated machine learning techniques to their research which helped identify association of PPAR-G pathway with BD.

Impairments in social interaction and the appearance of constrained, repetitive activities or interests are the hallmarks of autism spectrum disorder (ASD), a neurodevelopmental condition with a significant hereditary basis [63]. ASD is extensively studied utilizing microarray techniques, like many other health conditions. Fajarda and colleagues attempted to develop a strategy for combining microarray datasets in hopes of determination of differentially expressed marker genes for ASD [64]. They used machine learning algorithms in conjunction with statistical analysis of the microarray data. Their method identified ASD marker genes with 98 % accuracy. In another study, Sevimoglu evaluated ASD utilizing microarray data on DNA methylation and gene expression concurrently [65]. 42 genes were found to be differently regulated and methylated as a result of the research, the majority of which had not previously been linked to ASD.

Attention deficit hyperactivity disorder (ADHD) is a developmental condition where patients demonstrate continual patterns of lack of attention, hyperactivity, and/or restlessness. Relationships and daily activities of these individuals might be substantially impacted by ADHD symptoms. Cabana-Domínguez and coworkers carried out microarray analysis of ADHD where they identified seven modules associated with the disorder as well as significantly altered signaling pathways using peripheral blood [66]. Another study done by Mortimer and coworkers assessed gene expression profiles of ADHD patients and healthy counterparts blood samples [67]. Their study determined eight candidate genes which were previously unidentified.

8.5.2 RNA-seq Studies

Determining the genetic causes of brain illnesses and disorders has also been made possible by this relatively new method of detecting and examining the transcriptome. The development of research in the area has greatly accelerated through the use of NGS technologies. Once again, this demonstrates how researchers used these experiments to try and elucidate every facet of the complex genetic system.In this section recent RNA-seq studies of brain diseases and disorders mentioned previously were presented.

Darmanis and colleagues performed single cell RNA-seq on tumor core and surrounding tissue of four patients with GBM [68]. A total of 3,589 cells were analyzed. In the tissue encircling the GBM tumor core, they were able to identify and characterize specific invading tumor cells. Additionally, they inferred minor genomic variants like insertions or deletions as well as genomic variation at the level of severe chromosomal abnormalities. Wan and colleagues examined the tumor immune environment of glioma and normal tissue samples using both RNA-seq and single cell RNA-seq [69]. The high necroptosis-related signature glioma patient group had a poor prognosis and a significant involvement of immunosuppressive cells, according to their research. Additionally, glioma showed elevated expression of the necroptosis suppressor CASP8, which was linked to a bad prognosis.

Brastionas and colleagues analyzed meningioma tissue samples using whole genome and whole exome sequencing [70]. AKT1 and SMO mutations that are frequently oncogenic were found in a fraction of meningiomas that did not have NF2 changes, and these meningiomas also showed immunohistochemistry evidence that their pathways had been activated. Using RNA-seq, Abedalthagafi and colleagues found that PI3K mutations were similarly frequent in meningiomas in a different study [71].

Zhou and collegues analyzed tissue samples of primary CNSL patients using next generation sequencing [72]. According to their study, recurring alterations in the NF-B pathway's KMT2D and CD79B components comprised 65 % of all mutations in PCNSL cases. In another RNA-seq study, Zhang et al. analyzed tumor and adjacent normal tissues and PBMCs of Chinese primary PCNSL patients using whole exome sequencing [73]. They revealed that MYD88 had the highest alteration rate, which had an impact on the NF-B pathway's activity. Furthermore, compared to samples with wild-type LRP1B, PCNSL samples with LRP1B mutations exhibited a greater mutation rate.

RNA-seq studies on AD are also in rise. Guennewig and colleagues used RNA-seq to uncover differentially elevated genes in post-mortem brains from AD patients and healthy controls in the primary visual cortex and precuneus [74]. Shigemizu and collegues performed analysis using whole genome sequencing data using blood of AD patients and their healthy counterparts [75]. They discovered a missense mutation in OR51G1 and a stop-gain variant in MLKL as potential candidates for AD link. Furthermore, through gene-based association analyses of uncommon variations, they also discovered additional candidate genes for AD. Using these candidates, they identified NCOR2, PLEC, DMD, and NEDD4 as functionally significant hub genes.

Eitan and colleagues recently carried out a whole genome sequencing investigation using microglia of ALS patients and their healthy counterparts [76]. Their findings highlight the value of non-coding genetic association studies and showed that different genetic variations protect against ALS via lowering neuroinflammation. In another study Brusati and coworkers performed whole genome sequencing on patients with ALS [77]. They detected 86 uncommon variations in 77 different miRNAs, spread throughout the miRNA precursors in various locations.

Novak et al employed single cell transcriptomics using human IPSC (Induced pluripotent stem cells) and identified a core network which interacts with all 19 PD genes [78]. They also showed that this core network is associated with key PD signaling pathways. Hemmings and coworkers identified common and distinct biological pathways for posttraumatic stress disorder, PD and SCZ in a South African sample using RNA-seq analysis [79].

In a study by Hensman Moss and colleagues, whole blood from two HD groups was used for RNA-Seq transcriptomic analysis, which discovered dysregulated gene sets in the blood of these individuals [80]. Their findings indicate that transcription is disturbed in peripheral cells in HD by similar mechanism of actions as those in the brain. Using single nucleus RNA-seq, Lim and colleagues conducted a transcriptome-wide association research for HD [81]. Their data reveal PRKCE and TPK1 as key genes and link aberrant cell maturation to glucose and lipid metabolism.

Rare mutations may be partially to blame for the absent MS heritability. Mescheriakova and colleagues performed whole exome sequencing in hopes of identifying rare variants associated with the disease [82]. They discovered an uncommon missense variation in the FKBP6 gene. Esposito and colleagues performed a whole genome sequencing study of MS patients and healthy controls using DNA and blood samples [83]. They found that in response to inflammatory triggers in peripheral monocytes, the activity of GRAMD1B was reduced in vessel-associated astrocytes of MS lesions, suggesting a potential role in the modulation of inflammatory response and disease development.

The field of RNA-seq research has also included neuropsychiatric disorders. Mostafavi and coworkers performed whole blood RNA-seq in MDD revealing that there was no substantial single-gene connection [84]. They discovered correlation between MDD and elevated gene expression in the interferon signaling pathway. Their findings are consistent with the theory that alterations in immunological signaling contribute to the advancement, appearance and persistence of MDD. A more recent study by Fabbri and colleagues employed whole exome sequencing and genome-wide genotyping to examine treatment-resistant depression (TRD), which affects 30 % of MDD patients [85]. They proposed pertinent biological pathways linked to TRD as well as a fresh methodological strategy for TRD prediction.

As stated before, for some brain disease and disorders a special effort was made to investigate blood biomarkers. Through the simultaneous measurement of mRNAs, long noncoding RNAs (lncRNAs), miRNAs, and circular RNAs (circRNAs) in a group of patients, Yang et al. carried out a whole transcriptome investigation using whole blood to identify the molecular networks in SZC [86]. Their comprehensive analysis identified dysregulated networks and pathways in SZC. There are also SZC studies that combine microarray and RNA-seq technologies. For instance, Bakewell and colleagues performed exome sequencing and SNP (single nucleotide polymorphism) array to determine rare copy number variants that effect patients with SZC [87]. Their results indicated that combining technologies enables the detection of variants that are too small (<100KB) to be accurately observed in only array data.

Palmer and colleagues performed analysis on curated whole exome sequencing data from patients with BD [88]. They discovered that AKAP-11 engages with GSK3B, which is assumed to be the target of lithium, the primary therapy for BD. Their findings show that uncommon coding variation is a major risk contributor in the etiology of BD, supporting the polygenicity of BD. In order to study the exonic variation in BD, Jia and colleagues did whole genome and whole exome sequencing in a variety of cohorts [89]. In their work, which was the broadest investigation of exonic variation in BD, they discovered that there is no consistent enrichment of rare pathogenic/likely pathogenic (P-LP) changes in the exome or in any of the numerous gene families with biological significance in BD patients. Furthermore, despite a significant shared vulnerability between BD and SCZ due to similar genetic variation, a connection among BD risk and infrequent P-LP coding mutations in genes known to affect SCZ risk was not discovered. In an interesting study Kathuria et al generated 3D organoid model from human induced pluripotent stem cells (IPSCs) and analyzed them by designing an RNA-seq experiment with BD and healthy individuals [90]. Their findings demonstrated that neurocan plays a critical role in the biology of BD. They offered evidence of aberrant neurotransmission, and they revealed dysregulation in genes associated to cell adhesion, immunological signaling, and endoplasmic reticulum biology.

A growing resource for the autism research community, SFARI gene is focused on curated genes thought to play a role in autism susceptibility (https://gene.sfari.org). Other ASD scoring approaches and even data regarding other neurodevelopmental diseases are influenced by the SFARI gene scoring system's impact. Arpi and colleagues carried out research to determine the relationship between ASD-specific transcriptomic data and SFARI genes using RNA-seq data [91]. Their findings suggested that in order to effectively analyze the link between SFARI genes and ASD-specific RNAseq transcriptomic data, information drawn from the entire gene co-expression network is necessary. Furthermore, they have demonstrated that SFARI genes are not significantly connected with either differential expression results or co-expression modules with a high connection to diagnostic state. Rather, for the novel candidate gene prediction strategy described in the research, thorough systems-level network analysis and the use of machine learning models to combine different data sources in disease scenarios may out to be extremely beneficial. In another study, RNA sequencing was carried out by Tomaiuolo and colleagues on the peripheral blood of children with ASD and their unaffected siblings [92]. In addition to providing more proof that neurodevelopment, innate immunity, and transcriptional control are important factors in the etiology of ASD, their findings showed that transcriptome signatures can help increase the sensitivity of an intra-familial multimarker screening for the disorder.

Wang and coworkers performed NGS using whole blood samples from ADHD patients and their healthy counterparts [93]. 13 miRNAs were discovered as possible indicators for ADHD. In another study, Mccaffrey and associates performed whole blood RNA sequencing on ADHD patients under case-control [94]. They identified putative functions for a number of genes with differential expression, including ABCB5, RGS2, GAK, and GIT1, which have been linked mechanistically to molecular pathways associated with behavioral control and ADHD in the past.

8.6 Integration of Brain Transcriptomics and Imaging Data

There comes a time where data from only one source is not enough to understand the big picture anymore and integration of several types of data is necessary to move forward. Integrating brain transcriptomics with neuroimaging data advanced with the public unveiling of the Allen Human Brain Atlas (AHBA) dataset in 2012. This dataset contained histology data, structural MRI (sMRI), and whole-brain microarray transcriptome data collected from healthy mature human subjects [95]. Since then, attempts were made to integrate imaging with transcriptomics to shed more light into the etiology and progression of these brain diseases and disorders as well as diagnostic and therapeutic studies. For instance, Adewale and coworkers proposed a spatiotemporal brain model that takes into consideration the direct interaction between numerous RNA transcripts and macroscale imaging techniques like MRI and PET [96]. In another study, Wu and coworkers worked on a so-called federated model in detection of genomic and transcriptomic factors associated with AD using sMRI, GWAS (genome-wide association studies), and transcriptomics data [97]. It is important to interpret the interplay of biological factors at various spatial resolutions. This area is also called imaging genetics, which is the application of neuroimaging tools to examine how genetic differences affect brain structure or function in order to gain an insight into how these variations affect behavior and disease phenotypes [98]. Research in this field has been gaining momentum in recent years [99–107]. There are also online tools specialized in this area. One example of such tools is the Neuroimaging Informatics Tools and Resources Clearinghouse (www.nitrc.org), often known as NITRC-R. It is a collection of resources for neuroimaging, including data sets, software for analysis, and computer power. The research focus of NITRC comprises software tools, data, and computational resources for MR, PET/SPECT (Single-photon emission computed tomography), CT (computerized tomography), EEG (electroencephalogram)/MEG (Magnetoencephalography), optical imaging, clinical neuroimaging, computational neuroscience, and imaging genomics.

The abovementioned techniques and resources will assist in less invasive understanding of the researched diseases since both microarray and RNA-seq experiments on brain diseases mostly depend on data obtained through invasive sampling such as tissue from different areas of the brain which obviously is usually taken from a deceased person/animal.

The swift rise of various big data analysis methodologies, including artificial intelligence tools, may result in the creation of personalized patient-tailored diagnoses. In the future, in silico diagnostics is anticipated to be similar, reliable, less subject to variation, objective, and error-free [108].

8.7 Future Perspectives

Understanding the microscopic and macroscopic phenotypes of the healthy and the diseased brain and integrating them is difficult but necessary. Using microarray and RNA-seq high throughput technologies helped us move faster than ever before in elucidating the abovementioned neurological conditions. Nonetheless, both techniques have limitations that prevent us from establishing a solid genetic mechanism for the studied diseases and disorders. For instance, brain tissue samples are collected postmortem hence there may be a small sample size for each experiment. Another issue we may face is that every microarray platform has its own probe sets and annotations so comparing them also means annotation conversions are necessary. Some of the information may be lost during these conversions. Even in the same platform a gene may be assigned multiple probes, and this may cause wrongful identification of a gene, miRNA etc. RNA-seq does not rely on specific probes so this issue may be non-existent while using this technique. Still quality control issues surrounding the samples in the first place plus the cost of running an experiment with RNA-seq are two major issues currently dealt with. In addition, the data obtained from both high-throughput technologies as well as other technologies are increasing so maybe making good use of the information at hand is the best we can do currently. Knowing the limitations of the current technology will guide us in making better technologies in the future.

We may be able to accomplish our goal of deciphering the genetic mechanisms more quickly by combining new techniques with the recent discoveries, like imaging techniques and artificial intelligence systems. Since it is challenging to collect tissue samples before the patient passes away, the utilization of human organoids that develop in vitro environments with organ complexity similar to that found in vivo may be another potential new area of research especially for diseases and disorders of the brain. The rapidly changing innovative technologies give us hope that someday we will have deciphered the mechanisms that mediate our brain and present personalized therapeutics for each individual without any invasive experiments.

8.8 Conclusion

In this chapter, the methods for analyzing the brain transcriptome, the repositories utilized to store the information obtained using these high throughput methods, as well as the tools for data processing and visualization, have been covered. The advantages and disadvantages of each technique have been put forward. Furthermore, examples of recent microarray and RNA-seq studies on the disorders discussed in this book are given. A number of recommendations have been made that could aid researchers in better understanding the data now available on brain disease and disorders, including merging various methodologies (imaging techniques, transcriptomics data, and artificial intelligence techniques). Future viewpoints have also been presented to guide the research in this area.

Bibliography

[1] A. Bayat, "Science, medicine, and the future: Bioinformatics," *BMJ*, vol. 324 7344, pp. 1018–22, 2002.

[2] L. Hunt, "Margaret o. dayhoff 1925-1983," *DNA*, vol. 2 2, pp. 97–8, 1983.

[3] T. M. Morse, "Neuroinformatics: From bioinformatics to databasing the brain," *Bioinformatics and Biology Insights*, vol. 2, pp. 253–264, 2008.

[4] F. M. Giorgi, C. Ceraolo, and D. Mercatelli, "The r language: An engine for bioinformatics and data science," *Life*, vol. 12, 2022.

[5] M. Fourment and M. R. Gillings, "A comparison of common programming languages used in bioinformatics," *BMC Bioinformatics*, vol. 9, pp. 82–82, 2008.

[6] R. G. T. Lowe, N. J. Shirley, M. R. Bleackley, *et al.*, "Transcriptomics technologies," *PLoS Computational Biology*, vol. 13, 2017.

[7] T. Lenoir and E. Giannella, "The emergence and diffusion of dna microarray technology," *Journal of Biomedical Discovery and Collaboration*, vol. 1, pp. 11–11, 2006.

[8] R. Govindarajan, J. Duraiyan, K. Kaliyappan, *et al.*, "Microarray and its applications," *Journal of Pharmacy & Bioallied Sciences*, vol. 4, pp. S310–S312, 2012.

[9] U. R. Müller and D. V. Nicolau, "Microarray technology and its applications," *Springer*, Berlin, 2005.

[10] R. E. Bumgarner, "Overview of dna microarrays: types, applications, and their future," *Current protocols in molecular biology*, vol. Chapter 22, p. Unit 22.1., 2013.

[11] J. Chen, V. Agrawal, M. Rattray, *et al.*, "A comparison of microarray and mpss technology platforms for expression analysis of arabidopsis," *BMC Genomics*, vol. 8, pp. 414–414, 2007.

[12] S. Maouche, O. Poirier, T. Godefroy, *et al.*, "Performance comparison of two microarray platforms to assess differential gene expression in human monocyte and macrophage cells," *BMC Genomics*, vol. 9, pp. 302–302, 2008.

[13] R. Jaksik, M. Iwanaszko, J. Rzeszowska-Wolny, *et al.*, "Microarray experiments and factors which affect their reliability," *Biology Direct*, vol. 10, 2015.

[14] A. Haque, J. A. Engel, S. A. Teichmann, *et al.*, "A practical guide to single-cell rna-sequencing for biomedical research and clinical applications," *Genome Medicine*, vol. 9, 2017.

[15] K. R. Kukurba and S. B. Montgomery, "Rna sequencing and analysis," *Cold Spring Harbor protocols*, vol. 2015 11, pp. 951–69, 2015.

[16] D. Deshpande, K. Chhugani, Y. Chang, *et al.*, "Rna-seq data science: From raw data to effective interpretation," *Frontiers in Genetics*, vol. 14, 2023.

[17] E. Korpelainen, J. Tuimala, P. Somervuo, *et al.*, "Rna-seq data analysis: A practical approach," 2014.

[18] X. Li, A. A. Nair, S. Wang, *et al.*, "Quality control of rna-seq experiments," *Methods in Molecular Biology*, vol. 1269, pp. 137–46, 2015.

[19] Q. Zhou, X. Su, G. Jing, *et al.*, "Rna-qc-chain: comprehensive and fast quality control for rna-seq data," *BMC Genomics*, vol. 19, 2018.

[20] S. Zhao, W.-P. Fung-Leung, A. Bittner, *et al.*, "Comparison of rna-seq and microarray in transcriptome profiling of activated t cells," *PLoS ONE*, vol. 9, 2014.

[21] A. Athar, A. Füllgrabe, N. George, *et al.*, "Arrayexpress update – from bulk to single-cell expression data," *Nucleic Acids Research*, vol. 47, pp. D711–D715, 2018.

[22] Y. Tanizawa, T. Fujisawa, Y. Kodama, *et al.*, "Dna data bank of japan (ddbj) update report 2022," *Nucleic Acids Research*, vol. 51, pp. D101–D105, 2022.

[23] R. Gentleman, V. J. Carey, D. M. Bates, *et al.*, "Bioconductor: open software development for computational biology and bioinformatics," *Genome Biology*, vol. 5, pp. R80–R80, 2004.

[24] M. E. Ritchie, B. Phipson, D.-L. Wu, *et al.*, "limma powers differential expression analyses for rna-sequencing and microarray studies," *Nucleic Acids Research*, vol. 43, pp. e47–e47, 2015.

[25] S. Liu, Z. Wang, R. hui Zhu, *et al.*, "Three differential expression analysis methods for rna sequencing: limma, edger, deseq2," *Journal of visualized experiments: JoVE*, vol. 175, 2021.

[26] M. D. Robinson, D. J. McCarthy, and G. K. Smyth, "edger: a bioconductor package for differential expression analysis of digital gene expression data," *Bioinformatics*, vol. 26, pp. 139–140, 2009.

[27] M. I. Love, W. Huber, and S. Anders, "Moderated estimation of fold change and dispersion for rna-seq data with deseq2," *Genome Biology*, vol. 15, 2014.

[28] S. P. Lloyd, "Least squares quantization in pcm," *IEEE Trans. Inf. Theory*, vol. 28, pp. 129–136, 1982.

[29] S. C. Johnson, "Hierarchical clustering schemes," *Psychometrika*, vol. 32, pp. 241–254, 1967.

[30] P. Shannon, A. Markiel, O. Ozier, N. S. Baliga, J. T. Wang, D. Ramage, N. Amin, B. Schwikowski, and T. Ideker, "Cytoscape: a software environment for integrated models of biomolecular interaction networks," *Genome research*, vol. 13 11, pp. 2498–504, 2003.

[31] K. Tomczak, P. Czerwińska, and M. Wiznerowicz, "The cancer genome atlas (tcga): an immeasurable source of knowledge," *Contemporary Oncology*, vol. 19, pp. A68–A77, 2015.

[32] M. Kanehisa and S. Goto, "Kegg: Kyoto encyclopedia of genes and genomes," *Nucleic acids research*, vol. 28 1, pp. 27–30, 2000.

[33] P. D. Thomas, D. Ebert, A. Muruganujan, *et al.*, "Panther: Making genome-scale phylogenetics accessible to all," *Protein Science*, vol. 31, pp. 22–8, 2021.

[34] A. Subramanian, P. Tamayo, V. K. Mootha, *et al.*, "Gene set enrichment analysis: A knowledge-based approach for interpreting genome-wide expression profiles," *Proceedings of the National Academy of Sciences of the United States of America*, vol. 102, pp. 15545–15550, 2005.

[35] B. T. Sherman, M. Hao, J. Qiu, *et al.*, "David: a web server for functional enrichment analysis and functional annotation of gene lists (2021 update)," *Nucleic acids research*, 2022.

[36] K. G. Becker, K. C. Barnes, T. J. Bright, *et al.*, "The genetic association database," *Nature Genetics*, vol. 36, pp. 431–432, 2004.

[37] J. S. Amberger, C. A. Bocchini, A. F. Scott, *et al.*, "Omim.org: leveraging knowledge across phenotype–gene relationships," *Nucleic Acids Research*, vol. 47, pp. D1038–D1043, 2018.

[38] A. Bauer-Mehren, M. Bundschus, M. Rautschka, *et al.*, "Gene-disease network analysis reveals functional modules in mendelian, complex and environmental diseases," *PLoS ONE*, vol. 6, 2011.

[39] N. Grech, T. A. Dalli, S. Mizzi, *et al.*, "Rising incidence of glioblastoma multiforme in a well-defined population," *Cureus*, vol. 12, 2020.

[40] K. M. Bhawe and M. K. Aghi, "Microarray analysis in glioblastomas," *Methods in molecular biology*, vol. 1375, pp. 195–206, 2016.

[41] S. Wang, F. Liu, Y. Wang, *et al.*, "Integrated analysis of 34 microarray datasets reveals cbx3 as a diagnostic and prognostic biomarker in glioblastoma," *Journal of Translational Medicine*, vol. 17, 2019.

[42] Y. Zhang, J. Xu, and X. Zhu, "A 63 signature genes prediction system is effective for glioblastoma prognosis," *International Journal of Molecular Medicine*, vol. 41, pp. 2070–2078, 2018.

[43] M. A. Wedemeyer, I. S. Muskens, B. A. Strickland, *et al.*, "Epigenetic dysregulation in meningiomas," *Neuro-Oncology Advances*, vol. 4, 2022.

[44] F. Menghi, F. Orzan, M. Eoli, *et al.*, "Dna microarray analysis identifies cks2 and lepr as potential markers of meningioma recurrence," *The oncologist*, vol. 16 10, pp. 1440–50, 2011.

[45] D. Villa, K. L. Tan, C. Steidl, *et al.*, "Molecular features of a large cohort of primary central nervous system lymphoma using tissue microarray," *Blood advances*, vol. 3 23, pp. 3953–3961, 2019.

[46] Y. Takashima, A. Kawaguchi, Y. Iwadate, *et al.*, "mir-101, mir-548b, mir-554, and mir-1202 are reliable prognosis predictors of the mirnas associated with cancer immunity in primary central nervous system lymphoma," *PLoS ONE*, vol. 15, 2020.

[47] H. Takei, L. W. Buckleair, A. L. Rivera, *et al.*, "Brain tissue microarrays in neurodegenerative diseases: Validation of methodology and immunohistochemical study of growth-associated protein-43 and calretinin," *Pathology International*, vol. 57, 2007.

[48] C. Blauwendraat, O. Pletnikova, J. T. Geiger, *et al.*, "Genetic analysis of neurodegenerative diseases in a pathology cohort," *Neurobiology of Aging*, vol. 76, pp. 214.e1–214.e9, 2019.

[49] M. K. Sakharkar, S. K. K. Singh, K. Rajamanickam, *et al.*, "A systems biology approach towards the identification of candidate therapeutic genes and potential biomarkers for parkinson's disease," *PLoS ONE*, vol. 14, 2019.

[50] Y. Miki, S. Shimoyama, T. Kon, *et al.*, "Alteration of autophagy-related proteins in peripheral blood mononuclear cells of patients with parkinson's disease," *Neurobiology of Aging*, vol. 63, pp. 33–43, 2018.

[51] Z. Zhou, S. Zhong, R. Zhang, *et al.*, "Functional analysis of brain derived neurotrophic factor (bdnf) in huntington's disease," *Aging (Albany NY)*, vol. 13, pp. 6103–6114, 2021.

[52] E. Marfil-Marín, M. Santamaría-Olmedo, A. PerezGrovas-Saltijeral, *et al.*, "circrna regulates dopaminergic synapse, mapk, and long-term depression pathways in huntington disease," *Molecular Neurobiology*, vol. 58, pp. 6222–6231, 2021.

[53] W. van Rheenen, F. P. Diekstra, O. Harschnitz, H.-J. Westeneng, *et al.*, "Whole blood transcriptome analysis in amyotrophic lateral sclerosis: A biomarker study," *PLoS ONE*, vol. 13, 2018.

[54] W. R. Swindell, C. Kruse, E. O. List, *et al.*, "Als blood expression profiling identifies new biomarkers, patient subgroups, and evidence for neutrophilia and hypoxia," *Journal of Translational Medicine*, vol. 17, 2019.

[55] H. Li, H. Wu, W. Li, *et al.*, "Constructing a multiple sclerosis diagnosis model based on microarray," *Frontiers in Neurology*, vol. 12, 2022.

[56] E. Lin and S.-J. Tsai, "Genome-wide microarray analysis of gene expression profiling in major depression and antidepressant therapy," *Progress in Neuro-Psychopharmacology and Biological Psychiatry*, vol. 64, pp. 334–340, 2016.

[57] S. qian Yu, G. Wang, B. Yao, *et al.*, "Arc and homer1 are involved in comorbid epilepsy and depression: A microarray data analysis," *Epilepsy & Behavior*, vol. 132, 2022.

[58] J. Feng, Q. Zhou, W. Gao, Y. Wu, *et al.*, "Seeking for potential pathogenic genes of major depressive disorder in the gene expression omnibus database," *Asia-Pacific Psychiatry*, vol. 12, 2019.

[59] V. V. Wagh, P. Vyas, S. Agrawal, *et al.*, "Peripheral blood-based gene expression studies in schizophrenia: A systematic review," *Frontiers in Genetics*, vol. 12, 2021.

[60] J. quan Wang, Y. ru Liu, Y. Gao, J. Liang, *et al.*, "Comprehensive bioinformatics analysis and molecular validation of lncrnas-mediated cernas network in schizophrenia," *Life sciences*, p. 121205, 2022.

[61] I. S. Piras, M. Manchia, M. J. Huentelman, *et al.*, "Peripheral biomarkers in schizophrenia: A meta-analysis of microarray gene expression datasets," *International Journal of Neuropsychopharmacology*, vol. 22, pp. 186–193, 2018.

[62] J. Choi, D. F. Bodenstein, J. Geraci, *et al.*, "Evaluation of postmortem microarray data in bipolar disorder using traditional data comparison and artificial intelligence reveals novel gene targets," *Journal of psychiatric research*, vol. 142, pp. 328–336, 2021.

[63] H. Hodges, C. Fealko, and N. Soares, "Autism spectrum disorder: definition, epidemiology, causes, and clinical evaluation," *Translational Pediatrics*, vol. 9, pp. S55–S65, 2020.

[64] O. Fajarda, J. R. Almeida, S. Duarte-Pereira, *et al.*, "Methodology to identify a gene expression signature by merging microarray datasets," *Computers in biology and medicine*, vol. 159, p. 106867, 2023.

[65] T. Sevimoglu, "In silico analysis of autism spectrum disorder through the integration of dna methylation and gene expression data for biomarker search," *Minerva Biotechnology and Biomolecular Research*, vol. 35, no. 2, pp. 73–80, 2023.

[66] J. Cabana-Domínguez, M. S. Artigas, L. Arribas, *et al.*, "Comprehensive analysis of omics data identifies relevant gene networks for attention-deficit/hyperactivity disorder (adhd)," *Translational Psychiatry*, vol. 12, 2022.

[67] N. Mortimer, C. Sánchez-Mora, P. Rovira, *et al.*, "Transcriptome profiling in adult attention-deficit hyperactivity disorder," *European Neuropsychopharmacology*, vol. 41, pp. 160–166, 2020.

[68] S. Darmanis, S. A. Sloan, D. Croote, *et al.*, "Single-cell rnaseq analysis of infiltrating neoplastic cells at the migrating front of human glioblastoma," *bioRxiv*, 2017.

[69] S. Wan, U. A. E. Moure, R. Liu, and C. L. others, "Combined bulk rna-seq and single-cell rna-seq identifies a necroptosis-related prognostic signature associated with inhibitory immune microenvironment in glioma," *Frontiers in Immunology*, vol. 13, 2022.

[70] P. K. Brastianos, P. Horowitz, S. Santagata, *et al.*, "Genomic sequencing of meningiomas identifies oncogenic smo and akt1 mutations," *Nature genetics*, vol. 45, pp. 285–289, 2013.

[71] M. S. Abedalthagafi, W. L. Bi, A. A. Aizer, *et al.*, "Oncogenic pi3k mutations are as common as akt1 and smo mutations in meningioma," *Neuro-oncology*, vol. 18 5, pp. 649–55, 2016.

[72] Y. Zhou, W. Liu, Z. Xu, *et al.*, "Analysis of genomic alteration in primary central nervous system lymphoma and the expression of some related genes," *Neoplasia (New York, N.Y.)*, vol. 20, pp. 1059–1069, 2018.

[73] R. Zhang, B. yuan Wei, Y. Hu, *et al.*, "Whole-exome sequencing revealed the mutational profiles of primary central nervous system lymphoma," *Clinical lymphoma, myeloma & leukemia*, 2023.

[74] B. Guennewig, J. Lim, L. L. Marshall, *et al.*, "Defining early changes in alzheimer's disease from rna sequencing of brain regions differentially affected by pathology," *Scientific Reports*, vol. 11, 2021.

[75] D. Shigemizu, Y. Asanomi, S. Akiyama, *et al.*, "Whole-genome sequencing reveals novel ethnicity-specific rare variants associated with alzheimer's disease," *Molecular Psychiatry*, vol. 27, pp. 2554–2562, 2022.

[76] C. Eitan, A. Siany, E. Barkan, *et al.*, "Whole-genome sequencing reveals that variants in the interleukin 18 receptor accessory protein 3utr protect against als," *Nature neuroscience*, vol. 25, pp. 433–445, 2022.

[77] A. Brusati, A. Ratti, V. Pensato, *et al.*, "Analysis of mirna rare variants in amyotrophic lateral sclerosis and in silico prediction of their biological effects," *Frontiers in Genetics*, vol. 13, 2022.

[78] G. Novak, D. Kyriakis, K. Grzyb, *et al.*, "Single-cell transcriptomics of human ipsc differentiation dynamics reveal a core molecular network of parkinson's disease," *Communications Biology*, vol. 5, 2022.

[79] S. M. J. Hemmings, P. C. Swart, J. S. Womersely, *et al.*, "Rna-seq analysis of gene expression profiles in posttraumatic stress disorder, parkinson's disease and schizophrenia identifies roles for common and distinct biological pathways," *Discover Mental Health*, vol. 2, 2022.

[80] D. J. H. Moss, M. Flower, K. K. Lo, *et al.*, "Huntington's disease blood and brain show a common gene expression pattern and share an immune signature with alzheimer's disease," *Scientific Reports*, vol. 7, 2017.

[81] R. G. Lim, O. Al-Dalahmah, J. Wu, *et al.*, "Huntington disease oligodendrocyte maturation deficits revealed by single-nucleus rnaseq are rescued by thiamine-biotin supplementation," *Nature Communications*, vol. 13, 2022.

[82] J. Y. Mescheriakova, A. J. Verkerk, N. Amin, *et al.*, "Linkage analysis and whole exome sequencing identify a novel candidate gene in a dutch multiple sclerosis family," *Multiple Sclerosis (Houndmills, Basingstoke, England)*, vol. 25, pp. 909–917, 2018.

[83] F. Esposito, A. M. Osiceanu, M. Sorosina, *et al.*, "A whole-genome sequencing study implicates gramd1b in multiple sclerosis susceptibility," *Genes*, vol. 13, 2022.

[84] S. Mostafavi, A. J. Battle, X. Zhu, *et al.*, "Type i interferon signaling genes in recurrent major depression: increased expression detected by whole-blood rna sequencing," *Molecular psychiatry*, vol. 19, pp. 1267–1274, 2013.

[85] C. Fabbri, S. Kasper, A. Kautzky, *et al.*, "A polygenic predictor of treatment-resistant depression using whole exome sequencing and genome-wide genotyping," *Translational Psychiatry*, vol. 10, 2019.

[86] J. Yang, Q. Long, Y. Zhang, *et al.*, "Whole transcriptome analysis reveals dysregulation of molecular networks in schizophrenia," *Asian journal of psychiatry*, vol. 85, p. 103649, 2023.

[87] J. P. Bakewell, L. Hubbard, S. E. Legge, *et al.*, "Combining exome sequencing and microarray data to identify rare cnvs impacting cognition in schizophrenia," *European Neuropsychopharmacology*, vol. 63, 2022.

[88] D. S. Palmer, D. P. Howrigan, S. B. Chapman, *et al.*, "Exome sequencing in bipolar disorder identifies akap11 as a risk gene shared with schizophrenia," *Nature Genetics*, vol. 54, pp. 541–547, 2022.

[89] X. Jia, F. S. Goes, A. E. Locke, *et al.*, "Investigating rare pathogenic/likely pathogenic exonic variation in bipolar disorder," *Molecular Psychiatry*, vol. 26, pp. 5239–5250, 2021.

[90] A. Kathuria, K. Lopez-Lengowski, M. Vater, *et al.*, "Transcriptome analysis and functional characterization of cerebral organoids in bipolar disorder," *Genome Medicine*, vol. 12, 2020.

[91] M. N. T. Arpi and I. Simpson, "Sfari genes and where to find them; modelling autism spectrum disorder specific gene expression dysregulation with rna-seq data," *Scientific Reports*, vol. 12, 2022.

[92] P. Tomaiuolo, I. S. Piras, S. B. Sain, *et al.*, "Rna sequencing of blood from sex- and age-matched discordant siblings supports immune and transcriptional dysregulation in autism spectrum disorder," *Scientific Reports*, vol. 13, 2023.

[93] L.-J. Wang, S.-C. Li, M.-J. Lee, *et al.*, "Blood-bourne microrna biomarker evaluation in attention-deficit/hyperactivity disorder of han chinese individuals: An exploratory study," *Frontiers in Psychiatry*, vol. 9, 2018.

[94] T. A. McCaffrey, G. I. S. Laurent, D. Shtokalo, *et al.*, "Biomarker discovery in attention deficit hyperactivity disorder: Rna sequencing of whole

blood in discordant twin and case-controlled cohorts," *BMC Medical Genomics*, vol. 13, 2020.

[95] M. J. Hawrylycz, E. S. Lein, A. Guillozet-Bongaarts, *et al.*, "An anatomically comprehensive atlas of the adult human brain transcriptome," *Nature*, vol. 489, pp. 391–399, 2012.

[96] Q. Adewale, A. F. Khan, F. Carbonell, *et al.*, "Integrated transcriptomic and neuroimaging brain model decodes biological mechanisms in aging and alzheimer's disease," *eLife*, vol. 10, 2021.

[97] J. Wu, Y. Chen, P. Wang, *et al.*, "Integrating transcriptomics, genomics, and imaging in alzheimer's disease: A federated model," *Frontiers in radiology*, vol. 1, 2021.

[98] K. E. Muñoz, L. W. Hyde, and A. R. Hariri, "Imaging genetics," *Journal of the American Academy of Child and Adolescent Psychiatry*, vol. 48 4, pp. 356–61, 2009.

[99] S. H. Ameis and P. Szatmari, "Imaging-genetics in autism spectrum disorder: Advances, translational impact, and future directions," *Frontiers in Psychiatry*, vol. 3, 2012.

[100] M. Fakhoury, "Imaging genetics in autism spectrum disorders: Linking genetics and brain imaging in the pursuit of the underlying neurobiological mechanisms," *Progress in Neuro-Psychopharmacology and Biological Psychiatry*, vol. 80, pp. 101–114, 2018.

[101] R. Hashimoto, K. Ohi, H. Yamamori, *et al.*, "Imaging genetics and psychiatric disorders," *Current Molecular Medicine*, vol. 15, pp. 168 –175, 2015.

[102] M. Huang, X. Chen, Y. Yu, *et al.*, "Imaging genetics study based on a temporal group sparse regression and additive model for biomarker detection of alzheimer's disease," *IEEE Transactions on Medical Imaging*, vol. 40, pp. 1461–1473, 2021.

[103] W. Jiang, T. Z. King, and J. A. Turner, "Imaging genetics towards a refined diagnosis of schizophrenia," *Frontiers in Psychiatry*, vol. 10, 2019.

[104] M. Klein, M. M. J. van Donkelaar, E. Verhoef, *et al.*, "Imaging genetics in neurodevelopmental psychopathology," *American Journal of Medical Genetics Part B: Neuropsychiatric Genetics*, vol. 174, pp. 485–537, 2017.

[105] B. D. Le and J. L. Stein, "Mapping causal pathways from genetics to neuropsychiatric disorders using genome-wide imaging genetics: Current status and future directions," *Psychiatry and Clinical Neurosciences*, vol. 73, 2019.

[106] C. Scharinger, U. Rabl, H. H. Sitte, *et al.*, "Imaging genetics of mood disorders," *NeuroImage*, vol. 53, pp. 810–821, 2010.

[107] Y. Xin, J. Sheng, M. Miao, *et al.*, "A review ofimaging genetics in alzheimer's disease," *Journal of Clinical Neuroscience*, vol. 100, pp. 155–163, 2022.

[108] I. Jovcevska, "Next generation sequencing and machine learning technologies are painting the epigenetic portrait of glioblastoma," *Frontiers in Oncology*, vol. 10, 2020.

9

Complex Brain Networks: A Graph-Theoretical Analysis

Kayhan Erciyes

Yaşar University, İzmir, Türkiye

Complex brain networks are large consisting of many functional nodes and many more connections between them. A complex brain network may be modeled by a graph enabling many results obtained in this field of mathematics to be applied to the analysis of these networks. The nodes in a graph representing a brain network denote regions of the brain and edges show the structural or functional connections between these regions. In this review, we first describe how to construct various brain networks from data obtained by neuroimaging methods. We then review the analysis processes of graphs representing brain networks and focus on three main areas of research in brain networks: module detection to find clusters in brain networks, motif search to detect frequent repeating subgraphs and network alignment to evaluate similarities between two or more brain networks. We also provide a review of brain network alterations in various neurological disorders.

9.1 Introduction

Analysis of the brain has been an active research area due to three main advancements in the last decades: advancement in neuroimaging technologies, development of high-performance computers and development of software, algorithms and methods to analyze data obtained from various neuroimaging processes [1] which may be visualized as a graph with nodes and edges connecting the nodes.

Complex networks are large, consisting of thousands of nodes and tens of thousands of edges between these nodes. These networks range from biological networks to the Internet and to social networks. Analysis of these seemingly

DOI: 10.1201/9781003461906-9

diverse networks shows that they have some common characteristics not found in randomly constructed networks of similar sizes. Firstly, distance between any two nodes in a complex network is small compared to the number of nodes and this effect is called *small-world* property. Another frequently observed structure in complex networks is the manifestation of very few nodes with high number of connections where the rest of the nodes have fewer connections in general, termed as *scale-free* feature. Brain networks are a class of complex networks exhibiting the aforementioned small-world and scale-free properties, moreover, hierarchical cluster structures are also present in these networks.

In this review, we first describe the construction of various brain networks using data from neuroimaging techniques. We then review fundamental large graph analysis parameters and then concentrate on three main areas of brain network analysis: module detection or clustering, network motif search, and network alignment. We also investigate the relationship between brain networks and diseases of the brain with emphasis on the alterations of the brain networks due to neurological disorders. We conclude by reviewing the benefits of using graph theory as a tool to investigate brain networks to understand functioning of the brain in health and disease.

9.2 Brain Network Construction

The main neuroimaging technologies are functional magnetic resonance imaging (fMRI), diffusion tensor imaging (DTI), and electroencephalography (EEG) which may be utilized effectively to build brain networks. Difficulty of building a network of neuron nodes and interactions between them only entails dividing the brain into coarser areas called *region of interest* (ROI) with edges representing the communication between the ROIs. Types of networks produced by various neuroimaging methods are as follows [1]:

- *Structural Brain Networks*: This type of brain network, is formed using neuron synaptic connections and tracks that connect a cluster of neurons to another cluster. Brain networks obtained this way are called *structural brain networks* (SBN). Structure of a SBN is stable with changes in time scales of seconds or minutes.

- *Functional Brain Networks* (FBN): This brain network is constructed using fMRI data which is obtained by evaluating the blood-oxygen-level-dependent (BOLD) signal that shows the neural activity in a brain region.

- *Morphological Brain Networks* (MBN): The morphological brain networks consider the size, the shape and structure of brain regions such as cortical thickness or grey matter volume, rather than the functions performed by them. Commonly, average cortical values are calculated for each region and the difference in these values between two regions is used to determine the edge weight of the edge between them to construct the overall graph.

- *Effective Brain Networks* (EBN): This type of connectivity shows the casual interactions between brain regions by considering the influence of one brain region to another.

We will focus on the construction of FBNs here and the analysis of these networks throughout this review as this type of brain network is the subject of various research studies to analyze brain functions. The main steps of building such a network are as follows: [2]:

1. *Defining the nodes*: Dividing the brain into large-scale homogeneous and non-overlapping regions is performed to define the nodes of the network. Selection of these regions is called *parcellation* which is the process of dividing the brain into distinct regions based on anatomical, morphological or topological criteria.
2. *Computation of Connection Matrix*: Estimating the network connectivity is commonly employed by correlation and partial correlation to quantify brain activity between the ROIs. These methods provide similarity information between the time series or frequency spectra of nodes which can be used to construct the connectivity matrix C. The wiring diagram of the brain regions obtained in this manner is commonly called the *connectome* which is formed by the matrix representation of all pairwise connections between ROIs.
3. Thresholding: This is the process of filtering the connectivity matrix C such that connectivity values below a certain parameter are deleted from this matrix. As a result, the connectivity matrix C is processed to yield a binary matrix A such that entry $a_{ij} = 1$ if node i is connected to node j. A fixed threshold or a fixed threshold node degree or a fixed edge density value may be used to filter the connection matrix [2].

The processing of these steps that results in the connectome of the brain is depicted in Figure 9.1. The connection matrix C provides the representation of an edge weighted graph $G = (V, E, w)$ where V is the set of nodes, E is the set of edges and function $f : E \rightarrow \mathbb{R}$ provides the weights associated with edges which can be directed or undirected, depending on the interpretations of interactions between the nodes. This graph may be considered as a complete graph by associating a null value for an edge between two nodes that are not related. The binary adjacency matrix A can be used to build an unweighted, undirected graph $G = (V, E)$ over which various analysis methods may be applied.

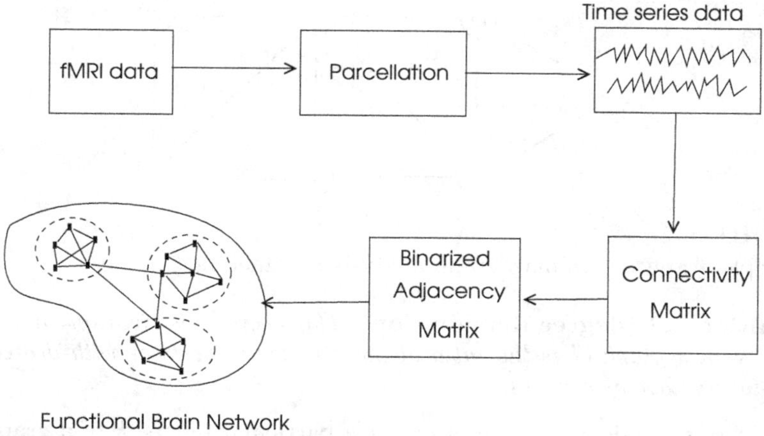

FIGURE 9.1
Functional brain network construction.

9.3 Analysis Parameters

We review basic parameters used in the analysis of brain networks which provide information on the local or global network structures, and in many cases, global network structures may be deduced from the local ones.

9.3.1 Density and Degree Distribution

The density of a graph shows how well it is connected; s *sparse graph* has very few connections between its nodes in the order of $O(n)$ where n is the number of nodes. A *dense graph* on the other hand has edges in the order of $O(n^2)$.

Definition 9.1 (graph density) *The density of a graph G denoted $\rho(G)$ is the ratio of the number of its edges to the maximum possible number of edges in G as below.*

$$\rho(G) = \frac{2m}{n(n-1)} \tag{9.1}$$

where $\rho(G)$ is between 0 and 1. The sum of degrees in an undirected graph G is $2m$, therefore, the average degree of G, $deg(G)$, is $2m/n$ resulting in the modification of Eqn. 9.1 as in Eqn. 9.2. The density of the graph of Figure 9.2 is 0.52 which means almost half of all possible edges exists in this graph.

$$\rho(G) = \frac{deg(G)}{(n-1)} \tag{9.2}$$

The *degree distribution* of a graph is another measure which shows the percentage of vertices of a given degree.

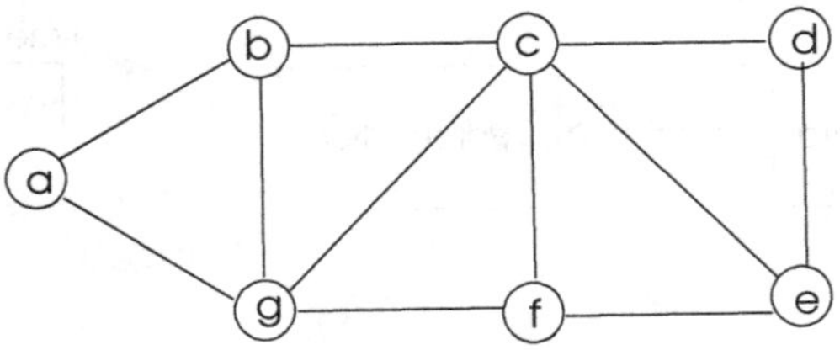

FIGURE 9.2
A sample graph to evaluate graph analysis parameters.

Definition 9.2 (degree distribution) *The degree distribution of a given degree k in a graph G is the ratio of the number of vertices with degree k to the total number of vertices.*

We can state degree distribution for a particular degree k of a graph formally as follows.

$$P(k) = \frac{n_k}{n} \tag{9.3}$$

where n_k is the number of vertices with degree k. $P(2) = 0.29$, $P(3) = 0.43$, $P(4) = 0.14$, and $P(5) = 0.14$ in the graph of Figure 9.2. Both graph density and degree distribution give us some idea on the overall global structure of a graph which may not be adequate for a finer analysis. Formally, the degree distribution shows the probability of a randomly selected vertex to have a degree k.

9.3.2 Clustering Coefficient

The clustering coefficient of a node in a graph is another measure of its importance in the network. A node with highly connected neighbors has a higher clustering coefficient than a node with sparsely connected neighbors.

Definition 9.3 (clustering coefficient) *The clustering coefficient $CC(v)$ of a node v is the ratio of total number of edges between the neighbors of v to the maximum number of edges possible between these neighbors.*

If a node v has k neighbors, the maximum possible number of connections among its neighbors is $k(k-1)/2$. The $CC(v)$ can now be stated as in Eqn. 9.4,

$$CC(v) = \frac{2x}{k(k-1)} \tag{9.4}$$

where x is the number of edges among neighbors of v. The average clustering coefficient of a graph G, $CC(G)$, is the arithmetic average of all these values as $CC(G) = \frac{1}{n}\sum_{v \in V} CC(v)$. The CC values of the vertices in the graph of Figure 9.2 are as follows: $CC(a) = 1$, $CC(b) = 0.67$, $CC(c) = 0.4$, $CC(d) = 1$, $CC(e) = 0.67$, $CC(f) = 0.67$, and $CC(g) = 0.5$. The characteristic path length of a network, L, is evaluated by calculating the average value of the length of all shortest paths between every node pair.

9.3.3 Matching Index

The matching index of a pair of nodes $\{u, v\}$ in a graph is determined by calculating the ratio of the number of their common neighbors to the number of the union of all of their neighbors. Matching indices for node pairs (a, b) and (b, c) of the graph in Figure 9.2 are 0.5 and 0.2 respectively.This parameter is used to determine how similar two nodes are, since two nodes with a high matching index have many common neighbors, thus, their main function in the network may be similar. For example, two proteins in a protein interface network with many common neighbors may have similar tasks to perform.

9.3.4 Centrality

Centrality is yet another measure to determine the importance of nodes or edges in a complex network. This parameter is evaluated by calculating shortest paths over the nodes or edges. Various centrality parameters provide significant importance of nodes or edges in a graph representing a complex brain network.

9.3.4.1 Closeness Centrality

The *closeness centrality* $C(v)$ of a node v in a graph provides information on how central that node is in the graph. It is determined for a node v by finding the sum of all distances from v to all other nodes and taking the reciprocal of this sum as in Eqn. 9.5 where $d(u, v)$ shows the distance between vertices u and v

$$C(v) = \frac{1}{\sum_{v \in V} d(u, v)} \tag{9.5}$$

The distances may be calculated using the breadth-first-search algorithm in an unweighted graph where edges do not have weights associated with them. Dijkstra's shortest path algorithm or Bellman-Ford algorithm [3] may be used to evaluate shortest paths between the nodes of a weighted graph with weights associated with edges commonly display the costs of transferring data over those edges. The closeness centrality values for the vertices in the graph of Figure 9.2 are as follows: $C(a) = 0.08$, $C(b) = 0.11$, $C(c) = 0.14$, $C(d) = 0.09$, $C(e) = 0.10$, $C(f) = 0.11$, and $C(g) = 0.13$. The node c has the highest value since it is more central than other nodes as can be seen.

9.3.4.2 Vertex Betweenness Centrality

The importance of a node v in a graph may be evaluated by finding the percentage of shortest paths that run through v called its vertex betweenness centrality $VC(v)$, since a high value of this parameter means node v is vital in transferring data among all nodes. The $VC(v)$ value of a vertex v may be determined using Eqn. 9.6 where σ_{st} shows the number of shortest paths between all nodes s and t other than node v, and $\sigma_{st}(v)$ is the number of shortest paths through node v.

$$VC(v) = \sum_{s \neq t \neq v} \frac{\sigma_{st}(v)}{\sigma_{st}} \tag{9.6}$$

9.3.4.3 Edge Betweenness Centrality

Analogous to vertex centrality, the importance of an edge e in a graph may be determined by calculating the percentage of shortest paths that run through e called betweenness centrality $BC(e)$. A relatively higher *BC(e)* value than other edges in a graph for an edge e means that this edge has a significant role in carrying data among all nodes in the network. Formally, *BC(e)* is defined as in Eqn. 9.7 where σ_{st} shows the number of shortest paths between all nodes s and t other than node v, and $\sigma_{st}(e)$ is the number of shortest paths through edge e. This parameter may be used for clustering in biological networks since clusters have a good probability of being connected with edges that have high BC values and removing these edges provides a method of isolating clusters.

$$BC(e) = \sum_{s \neq t \neq v} \frac{\sigma_{st}(e)}{\sigma_{st}} \tag{9.7}$$

9.3.5 Network Models

Complex networks can be classified based on their topological properties as follows:

- *Random Networks*: The basic assumption in forming these networks is that an edge (u, v) between the vertices u and v has the probability $p = 2m/(n(n-1))$. A random network is identified by a short average path length and a clustering coefficient that is inversely proportional to the size of the network [3].
- *Small-world Networks*: The distance between any two nodes in such a network is small, providing fast data transfer among all the nodes [4]. The diameter of a small-world network is proportional to $\log n$ where n is the number of nodes in the network. Brain networks exhibit this property providing efficient data transfer between separate brain regions.
- *Scale-free networks*: This kind of complex networks is characterized by few nodes with high degrees with the rest of the nodes having relatively low degrees. Many biological networks such as protein interaction networks, metabolic pathways and also complex brain networks exhibit this property. The degree distribution of these networks can be specified in Eqn. 9.8 where γ is known as the power-law exponent.

$$P(k) \approx k{-}\gamma, \gamma > 1 \tag{9.8}$$

A scale-free network can be constructed using the following steps [5]:

1. *Growth*: A new node is added to network at each step.
2. *Preferential Attachment*: A new node u is attached to any node v in the network with a probability proportional to the degree of v. Applying this rule ensures that higher degree nodes will have relatively more neighbors eventually. This mode of operation is known as "rich gets richer" principle.

- *Hierarchical Networks*: Analysis of complex brain networks reveals an interesting property: Dense clusters of low-degree nodes are connected by high-degree nodes called *hubs* providing a hierarchical network structure. The complex brain networks show small-world and scale-free properties in this hierarchical structure.

9.3.6 Network Analysis with Python

Complex networks can be analyzed, constructed and visualized using the programming language Python which provides a library called *networkx* for this purpose. Using this module, a random network may be constructed by the *erdos_renyi_graph* method and a small-world network by the *watts_strogatz_graph method*; and a scale-free network by the *albert_barabasi_graph* method as shown in the following Python code. Graphs with 20 nodes built using these algorithms are displayed in Figure 9.3 and Figure 9.4.

```
import networkx as nx
import matplotlib.pyplot as plt

G=nx.erdos_renyi_graph(20,0.4) # 0.4: probability of connection
nx.draw(G,with_labels=1)
plt.show()

G=nx.watts_strogatz_graph(20,5,0.5) # 5 connections, 0.5 probability
pos=nx.circular_layout(G)
nx.draw(G,pos,with_labels=True)
plt.show()

G=nx.barabasi_albert_graph(20,2) # Average 2 connections
nx.draw(G,with_labels=1)
plt.show()
```

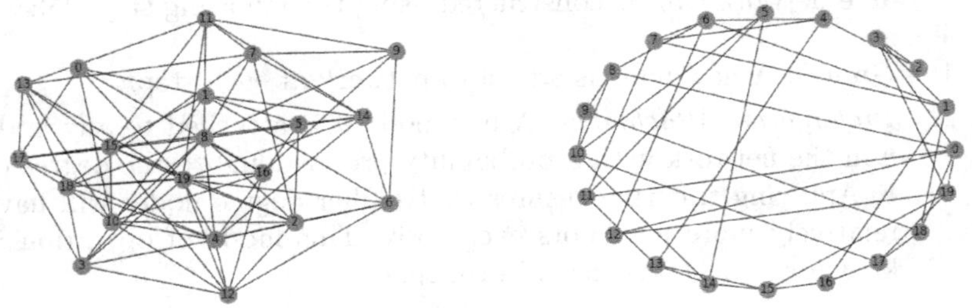

FIGURE 9.3
a Erdos-Renyi Network, **b** Watts-Strogats Network.

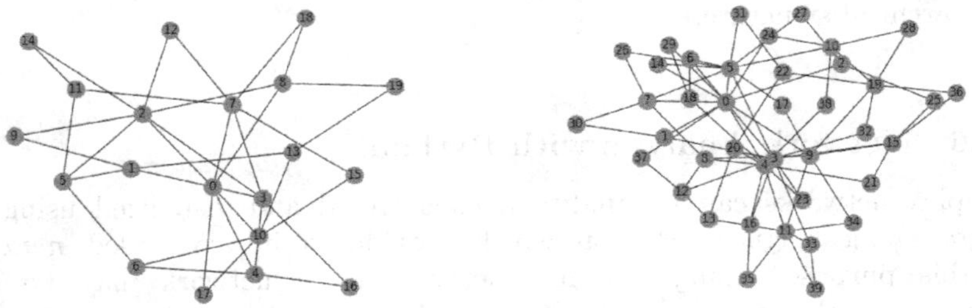

FIGURE 9.4
a Barabasi-Albert Network 20 nodes, **b** Barabasi-Albert Network 40 nodes.

9.4 Modules and Hubs

A general property of complex networks is the existence of densely connected subnetworks which are commonly called *modules*. This behavior can be observed in various real networks such as social networks and the Web. Yet another significant property of these networks is their hierarchical organization such that a number of modules may be contained in a larger module. Brain networks are no exception to these properties of complex networks; they are small-world, scale-free networks containing modules in a hierarchical structure.

9.4.1 Background

The problem of detecting such modules is commonly termed as *clustering* and when the brain networks is modelled by a graph, the problem is referred to as *graph clustering* which aims to find the densely connected regions of a brain network. A *hub* in a complex brain network is a node that is highly connected

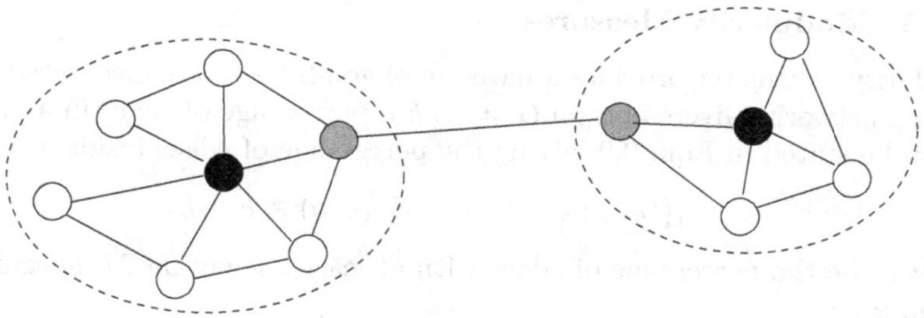

FIGURE 9.5
Modules and hubs. Modules are shown in dotted regions, central hubs are in black and gateway hubs are in gray.

to the other nodes as displayed in Figure 9.5 with *gateway hubs* connecting different regions and *central hubs* being the main connection point of the nodes in a region. Clustering algorithms in brain networks can be classified as hierarchical, density-based, flow-based and spectral algorithms as we review in the next sections.

9.4.1.1 Minimum Spanning Tree-based Clustering

Given a weighted and undirected graph $G = (V, E)$, the minimum spanning tree (MST) of G is a tree T of G that connects all vertices of G and has the minimum value of $\sum_{(u,v) \in T} d(u,v)$ where $d(u,v)$ is the weight associated with edge (u,v). Various linear-time algorithms to build MST of a weighted graph exist including Prim-Jarnik, Kruskal, and Boruvka [6].

MST-based clustering is a popular module detection algorithm to find clusters in biological networks [6]. An MST of the weighted graph is first constructed using any algorithm first and the heaviest edge weight is discarded from the MST at each iteration of the algorithm to form clusters. The main idea of this algorithm is that the heavy-weight edges have a high probability of joining clusters.

9.4.1.2 Edge Betweenness-based Clustering

The edge betweenness (EB) analysis of a graph may be used to detect modules in a brain network as proposed by Newman and Girvan [7] with the idea that clusters have a high probability of being connected by edges with large edge betweenness values. The steps of this algorithm may be stated as follows:

1. Calculate EB values of all edges in the network.
2. Remove the edge with the highest EB from the network.
3. Recalculate EB values of the network.
4. Repeat steps 1-3 until a clustering quality is satisfied.

9.4.1.3 Modularity Measures

Modularity parameter provides a measure of goodness of the discovered modules in a network. Given a graph $G = (V, E)$, percentage of edges in a module M_i can be stated in Eqn. 9.9, giving the percentage of edges inside a module

$$e_{ii} = |\{(uv) : u \in V_i, v \in V_i, (u, v) \in E|/|E| \tag{9.9}$$

Let a_i be the percentage of edges with at least one end in M_i specified as in Eqn. 9.10:

$$a_i = |\{(uv) : u \in V_i, v \in V \setminus V_i, (u, v) \in E|/|E| \tag{9.10}$$

Modularity of a complex network with k modules can now be defined as in Eqn. 9.11, providing the quality of all modules discovered in the network. In other words, we evaluate the ratio of edges totally contained in modules to the edges that have one end in a module.

$$Q = \sum_{i=1}^{k} (e_{ii} - a_i^2) \tag{9.11}$$

Based on the modularity parameter, modularity-based clustering algorithm proposed by Newman has the following steps. This algorithm with time complexity $O(m + n)n)$ is classified as agglomerative hierarchical clustering algorithm as it iteratively forms larger clusters.

1. Each node $v \in V$ is a cluster initially.
2. **Repeat**
    - Merge two clusters C_i and C_j that will increase modularity M by the largest amount.
3. **Until** merging any two clusters does not improve M.

9.4.1.4 Spectral Clustering

This method of graph clustering uses algebraic properties of the graph that represents the complex network. The Laplacian matrix of a graph $G = (V, E)$ is $L = D - A$ where D is the degree matrix with $d_i \in D$ is a diagonal element representing degree of vertex i and A is the adjacency matrix. In normalized form, $L = I - D^{1/2}AD{-}1/2$. The eigenvalues of L are real and symmetric and the second eigenvalue of L is called the *Fiedler value* and the corresponding eigenvector is denoted as *Fiedler vector*. The spectral bisection procedure using Fiedler vector is defined as follows. Having constructed the Fiedler vector, each entry is compared with a threshold value, commonly 0 or the median value of the Fiedler vector, and a vertex that has a smaller or equal value to the threshold is placed in cluster 1; any vertex with a larger value is stored in cluster 2. This algorithm may be implemented recursively to discover k clusters.

9.4.2 Modules in Brain Networks

Discovery of dense regions in brain networks may provide insight into understanding basic brain functions related to its topology [8]. These highly connected regions perform specialized functions cooperating and coordinating with each other to produce high-level cognitive tasks. Since detection of modules is an NP-hard problem with no algorithmic solutions in polynomial time, heuristics are commonly used.

Modularity maximization is widely used to find modules in brain networks due to its fast convergence and efficient use in large networks. A heuristic called *Louvian heuristic* is used in [9] to provide a fast modularity maximization in large networks. Each node is a cluster initially and moving nodes between clusters is evaluated in terms of modularity gains achieved. The authors report that the quality of the communities discovered using their method is very good with fast computation time.

Dynamic community structure in multilayer networks is considered in [10] by analysing the behavior of several null models used for optimizing quality functions such as modularity. Although modularity maximization proves to be a favourable heuristic to detect communities in networks, it is difficult to use it directly to find clusters in hierarchical networks making it unsuitable to find these dense regions in brain networks. A weighted modularity maximization(WMM) method that uses the weighted adjacency matrix is proposed in [11] to be used in functional brain networks to overcome the difficulties of applying the modularity maximization method directly in these networks. The authors present a two-step maximization method to detect hierarchical clusters in functional brain networks by testing hierarchy of the clusters using node attributes. Various clustering methods applied to neuroimaging data to discover clusters in brain networks include spectral clustering [12] and bayesian community detection [13].

9.5 Motifs of the Brain

A network motif is a frequently found subnetwork of a given brain network. Such a repeating structure may indicate some basic function performed by that motif. Moreover, detection of similar motifs in various BFNs may indicate similarity which may be useful in the diagnose of diseases.

9.5.1 Background

Discovery of a subgraph within a larger graph is an NP-Hard problem, thus, approximation algorithms or more commonly, heuristic algorithms are needed. Some common directed network motifs of three nodes found in brain networks

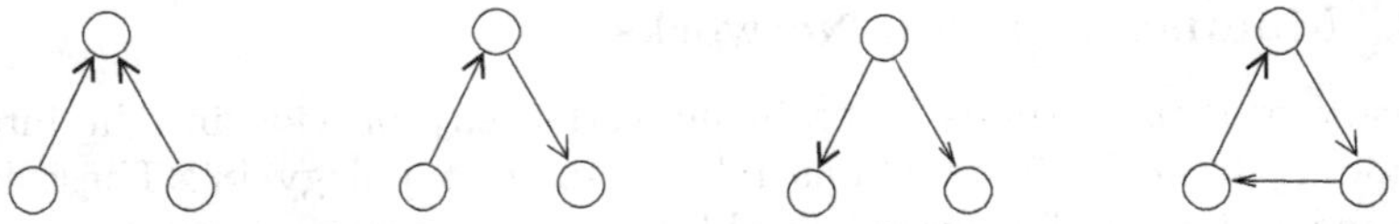

FIGURE 9.6
Some motifs of three nodes found in brain networks.

are depicted in Figure 9.6 as re-organization of 3-node motifs during loss and recovery of consciousness is explored in [14].

Motifs of a brain network may be discovered using either *network-centric* or *motif-centric* methods. All subgraphs of given size are searched in network-centric methods whereas the motif m_k of size k is input to a motif-centric method. Evaluation of motifs in a given network involves implementation of the following steps:

1. *Motif Discovery*: Motifs can be found either by exact counting methods which require high computational times, or by sampling in which random small samples from the large complex graph may be extracted and motifs search is carried in these samples. The results obtained are then projected to the whole graph to estimate its overall structure.
2. *Isomorphic Classes*: Motifs of equivalent isomorphic class found are placed in the same group to simplify processing since they are of the same structure.
3. *Statistical Significance*: The evaluation of the discovered motifs is performed in this step, commonly by generating a set of random graphs of similar structures to the original graph and applying the above two steps to this set. Then, statistical significance of the discovered motifs in both cases is evaluated to determine the validity of the motifs found in the original graph.

Two main methods of motif search are *network-centric* and *motif-centric.* All subgraphs of size k is searched in the former and a certain motif m_k of size k is investigated in the latter. Statistical significance of the discovered motifs can be evaluated using *P-score*, *Z-score* or *motif significance profile* [6].

9.5.2 Motifs of the Brain Networks

Detection of motifs which are recurring subgraph patterns in connectome may provide crucial information on the functioning of the human brain. These motifs are assumed to perform some important function whereas infrequent subgraph patterns across a number of connectomes may be associated with individual variability.

DotMotif is a tool that combines graph database and analysis libraries providing a query interface to search subgraphs in connectome [15]. The authors show the implementations searching for motifs on simulated data and real public datasets. Considering that exact enumeration is computationally expensive and the need to distinguish the types of edges which may have an effect on the functioning of a motif, a parallel, general-purpose subgraph enumeration method to count motifs in connectome is proposed in [16]. The authors also describe a divide-and-conquer community-based subgraph enumeration method that provides enumeration per brain region.

Frequent complete subgraphs of the connectome are mapped by also examining sex differences in [17]. The results display complete subgraphs of the connectome of 238 women and 175 men each with 463 nodes. The authors report that 812 complete subgraphs are more frequent in men connectomes and 224 complete subgraphs are more frequent in women connectomes. The motifs of the human brain having at most six edges is described and analyzed in [18]. The authors provide sex differences in these motifs for 426 human subjects and conclude that for k edge connected subgraphs; male samples have slightly more frequent motifs when k=1 or 2 whereas female samples have many more motifs than males when k=6.

Motif search can be viewed as a frequent subgraph mining problem which generally consists of two steps: generating a candidate subgraph and identifying its isomorphism in the input graph. Subgraph mining problem is introduced and various subgraph mining algorithms from a bioinformatics perspective are reviewed in [19].

9.6 Brain Network Alignment

The aim of *network alignment* is to find the similar structures among two or more networks by comparing them. This problem is closely related to the subgraph and graph isomorphism problem and heuristic algorithms are commonly used.

9.6.1 Background

Network alignment can be performed *pairwise* in which two networks are compared or *multiple* where a number of networks are evaluated for similarity. It is also possible to search subnetworks in *local alignment* whereas *global alignment* aims to find similarities between two or more networks as a whole. When applied to biological networks, global alignment is performed to evaluate similarities between similar species whereas local alignment is commonly preferred when comparing diverse species.

The internal structures of the nodes of the networks such as the amino acid sequences of proteins in a PPI network is evaluated in *node similarity* method. On the other hand, the network structure is the main parameter of similarity search in *topological similarity* method of network alignment. Commonly, both of these methods are used with different weights to evaluate similarity of networks [6].

9.6.1.1 Relation to Bipartite Graph Matching

A matching of a graph $G = (V, E)$ is the set $E' \in E$ such that any edge $(u, v) \in E'$ does not share any endpoints with any other edge in E' and a maximal matching can not be enlarged. A weighted maximal matching attempts to find the maximal weighted matching with total weights of matched edges in a weighted graph where edges have weights associated with them. A detailed survey of graph matching methods can be found in [20].

A bipartite graph $G = (V_1 \cup V_2, E)$ has edges only between vertices in V_1 and vertices in V_2. Matching, unweighted or weighted in a bipartite graph is similar, edges that are not adjacent are included in the matching. Global alignment problem can be related to weighted bipartite graph matching problem as follows. Let G_1 and G_2 be the two graphs that are searched for similarity. A similarity matrix R is built with elements r_{ij} showing the weights of similarity, using node or topological similarities or both, between the node i in G_1 and node j in G_2. Thus, evaluating the similarity of G_1 and G_2 is reduced to finding the maximal matching in $G = G_1 \cup G_2$ using a suitable algorithm. Fortunately, finding maximum unweighted or weighted matching in a graph is one of the rare graph problems that can be solved in polynomial time.

9.6.1.2 Alignment Quality Evaluation

Quality of the discovered similarity may be evaluated using edge correctness and induced conserved structure parameters. Edge correctness (EC) parameter to evaluate the alignment method of two graphs G_1 and G_2 is given in Eqn. 9.12 [21].

$$EC(G_1, G_2, f) = \frac{|f(E_1) \cap E_2|}{|E_1|} \tag{9.12}$$

where f is the function to relate edges of graph G_1 to the edges of graph G_2. This parameter shows the percentage of correctly aligned edges to evaluate the goodness of the function. The induced conserved structure (ICS) parameter is a generalization of the EC parameter as given in Eqn. 9.13 [22]. The denominator in this equation denotes the size of edges induced in graph G_2 by the mapped vertices.

$$ICS(G_1, G_2, f) = \frac{|f(E_1) \cap E_2|}{|E_{G_2[f(V_1)]}|} \tag{9.13}$$

9.6.2 Alignment of Brain Networks

Graph matching is used in [23] to form a similarity parameter called the swap distance to quantify the distance between partial functional connectomes of individuals. The authors used 997 samples from the Human Connectome Project and concluded that the swap distance is directly proportional to the familial distances and ages of the subjects. They also found that this distance is lower in females compared to males and is greater for females with lower cognitive scores compared to females with larger cognitive scores. Regions that affected swap distances significantly were in higher-order networks which are default-mode and fronto-parietal which perform executive function and memory.

Choosing an atlas for parcellation of the brain to yield connectome is a crucial task in the graph-theoretical analysis of the brain. The robustness of a built atlas in constructing network topology may be determined by finding the similarity across a number of connectomes. Graph matching to assess the similarity of connectomes built from atlases is used in [24] by introducing the graph Jaccard index (GJI) based on the Jaccard index. The authors also propose WL-align method derived from the Weisfeiler-Leman (WL) graph-isomorphism test to align connectomes. Subjects from the Human Connectome Project database are used to validate the proposed GJI and WL-align method and a strategy is proposed to choose a suitable parcellation scheme for structural connectivity. Brain parcellation may be performed in network domain using a suitable network alignment algorithm, without using an atlas as described in [25]. The authors implement and compare six global network alignment algorithms in brain networks: MAGNA [26], NETAL [27], GHOST [22], GEDEVO [28], WAVE [29], and Natalie2.0 [30]. They conclude that the best results in terms of edge conservation were obtained when MAGNA++ which is an extension to MAGNA as global aligner was used. MAGNA is a global network aligner based on a genetic algorithm that uses the evolution of a population of alignments over time.

An unsupervised graph matching method is used in [31] to align structural connectomes of a set of healthy subjects with parcellations of varying granularities. Four different algorithms are used for initialization: Spatial Adjacency, Identity, Barycenter, and Random. The resulting permutations indicate that applying the alignment methods improve the similarity of subjects when the number of parcels is greater than 100 and when Spatial Adjacency and Identity initializations are used. The authors also state that permutations are observed mostly among neighbor parcels and that the spatial distribution of the permutations indicate all the regions across the context are mostly permuted with first and second-order neighbors.

9.7 Disease Networks of the Brain

Diagnosis of a brain disease traditionally is commonly performed by self-reported symptoms and clinical signs of the patient. Investigation of the brain networks for the diagnose of neurological diseases such as Alzheimer's disease

(AD), Autism, Bipolar Disorder (BD), Parkinson's Disease (PD), Multiple Sclerosis (MS), and schizophrenia is a current functional connectome research area in neuroscience attracting many researchers.

The topological properties of a normal brain network are characterized by being a small-world, scale-free network with a hierarchical structure consisting of modules connected by hubs as outlined. On the other hand, neurological disorders result in structural and functional brain network changes as shown in various clinical research studies [32–34]. Neurological disorders such as AD, schizophrenia and PD result in deviation from these properties as outlined in the following sections. The organization of normal structural and functional brain networks is described and the network studies of neurological disorders with a focus on AD, MS, and epilepsy to discover possible common patterns in the analysis of diseases are presented in [35]. The author proposes that hub overload and failure which results in the separation of the hierarchical brain network structure may be a common characteristic of several neurological disorders.

9.7.1 AD Connectome

AD is a progressive neurological disorder prevalent mostly in elderly populations. The structure of a connectome in AD is affected resulting in the loss of small-world, scale-free and hierarchical modular structure of normal brain networks as shown in various studies.

Functional brain networks of 15 AD patients and 13 control subjects were investigated in [36] by forming connectivity matrices of beta band-filtered electroencephalography (EEG) channels and then analyzing the equivalent graphs for characteristic path length L and cluster coefficient C. The authors report that for various threshold values in converting the matrices to graphs, L was significantly longer in AD patients than normal subjects although clustering coefficients were similar and concluded that these results indicate the loss of small-world feature in AD which may be used to diagnose this disease.

A sub-network kernel to validate the similarity between a pair of connectomes to classify brain diseases is presented in [37]. The local to global topological properties of brain network nodes are considered to evaluate similarities of connectomes. The proposed method is tested on subjects with baseline functional magnetic resonance imaging (fMRI) data obtained from the Alzheimer's Disease Neuroimaging Initiative (ADNI) database. The authors state that the results indicate that their method outperforms several graph-based methods in mild cognitive impairment classification.

The effective connectivity of default mode network in AD patients and normal controls is investigated in [38] to find that the intensity and quantity of connections in AD were decreased when compared to the control subjects. In particular, the authors note that posterior cingulated cortex (PCC) was strongly connected to most of the default mode network regions in control subjects whereas the connections of PCC were reduced in AD patients. According to the authors, decline in memory functions may be attributed to this effect and thus, the activity in PCC may be used to determine the level of AD progression in patients providing a potential biomarker.

Local network connectivity changes in AD patients using graph analysis in fMRI were searched in [39]. 18 mild AD patients and 21 healthy age-matched control subjects were tested to find that the characteristic path length of AD functional networks is closer to that of random networks whereas the clustering coefficient values were similar to that of control subjects. The average synchronization of the brain in both groups were similar, however, increased synchronization related to frontal cortices and decreased synchronization at the parietal and occipital regions were detected in Ad patients. The authors conclude that long distance connectivity is affected and the randomization of functional brain network structure is observed which probably is responsible for the loss of global information integration in AD.

The default mode network (DMN) is a canonical large-scale brain network consisting of distributed nodes that show increased and correlated BOLD response during wakeful rest. The characteristics of brain networks in subjects with AD is observed as the loss of small-world features and tendency to change into a randomized and/or regular network topology; change in hub regions especially in the DMN and medial temporal lobe [40].

9.7.2 Schizophrenia Connectome

Schizophrenia is a psychiatric disorder with heterogeneous symptoms among affected individuals. The cause of this disease which generally starts at early adulthood is not known. Schizophrenia is often characterized by delusions, hallucinations, disorganized thinking and behavior and impairment of cognitive functions. Schizophrenia is commonly considered as a disorder of connectivity between large-scale brain network regions and as with other neurological disorders, this disease is associated with impairment of brain connectivity [41].

Structural brain networks were found to be less strongly integrated in patients with schizophrenia in [42] with key frontal hubs having a reduced central role. Also, the network connectivity of frontal and temporal areas was significantly reduced and the path length was substantially increased in of olfactory, medial, and superior frontal regions, anterior cingulate, medial temporal pole, and superior occipital regions preventing efficient transfer between these regions.

In a review of brain networks in schizophrenia [43], reduced structural connectivity is reported with white matter projections linking frontal, temporal and parietal regions being the most affected. The authors state that the average path length is increased and the communication between segregated regions of the brain is reduced as verified in various studies. Moreover, it is reported that a main characteristic of schizophrenia may be the pathology of mostly frontal hub regions. The authors conclude that dsyconnectivity of brain regions in this disease is a general finding reported by many researchers and highly connected hub regions display abnormalities.

Functional brain networks in schizophrenia are investigated in [44] to reveal localized functional connectivity abnormalities at three different levels: either in regional connectivity strength or node degrees; edge strengths and interconnected subnetworks. Abnormalities of the prefrontal cortex (PFC) in this disease have been reported in various studies.

Structure of hubs in schizophrenia is studied in [45] where the authors report strong evidence for network abnormalities of prefrontal hubs, and moderate evidence for network abnormalities of limbic, temporal, and parietal hubs. The authors also postulate that a wide range of symptoms of schizophrenia may be due to abnormalities of brain hubs.

Connectivity impairment between brain network regions in schizophrenia is investigated in [46] over 72 cerebral regions in 15 healthy subjects and 12 subjects with schizophrenia. Functional connectivity was found to be significantly reduced in patients with increased diversity of functional connections. Functional brain networks were found to have reduced clustering and small-world properties with fewer number of high-degree hubs in edial parietal, premotor and cingulate, and right orbitofrontal cortical nodes of functional networks of affected individuals than normal subjects.

In conclusion, the altered brain network structures in this disease may be summarized as reduced average path length, the existence of abnormal frontal hubs, reduced clustering and segregated brain regions with less connections than normal. These characteristics may prove to be decisive in diagnosing patients with schizophrenia.

9.7.3 Other Disease Networks

PD is a progressive neurological disorder that affects the nervous system, characterized by progressive neuronal loss in the brain. As with all other neurological disorders, alterations of connectome topology in patients with PD is observed in a number of studies. Changes in connectome in PD is surveyed in [47] to conclude that it is difficult to have clear-cut conclusions about the functional connectome changes associated with PD and parkinsonism.

Freezing of gait (FOG) is one of the disturbances developed in patients with PD. Resting-state fMRI values were investigated in [48] with 28 PD patients, 15 with FOG and 13 without it, to find that patients with FOG had reduced functional connectivity across many seeds. The authors conclude that alterations in the resting state functional connectivity of the opercular parietal cortex may be one of the substrates of FOG.

Global structural connectome properties in PD using meta-analysis were investigated in [49] in patients with PD and healthy subjects in to discover that the clustering coefficient is significantly reduced and characteristic path length is significantly increased in PD patients compared with the healthy subjects. The authors postulate that these findings imply that a shift from a balanced small-world structure to a weaker small-world occurs in PD.

Attention-deficit/hyperactivity disorder (ADHD) is a neurodevelopmental disorder with general symptoms of hyperactivity, inattention, impulsivity and emotional dysregulation. Individuals with ADHD have abnormal interactions in macro- and micro-scale functional networks of the brain. Functional motif patterns in patients with ADHD is investigated in [50] to validate information flow and interaction modes. The results showed that the interaction between right hippocampus and the right amygdala were significantly increased which may cause the mood disorders in patients. Changes in the information interaction of the bilateral thalamus were noted, influencing and modifying behavioral results.

Autism spectrum disorder (ASD) is a neurodevelopmental disorder with symptoms such as impairments in social interaction and restricted, repetitive patterns of behavior, interests, or activities. Graph-theoretic analysis of the weighted and unweighted structural brain networks of 14 adult male highly functioning ASD patients and 19 matching control subjects is investigated in [51]. The findings are that global efficiency was significantly decreased in both unweighted and weighted networks, normalized characteristic path length was significantly increased in the unweighted networks, and strength was significantly decreased in the weighted networks of ASD patients. Betweenness centrality of the right caudate was significantly increased in the weighted networks in local structure analyses, and the strength of the right superior temporal pole was significantly decreased in the unweighted ASD patient networks.

Primary Angle Closure Glaucoma (PACG) is a chronic optic neuropathy with a loss of retinal ganglion cells and their axons commonly affecting the elderly populations. Topological brain network properties of resting-state fMRI data in 33 patients with PACG and 33 healthy controls were investigated in [52]. The findings are that there are no significant differences between the global topological measures between the two groups. However, significant regional changes were detected in PACG patients within visual and nonvisual (somatomotor and cognition-emotion) regions.

A recent survey on the importance of brain network hubs in neurological disease formation is reviewed in [53]. The author notes that pathological hubs may play a role in spreading of seizure activity in patients with epilepsy and removal of such hubs may provide improved healing. It is also postulated that optimal network organization is damaged in multiple sclerosis possibly causing cognitive dysfunction and damaged hubs in stroke may be the reason for impaired cognitive recovery. Amyloid beta and tau pathology in AD are directly related to hyperactive hub nodes in this disorder as stated.

9.8 Conclusions

We have provided a graph-theoretical analysis of complex brain networks in this chapter. The brain network needs to be constructed using the neuroimaging process and then processing obtained data to yield the connectivity matrix first. The adjacency matrix is then formed by filtering the connectivity matrix over which the graph representing the connectivity of the brain nodes is constructed. This graph has the small-world and scale-free properties as various other complex biological networks such as protein interaction networks and metabolic pathways. We then reviewed main analysis parameters that can be used for the analysis of brain networks which are clustering coefficient, matching index, and centrality. A brain network has densely connected regions called modules or clusters and within each cluster, hubs are the nodes with very high number of connections to their neighbors. We provided basic module search algorithms that can be applied to brain networks with modularity maximization oriented algorithms commonly used for this purpose. A repeating subgraph of a larger graph is called a motif and brain networks have motifs which may represent some basic function performed by them. Discovery of motifs is a computationally hard problem and various heuristics are used to find them. We reviewed motif discovery in brain networks and various methods to evaluate the significance of the motifs found in brain networks. [54].

Network alignment aims to find similarity between two or more networks. Finding similarity between a brain network with a disease condition such as AD, ADHD, MS or autism and a suspected patient may guide health professionals to diagnose these diseases. We also surveyed the brain network structure alterations in neurological disorders with emphasis on AD, schizophrenia and PD. General findings in various studies outlined were reduced or abnormal connectivity of hubs which connect brain functional regions, reduced clustering coefficient and increased characteristic path length causing the loss of small-world and scale-free features of brain networks, thus implying the cause of the disorder.

Our general conclusion is that representing brain activities as a graph provides various graph algorithms, methods and tools to be readily available for the analysis of brain networks to aid our understanding of disease states and the cognitive processes of the brain. Research studies in this area, namely graph-theoretic analysis of brain networks, may lead to improved diagnosis and treatments of neurological disorders resulting in clinical outcomes.

Bibliography

[1] H. Tang, G. Ma, Y. Zhang, *et al.*, "A comprehensive survey of complex brain network representation," *Meta Radiology*, vol. 1, no. 3, p. 100046, 2023.

[2] S. Simpson, F. Bowman, and P. J. Laurienti, "Analyzing complex functional brain networks: Fusing statistics and network science to understand the brain," *Stat Surv*, no. 7, pp. 1–36, 2013.

[3] K. Erciyes, *Distributed Graph Algorithms for Computer Networks.* Springer Computer Communications and Networks Series, 2013.

[4] D. Watts and S. Strogatz, "Collective dynamics of 'small-world' networks," *Nature*, vol. 69, no. 6684, pp. 440–442, 1998.

[5] A. Barabasi and R. Albert, "Emergence of scaling in random networks," *Science*, no. 286, pp. 509–512, 1999.

[6] K. Erciyes, *Distributed and Sequential Akgorithms for Bioinformatics.* Springer Computational Biology Series, 2015.

[7] M. Newman and M. Girvan, "Finding and evaluating community structure in networks," *Phys Rev*, vol. 69, no. 2, p. 026113, 2004.

[8] O. Sporns and R. Betzel, "Modular Brain Networks," *Annu Rev Psychol*, no. 67, pp. 613–640, 2016.

[9] V. Blondel, J. Guillaume, R. Lambiotte, *et al.*, "Fast unfolding of communities in large networks," *Journal of Statistical Mechanics: Theory and Experiment*, vol. 2008, no. 10, p. P10008, 2008.

[10] D. Bassett, M. Porter, N. Wymbs, *et al.*, "Robust detection of dynamic community structure in networks," *Chaos*, vol. 23, no. 1, 2013.

[11] Z. Guo, X. Zhao, L. Yao, *et al.*, "Improved brain community structure detection by two-step weighted modularity maximization," *PLoS One*, vol. 18, no. 12, 2023.

[12] R. Craddock, G. James, P. Holtzheimer, *et al.*, "A whole brain fMRI atlas generated via spatially constrained spectral clustering," *Human Brain Mapping*, vol. 33, no. 8, pp. 1914–1928, 2012.

[13] K. Andersen, K. Madsen, H. Siebner, *et al.*, "Non-Parametric Bayesian Graph Models Reveal Community Structure in Resting State fMRIs," *Neuroimage*, no. 100, pp. 301–35, 2014.

[14] C. Duclos, D. Nadin, Y. Mahdid, *et al.*, "Brain network motifs are markers of loss and recovery of consciousness," *Sci Rep*, vol. 11, no. 1, p. 3892, 2021.

[15] J. Matelsky, E. Reilly, E. Johnson, *et al.*, "DotMotif: an open-source tool for connectome subgraph isomorphism search and graph queries," *Sci Rep*, vol. 11, no. 1, p. 13045, 2021.

[16] B. Matejek, D. Wei, T. Chen, *et al.*, "Edge-colored directed subgraph enumeration on the connectome," *Sci Rep*, vol. 12, no. 1, p. 11349, 2022.

[17] M. Fellner, B. Varga, and V. Grolmusz, "The frequent complete subgraphs in the human connectome," *PLoS One*, vol. 15, no. 8, p. e0236883, 2020.

[18] M. Fellner, B. Varga, and V. Grolmusz, "The frequent subgraphs of the connectome of the human brain," *Cogn Neurodyn*, vol. 13, no. 5, pp. 453–460, 2019.

[19] A. Mrzic, P. Meysman, W. Bittremieux, *et al.*, "Grasping frequent subgraph mining for bioinformatics applications," *BioData Min*, vol. 11, no. 20, 2018.

[20] D. Conte, P. Foggia, C. Sansone, *et al.*, "Thirty years of graph matching in pattern recognition," *International Journal of Pattern Recognition and Artificial Intelligence*, vol. 18, pp. 265–298, 2018.

[21] R. Singh, J. Xu, and B. Berger, "Pairwise global alignment of protein interaction networks by matching neighborhood topology," in Speed, T., Huang, H. (eds) *Research in Computational Molecular Biology. RECOMB 2007. Lecture Notes in Computer Science*, vol. 4453, pp. 16–31, Springer, Berlin, Heidelberg, 2007.

[22] R. Patro and C. Kingsford, "Global network alignment using multiscale spectral signatures," *Bioinformatics*, vol. 28, no. 23, pp. 3105–3114, 2012.

[23] H. Bukhari, C. Su, E. Dhamala, *et al.*, "Graph-matching distance between individuals' functional connectomes varies with relatedness, age, and cognitive score," *Hum Brain Mapp*, vol. 44, no. 9, pp. 3541–3554, 2023.

[24] M. Frigo, E. Cruciani, D. Coudert, *et al.*, "Network alignment and similarity reveal atlas-based topological differences in structural connectomes," *Netw Neurosci*, vol. 5, no. 3, pp. 711–733, 2021.

[25] M. Milano, P. Guzzi, O. Tymofieva, *et al.*, "An extensive assessment of network alignment algorithms for comparison of brain connectomes," *BMC Bioinformatics*, vol. 18, no. 6, p. 235, 2017.

[26] V. Saraph and T. Milenkovic, "MAGNA: Maximizing accuracy in global network alignment," *Bioinformatics*, vol. 30, pp. 2931–2940, 2014.

[27] B. Neyshabur, A. Khadem, S. Hashemifar, *et al.*, "Netal: a new graph-based method for global alignment of protein–protein interaction networks," *Bioinformatics*, vol. 29, no. 13, pp. 1654–1662, 2013.

[28] R. Ibragimov, M. Malek, J. Guo, *et al.*, "GEDEVO: An evolutionary graph edit distance algorithm for biological network alignment," *GCB*, pp. 68–79, 2013.

[29] Y. Sun, J. Crawford, J. Tang, *et al.*, "Simultaneous optimization of both node and edge conservation in network alignment via wave," in *International Workshop on Algorithms in Bioinformatics*, pp. 16–39, Netherland: Springer, 2015.

[30] M. El-Kebir, J. Heringa, and G. Klau, "Lagrangian relaxation applied to sparse global network alignment," in *IAPR International Conference on Pattern Recognition in Bioinformatics*, pp. 225–236, Netherlands: Springer, 2011.

[31] A. Calissano, T. Papadopoulo, X. Pennec, *et al.*, "Graph-matching distance between individuals' functional connectomes varies with relatedness, age, and cognitive score," *Hum Brain Mapp*, vol. 45, no. 1, p. e26554, 2024.

[32] Y. He and A. Evans, "Graph theoretical modeling of brain connectivity," *Curr Opin Neurol*, vol. 23, no. 4, pp. 341–350, 2010.

[33] D. Bassett and E. Bullmore, "Human brain networks in health and disease," *Curr Opin Neurol*, vol. 22, no. 4, pp. 340–347, 2009.

[34] M. Guye, G. Bettus, F. Bartolomei, *et al.*, "Graph theoretical analysis of structural and functional connectivity MRI in normal and pathological brain networks," *Magn Reson Mater Phy*, vol. 23, pp. 409–421, 2010.

[35] C. J. Stam, "Modern network science of neurological disorders," *Nat Rev Neurosci*, vol. 15, no. 10, pp. 683–695, 2014.

[36] C. Stam, B. Jones, G. Nolte, *et al.*, "Small-world networks and functional connectivity in Alzheimer's disease," *Cereb Cortex*, vol. 17, no. 1, pp. 92–99, 2007.

[37] B. Jie, M. Liu, D. Zhang, *et al.*, "Sub-Network Kernels for Measuring Similarity of Brain Connectivity Networks in Disease Diagnosis," *IEEE Trans Image Process*, vol. 27, no. 5, pp. 2340–2353, 2018.

[38] Y. Zhong, L. Huang, S. Cai, *et al.*, "Alzheimer's Disease Neuroimaging Initiative. Altered effective connectivity patterns of the default mode network in Alzheimer's disease: an fMRI study," *Neurosci Lett*, no. 578, pp. 171–175, 2009.

[39] E. Sanz-Arigita, M. M. Schoonheim, J. S. Damoiseaux, *et al.*, "Loss of 'small-world' networks in Alzheimer's disease: graph analysis of FMRI resting-state functional connectivity," *PLoS One*, vol. 5, no. 11:e13788, 2010.

[40] M. Yu, O. Sporns, and A. Saykin, "The human connectome in Alzheimer disease - relationship to biomarkers and genetics," *Nat Rev Neurol*, vol. 17, no. 9, pp. 545–563, 2021.

[41] K. Narr and A. Leaver, "Connectome and schizophrenia," *Curr Opin Psychiatry*, vol. 28, no. 3, pp. 229–235, 2015.

[42] M. van den Heuvel, R. Mandl, C. J. Stam *et al.*, "Aberrant frontal and temporal complex network structure in schizophrenia: a graph theoretical analysis," *J Neurosci*, vol. 30, no. 47, pp. 15915–15926, 2010.

[43] M. van den Heuvel and A. Fornito, "Brain networks in schizophrenia," *Neuropsychol Rev*, vol. 24, no. 1, pp. 32–48, 2014.

[44] A. Fornito, A. Zalesky, C. Pantelis, *et al.*, "Schizophrenia, neuroimaging and connectomics," *Neuroimage*, vol. 62, no. 4, pp. 2296–2314, 2012.

[45] M. Rubinov and E. Bullmore, "Schizophrenia and abnormal brain network hubs," *Dialogues Clin Neurosci*, vol. 15, no. 3, pp. 339–349, 2013.

[46] M. Lynall, D. Bassett, R. Kerwin, *et al.*, "Functional connectivity and brain networks in schizophrenia," *J Neurosci*, vol. 30, no. 28, pp. 9477–9487, 2010.

[47] S. Tinaz, "Functional connectome in Parkinson's disease and Parkinsonism," *Curr Neurol Neurosci Rep*, vol. 24, 2021.

[48] A. Lenka, R. Naduthota, M. Jha, *et al.*, "Freezing of gait in Parkinson's disease is associated with altered functional brain connectivity," *PLoS One*, vol. 24, pp. 100–106, 2016.

[49] C. Zuol, X. Suol, H. Lanl, *et al.*, "Global alterations of whole brain structural connectome in Parkinson's disease: A Meta-analysis," *Neuropsychology Review*, vol. 33, pp. 783–802, 2023.

[50] X. Wu, Y. Guo, J. Xue, *et al.*, "Abnormal and changing information interaction in adults with Attention-Deficit/Hyperactivity Disorder based on network motifs," *Brain Sci*, vol. 13, no. 9, p. 1331, 2023.

[51] U. Roine, T. Roine, J. Salmi, *et al.*, "Abnormal wiring of the connectome in adults with high-functioning autism spectrum disorders," *Molecular Autism*, vol. 6, no. 65, 2015.

[52] D. Liu, J. Gao, T. You, *et al.*, "Brain Functional Network Analysis of Patients with Primary Angle-Closure Glaucoma," *Dis Markers*, no. 2731007, 2022.

[53] C. Stam, "Hub overload and failure as a final common pathway in neurological brain network disorders," *Network Neuroscience*, vol. 8, no. 1, pp. 1–34, 2023.

[54] K. Erciyes, *Guide to Graph Algorithms Sequential, Parallel and Distributed.* Springer Texts in Computer Science Series, 2015.

10

Brain Proteomics

Saime Sürmen and Mustafa Gani Sürmen

University of Health Sciences, İstanbul, Türkiye

With the development of high-resolution mass spectrometry systems, proteomic research has reached a much more advanced level. Next-generation MS-based proteomic approaches have enabled the robust and large-scale identification and quantification of biological macromolecules such as proteins. Defining a biological condition through thousands of proteins is promising in terms of taking current evaluations of diseases much further. Another important aspect in performing these MS-based studies is the advanced algorithms that enable the processing of tens of gigabytes of raw data obtained from analyzes and the bioinformatics programs that use them. Thus, proteomics has paved the way for studies to reconsider many chronic diseases that negatively affect human life. Proteomics offers a powerful molecular perspective, especially in generating new data on the early diagnosis and characterization of chronic diseases such as Alzheimer's disease (AD), Parkinson's disease (PD), and schizophrenia, and thus obtaining more comprehensive diagnosis and treatment approaches.

10.1 Introduction

Over the past decade, mass spectrometry-based approaches have enabled great advancements in identification and quantification of thousands of proteins. On the other hand, new informatics tools continue to be developed that make it easier for researchers to interpret and present increasingly complex data sets. Therefore, MS-based proteomics hold promises as powerful approaches to better understand various neurodegenerative diseases such as Alzheimer's disease (AD), Parkinson's disease (PD), and schizophrenia [1–3]. In this chapter, MS-based proteomic studies on common neurological diseases will be discussed to provide an overview of the field of brain proteomics . The majority of MS-based

DOI: 10.1201/9781003461906-10

studies present extensive proteomic data, including a large number of differentially expressed proteins. However, the results of these analysis may vary depending on the biological materials, instruments, sample preparation and analysis methods to be selected [1, 4, 5]. The diversity in the studies is too great to explain each method and summarize the studies here. Therefore, the scope of this study is only limited to the presentation of shotgun proteomics . In the following headings, information will be given about the programs used to process the raw data, and then the databases and tools used to visualize the data in these studies. A significant portion of these tools are utilized to perform enrichment analyses that reveal the biological significance of identified proteins. These analyses classify proteins and reveal possible molecular mechanisms in which the proteins play a role. Some other informatics tools provide networks depicting protein interactions and these will also be mentioned. Finally, MS-based proteomic studies using these technologies in the investigation of neurodegenerative diseases will be discussed. We believe that this chapter will provide important clues about new developments for those who want to carry out research in the field of proteomics using high-throughput technologies.

10.2 The Importance of Proteomics in Brain Research

The field of proteomics, which brings together different disciplines and aims to analyses all proteins in a given sample, has made great progress in the last decade. During this period, advances in methodological, technological, and bioinformatics greatly facilitated researchers' efforts to uncover how the brain proteome is dynamically regulated. Proteins, as functional molecules of the cell, exhibit a highly dynamic profile. The fact that the human brain is more difficult to obtain than other tissues has made mass spectrometry-based proteomics studies, which provide the opportunity for large-scale analysis, very valuable compared to gel electrophoresis and antibody-dependent protein analyses that provide limited information. In this regard, MS systems, which have a high scanning speed and allow the measurement of thousands of proteins and peptides even in complex biological samples, contribute to the creation of proteome catalogs of the nervous system and the discovery of processes related to neurological diseases. Moreover, these catalogs are important data sources for understanding protein-protein, protein-DNA or protein-small molecule interactions [6].

Therefore, large-scale proteomic studies conducted to understand the molecular pathophysiology of the human brain encourage researchers to develop early diagnosis and treatment strategies for neurodegenerative diseases such as Alzheimer's and Parkinson's for the near future. For this purpose, there are various studies in which comprehensive protein profiles are obtained in various biological materials such as cerebrospinal fluid (CSF), serum, plasma and brain tissue. However, finding robust biomarkers that meet expectations for these diseases remains a challenging aspect of the field of proteomics. In a significant portion of studies, further analysis of biomarker candidates cannot be performed due to sample size and technical difficulties in the sample collection procedures, device and informatics analysis, and thus candidate markers cannot progress to the clinic.

Constructing a strong study design is one of the main challenges, and a successful proteomic study requires choosing the most appropriate one among many methods and instruments that have their own strengths and weaknesses [3, 4]. Recently, bioinformatics tools used in the evaluation of big data have become widespread, making it easier to interpret many data sets together and visualize these data [7, 8]. In this context, integrating various proteomic approaches with each other and with other omics platforms has the potential to find biomarker panels that are more clinically reliable and robust.

10.3 The Importance of Sample Selection for Proteomics Research

Sample selection and preparation in a proteomics study affects the entire process, from the first step to the last step of the workflow. Despite the great selectivity and sensitivity of MS approaches, a major drawback is that abundant proteins obscure low-abundance proteins during analysis, preventing their detection. Accordingly, the biggest effort spent in the sample preparation process is to reduce sample complexity. However, this difficulty cannot be overcome by a single method but can be achieved with a combination of several methods [9, 10]. An ideal sample preparation procedure that will increase the analysis power of MS and reveal the highest protein coverage therefore requires meticulousness in every aspect. The most commonly used samples to investigate neurodegenerative diseases include brain tissue, serum/plasma, and CSF [11–13]. In this context, knowing some of the characteristics of the samples planned to be examined that will shape the study design and choosing the method accordingly will make the study valuable.

10.4 Shotgun Proteomics

To date, various methods such as ELISA, western-blot, 2D-PAGE, 2D-DIGE, protein microarray and mass spectrometry techniques have been used for protein analysis in brain research [4, 14]. However, the evolution and widespread use of MS systems has caused changes in the intended use of these methods. For example, gel systems, which were previously widely used in quantitative protein detection, are now preferred to reduce protein complexity before MS analysis, while antibody-based methods such as ELISA and western blot are used to confirm the findings obtained after MS analysis.

There are two main approaches to proteomics: top-down and bottom-up, which differ depending on the stage of preparation of samples before MS analysis (Figure 10.1). Among these approaches, shotgun (bottom-up) proteomics has a wide application for neurodegenerative diseases. Therefore, the focus of this chapter will be on liquid chromatography-mass spectrometry-based (LC-MS) methods from the perspective of shotgun proteomics. In the shotgun proteomics workflow, peptides are first obtained from extracted proteins through denaturation, alkylation, and enzyme digestion. After this step, the peptide mixture is usually separated by high-performance liquid chromatography and ionized via an ion source integrated into the MS. Although there are several techniques for ionization of peptides, the best known are ESI (Electrospray ionization) and MALDI (Matrix-assisted laser desorption ionization), and ESI is used combined with liquid chromatography for peptide separation in shotgun proteomics. With the ESI technique, ionized peptides are sprayed into a high-resolution tandem mass spectrometer to measure the mass/charge (m/z) ratios followed by their fragmentation in the collision cell for the acquisition of mass spectra.

Finally, raw data files of several GB in size are processed by loading them into software programs that use various algorithms for peptide-spectrum matching. Global analysis of proteins by the high-resolution mass spectrometry provides us with information not only about the expression differences of proteins, but also the amino acid sequence of that protein and what modifications there are on it [15–17]. There are variety of methods used in this approach, each with their pros and cons (Figure 10.2). Therefore, each step in these methods requires meticulous work.

10.5 Processing and Visualizing Proteomics Data

Nowadays, the shotgun proteomics approach offers the opportunity to simultaneously examine over ten thousand proteins in brain tissue and over 1000 proteins in cerebrospinal fluid [18, 19]. In this process, successful sample preparation and LC-MS/MS analysis is followed by processing of large amounts of proteomic data. However, processing and interpretation of data is a critical step of the proteomics workflow and is as labor intensive as the other steps. At this step, programs using special software are needed to process several GB of data obtained by LC-MS/MS analysis. Progenesis QI (Waters), Protein Lynx Global Server (Waters), MaxQuant

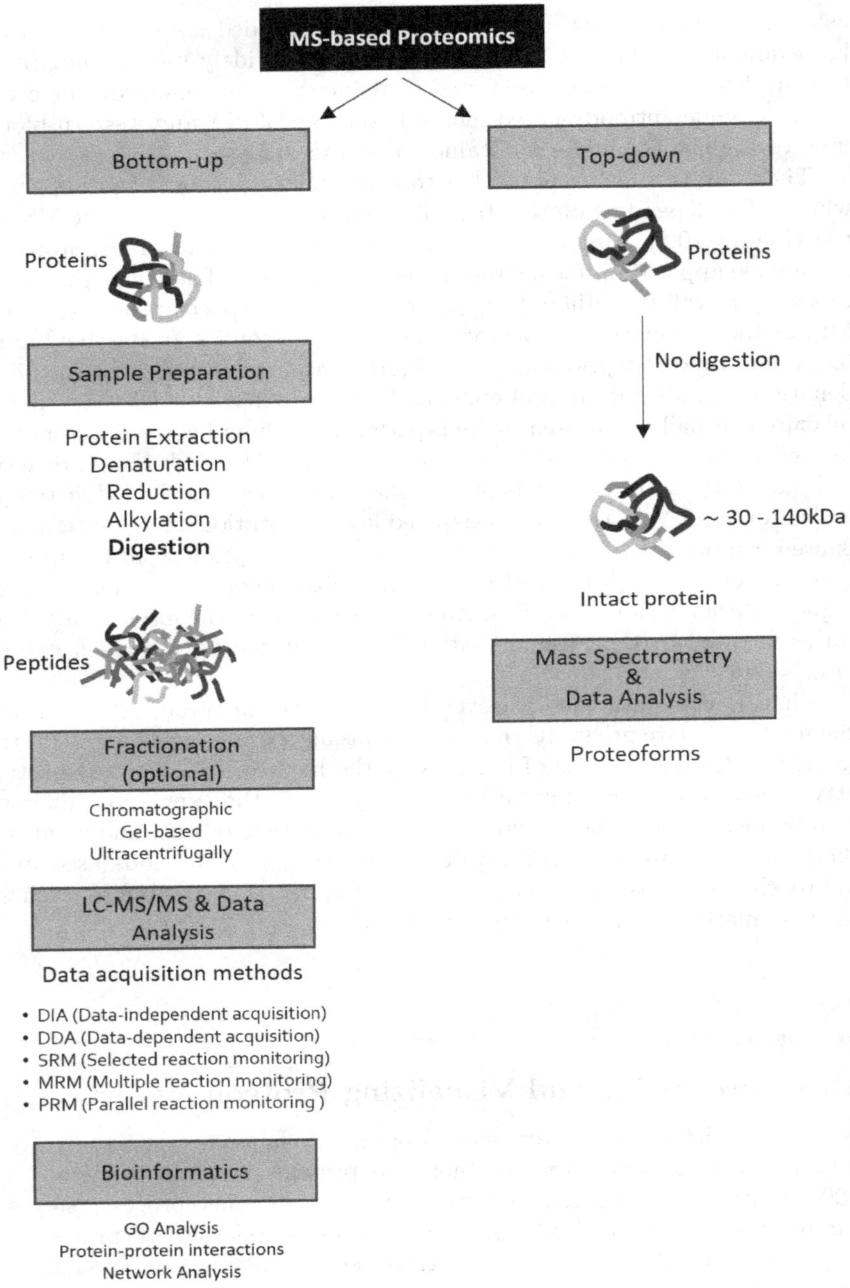

FIGURE 10.1
A typical workflow of MS-based proteomics.

Digestion strategies

In-solution digestion
In-gel digestion
FASP (Filter-aided Sample Preperation)

Peptide enrichment strategies

Metal Oxide Affinity Chromatography (MOAC)
Immobilized Metal Affinity Chromatography (IMAC)
Phos-tag
Lectin-affinity chromatography

Depletion strategies

Immunoaffinity
Precipitation
Affinity chromatography

Fractionation strategies

High pH reverse phase chromatography
Strong Anion Exchange (SAX)
Strong Cation Exchange (SCX)
Hydrophilic Interaction Liquid Affinity (HILIC)

Quantification strategies (Labeled & Unlabeled)

Stable Isotope Labeling with Amino acids in Cell Culture (SILAC)
Isobaric Tag for Relative and Absolute Quantitation (iTRAQ)
Isotope-Coded Affinity Tag (ICAT)
Tandem Mass Tag (TMT)
Spectral counting
Peak intensity
SWATH-MS

Some online tools for bioinformatics

STRING	(https://string-db.org)
PANTHER	(https://www.pantherdb.org/)
KEGG	(https://www.genome.jp/kegg/)
REACTOME	(https://reactome.org/)
DAVID	(https://david.ncifcrf.gov/)
PhosphoSitePLus	(https://www.phosphosite.org)

FIGURE 10.2
An overview of proteomics methods and applications.

(https://www.maxquant.org/), Proteome Discoverer (Thermo Scientific) and Skyline (https://skyline.ms/project/home/software/Skyline/begin.view) are among the programs frequently used in these studies. Additionally, various search engines such as MASCOT (www.matrixscience.com), SEQUEST, X!Tandem, OMSSA (Open Mass Spectrometry Search Algorithm) and Andromeda are used for peptide and protein identifications [20–24]. While raw data processing, statistical analysis and visualizations can be done in a single program, they have limited use. However, for further analysis, proteomic data can be exported to different formats (e.g., mzML mzIdentML and pepXML) and visualized using various online tools, programs or programming languages [25, 26]. It is possible to group the figures used in a proteomic study under several headings for the purpose. The first involves assessing MS data quality. Quality control of MS data is crucial for early detection of faults in the sample collection or preparation process and problems such as sample overload, contamination, and uneven spraying. For this purpose, it would be very useful to visualize the raw data at the precursor and fragment level and evaluate it using a reference extracted ion chromatogram and total ion chromatogram images.

The next step is to look at the distribution of examples and similarities between groups. The distribution of identified peptides and proteins can be evaluated by histogram and PCA analyses. Additionally, box-whisker plots can be used to see differences between sample abundances. In terms of protein coverage, common or unique proteins between groups can be represented by a Venn diagram using accession numbers. Heat maps and volcano-plot graphics, in which proteins whose expression changes are evaluated quantitatively, are constructed based on fold change and p-values in terms of statistical and biological significance. Normalization of protein abundances is very important before drawing such graphs. Rows and columns with similar abundance values in heat maps generated by calculating the distance between protein amounts are clustered using Distance Function methods such as Euclidean, Manhattan and Pearson [25, 27, 28].

In addition, further analyses are required to understand and interpret the thousands of protein lists obtained by processing raw data and to reveal their biological significance. Page-long protein lists are translated into more understandable visuals thanks to the increasing number of enrichment tools. Online databases such as Panther (https://www.pantherdb.org/), STRING (https://string-db.org/) and DAVID (https://david.ncifcrf.gov/) are widely used for gene ontology analyses. In addition, the Cytoscape software platform (https://apps.cytoscape.org/apps/all_#downloads), which supports a wide range of plug-ins such as ClueGO, CluePedia, PiNGO, BINGO and Cyto-Cluster, provides researchers with more options for enrichment analyses and greater flexibility for figures. Various databases are utilized for functional enrichment analyses. KEGG (https://www.genome.jp/kegg/) and REACTOME (https://reactome.org/) are the most frequently referenced databases for molecular networks of diseases and a graphical map of biological processes and pathways.

STRING database, which contains protein information of a wide variety of organisms from the human proteome to *Blastomyces parvus*, is the most preferred address for displaying known and predicted protein-protein interactions. Although this platform offers limited color and features for PPI, the existing network can be exported. However, the fact that each program or tool allows importing files in different formats for processing can sometimes increase the workload.

The recently introduced STRINGApp tool also provides ease of transferring the network and enrichment results performed on STRING to Cytoscape and allows more analysis opportunities [29]. Additionally, following the Perseus software platform (https://maxquant.net/perseus/) used for both statistical analysis and data visualization, a new network module, PerseusNet, was recently introduced to facilitate graph analysis of proteome interaction [30].

Moreover, the use of R and Python programming languages with various interfaces has ensured researchers with great flexibility in this process. In this context, the use of programming languages has become more common in recent studies. Studies explaining how to visualize proteomic data using these programming languages are also very useful for scientists who do not have programming experience. See Ref [27, 31] for more information.

10.6 Proteomic Studies on Neurological Diseases

Alzheimer's and Parkinson's diseases, which cause progressive neurodegeneration, affect a significant portion of the elderly population worldwide. Schizophrenia is a psychiatric disease that seriously affects both the individual and the people around him. However, it may include neurological findings in which physical damage to the brain tissue can be observed. Further investigation of these three diseases, which seriously affect public health, with proteomic approaches is very interesting as it can provide depth at the molecular level regarding the definitions and treatment practices of these diseases. Here we review recent proteomic studies in a variety of, but not all, clinical samples and animal models.

10.6.1 Alzheimer's Disease (AD)

AD is a neurodegenerative disease characterized by progressive cognitive impairment. Amyloid β (Aβ) peptide accumulation and neurofibrillary tangles due to tau hyperphosphorylation, seen in advanced stages, are the two known basic pathological features of the disease. Although clinical symptoms and neuroimaging are used for diagnosis, significant findings are usually obtained in the late stages. Finding robust biomarkers is essential for early-stage diagnosis and effective treatment protocol. The first studies focused mostly on these two molecular pathological processes that result in neuron loss. However, the lack of an effective treatment protocol yet has increased the number of studies aimed at elucidating the molecular changes that direct the pathogenesis of the disease and finding new biomarkers.

While AD studies conducted in recent years offer new perspectives on AD using various omics approaches, there is great interest in proteomic approaches that comprehensively reveal pathogenesis-related protein differences [32, 33]. Redox and organelle proteomics have revealed the dysregulation of a number of proteins related to oxidative stress, impaired energy metabolism, and mitochondrial and synaptic dysfunctions that occur in the neurodegenerative process [34–38].

In fact, there are many studies aimed at identifying AD-specific markers in brain tissue and CSF. Due to the heterogeneous nature of the brain, some studies have focused on specific brain regions or specific cell populations and used localized proteomics approaches [39–42]. Frontal cortex and Hippocampus are the regions of the brain most affected by AD. A recent study examining brain regions affected early (entorhinal and parahippocampal cortices) and late (temporal and frontal cortices) by tau pathology showed that synaptic proteins are altered in the early B/B stages, whereas proteins indicating translation dysregulation are mainly down-regulated in the frontal, entorhinal, and parahippocampal cortices [40]. Sathe et al. conducted both exploratory and targeted proteomic analyses between post-mortem patients with AD and cognitively normal and age-matched individuals. Using TMT labeling, researchers identified 8066 proteins in medial frontal gyrus tissues, 432 of which showed significant changes [41]. In another proteomic study conducted on fresh frozen brain tissue samples from the dorsolateral prefrontal cortex, more than six thousand proteins were identified using prefractionation and TMT labeling methods, and it was reported that there were changes in 350 proteins, including RNA-binding proteins, between AD and asymptomatic AD [43].

On the other hand, as an alternative to fresh human tissue, FFPE (formalin-fixed, paraffin-embedded) tissue may be a valuable source of information for clinical proteomic studies. Since it can be stored for a long time, it can also provide the opportunity to evaluate AD patients retrospectively. Drummond et al. reported a strategy that would be advantageous in evaluating very specific cell types in brain regions in their study in which they isolated neuronal cells from temporal cortex FFPE tissue blocks of patients with severe AD using the laser capture microdissection (LCM) method [44]. The same researcher also used the LCM method, which allows localized proteomics , for the isolation of amyloid plaques and neurofibrillary tangles [45]. Another study used LCM to compare the amyloid pathology of Rapidly progressive Alzheimer's disease (rpAD) and sporadic Alzheimer's disease (sAD) patient groups and found that the protein composition of the plaques was significantly different. In addition, findings regarding the abundance of synaptic proteins in rpAD plaques pointed to the importance of synaptic dysfunction in plaque development. [39]. Furthermore, the applicability of various strategies such as MACS, FACS, BONCAT and FUNCAT to proteomic studies will accelerate the creation of cell type-specific proteome catalogs [33, 46].

Consistent results of Aβ42, t-tau and p-tau measurements in CSF from various studies also indicate that they may be important in clinical practice for the early diagnosis of AD. A comprehensive meta-analysis evaluating these findings showed that lower Aβ42 and higher t-tau and p-tau levels in CSF can discriminate between disease-related mild cognitive impairment and stable mild cognitive impairment [47]. Another evaluation revealed that 48 proteins associated with steroid esterification and protein activation cascade processes were upregulated in CSF [10]. A recent deep proteomic analysis of brain and CSF samples allowed the identification of approximately 3500 proteins in 40 CSF samples and close to 12000 proteins in 27 brain tissues. Interestingly, 70% of the CSF proteome was shared with proteins in brain tissue, and some of the proteins were involved in synaptic, vascular, myelination, inflammatory and metabolic pathways [48]. The fact that cellular processes are reflected in the CSF, which is in direct contact with the brain, makes it a valuable resource in this respect. Sathe et al. also identified 2327 proteins, 139 of which showed significant changes in AD compared to control. Although a small number of CSF samples were used in the study, they were able to confirm that neuronal pentraxin 2 (NPTX2) and VGF nerve growth factor inducible (VGF) proteins decreased and 14-3-3 protein gamma (YWHAG) and pyruvate kinase (PKM) proteins increased with the targeted PRM method [49]. According to a review of CSF proteomic studies, nearly half of previously reported protein alterations showed consistent results. However, the fact that the study results are not directly comparable may have affected the number of common proteins. The same review showed enrichment of haemostasis, lipoprotein, and extracellular matrix for pathway outcomes of AD-related proteins. Additionally, while there are very few studies evaluating the impact of patients' demographic characteristics on the CSF proteome, further research in this direction may provide clues to explain the heterogeneity in AD [50].

Although they have not yet been reflected in the clinic other than plaque and tau pathology, candidate protein markers that can support the diagnosis in various body fluids are recommended. One research group has performed comprehensive proteome characterization in serum as well as human cerebral cortex and CSF. They also used TOMAHAQ-targeted MS analysis for validation in their study, which allowed direct profiling of human serum and CSF without depleting proteins for biomarker discovery. In the study, nearly 5000 serum proteins and nearly 6000 CSF proteins were identified, especially the altered proteins that were related to mitochondrial function [51–53].

Studies conducted in the saliva of individuals with mild cognitive impairment (MCI) and AD have also reported that salivary transthyretin (TTR), cystatin-C, interleukin-1 receptor antagonist, stratifin, matrix metalloproteinase 9 and haptoglobin protein levels vary compared to controls [54, 55].

In general, various studies conducted by different researchers have shown that serum, plasma, saliva and urine may also contain proteins that will provide information about disease pathogenesis [54–57]. However, these findings in proteomic studies have not yet become biomarker panels that will support clinical diagnosis due to the need for further validation in large samples.

10.6.2 Parkinson's Disease (PD)

PD, considered the second most common neurodegenerative disease, is characterized by the preferential degeneration of dopaminergic neurons extending from the substantia nigra to the striatum. Motor dysfunctions that occur in the middle and late stages of the disease are attributed to the loss of more than half of these neurons. Dopaminergic neurons are cells rich in mitochondria to meet high energy needs, and in many studies the pathogenesis of the disease has been associated with mitochondrial dysfunction [58]. Proteomic studies conducted with both human brain and model organisms have highlighted proteins related to neuroinflammation, oxidative stress, and the Ubiquitin-proteasome system, especially mitochondrial respiratory chain proteins. In this context, the substantia nigra has been the most studied region of the brain due to dopaminergic neuron losses [59–61]. The results of an in-depth proteomic analysis, in which more than ten thousand proteins were identified, also showed that the downregulated mitoribosome proteins in the substantia nigra were the most dysregulated proteins [59]. In the study characterizing the protein profile of synaptosomes isolated from neuronal cell bodies in this region, it was pointed out that mitochondrial Thymidine kinase 2 (TK2), 39S ribosomal protein L2, neurolysin and Methionine-tRNA ligase (MARS2) may have a stronger relationship with Parkinson's disease than known [61].

In addition to post-mortem brain tissue, the pathogenesis of the disease has also been investigated in animal models developed with toxin treatments that promote PD-like dopaminergic neuron loss. In some studies, proteomic, targeted proteomic and phosphoproteomic analyses were performed on various samples obtained from zebrafish that exhibited PD-like symptoms after exposure to rotenone, a neurotoxin. Interestingly, in addition to mitochondrial proteins altered by rotenone toxicity, it has been reported that proteins involved in the redox system, calcium and lipid transport activity, and energy metabolism were significantly improved after octanoic acid and erucic acid treatments [62–64].

On the other hand, biomarker studies have been conducted in various biological fluids for Parkinson's disease, as well as Alzheimer's. In a CSF proteomics study aiming to distinguish Parkinson's syndromes from healthy controls, 341 proteins were quantified using two different cohorts. Of the 13 proteins common to both cohorts, the importance of extended granin family proteins was highlighted [65]. Moreover, recently different workflow applications have greatly improved the protein profile in CSF. Despite the disadvantages of biofluid proteomics, such as low measurement sensitivity and limited proteome depth, 1400 CSF proteins were identified in a single analysis with very small amounts of CSF samples. Thus, with the high protein count and reproducibility in the study, a workflow is presented showing that MS-based proteomics is a powerful technology for biomarker discovery in biofluids [18].

Additionally, intense efforts have been directed towards plasma, serum exosome, urine, saliva, tears, and organelle proteomics in the hope of finding specific biomarkers [66–71]. Chitinase-3-like protein 1 (CHI3L1) and thymosin beta-4 (TMSB4X) were most significantly altered in the plasma proteome, while 14 targetable proteins were reported in the serum exosome, including Apolipoprotein J, pigment epithelium-derived factor (PEDF), and gelsolin [66, 67]. In the study investigating the salivary proteome, it was hypothesized that there may be protein markers reflected in saliva before the onset of motor symptoms in PD. In the light of the findings, it was reported that a decrease in the levels of proteins playing a role in inflammatory processes, exosome formation and adipose tissue formation, and it was suggested that the inflammation associated with PD pathology may be reflected in the saliva profile [69]. The protein profile results of tears, which are rarely investigated in proteomic studies, are also very interesting. In addition to the results supporting dry eye syndrome-like pathology in PD, it has been revealed that there are irregularities in proteins that play a role in lipid metabolism, oxidative stress, vesicle secretion and immune response, specific to PD [70].

Organelle proteomics studies, which provide more specific data, also provide important information about the pathogenesis of PD. A new strategy for Mitochondrial Degradoma has been developed in which the N-terminal peptides are enriched by the dimethylation-TAILS approach after isolating the mitochondrial subcellular fraction In the study showing the effects of changing dopamine homeostasis on the mitochondrial N-terminome using this strategy, it was reported that neprilysin may be a candidate for mitochondrial protease indicating mitochondrial dysfunction [71].

10.6.3 Schizophrenia

Schizophrenia is a serious neuropsychiatric disease that negatively affects social life. Since its diagnosis is based on the subjective evaluation of clinical symptoms, it can be confused with different types of diseases such as bipolar disorder. Although genomic studies reveal some rare mutations in schizophrenia, there are significant deficiencies in the diagnosis and classification of the disease [72]. Although fewer reports have been stated on schizophrenia compared to Alzheimer's and Parkinson's, proteomic studies provide important contributions to the molecular pathogenesis, diagnosis, and treatment of this disease. While the studies are generally based on comparisons between schizophrenia patients and healthy control groups, a significant portion of them were conducted in patients using medication [73].

Proteomic and phosphoproteomic analyses specific to different regions of the brain such as the cerebellum, caudate nucleus, posterior cingulate cortex, orbitofrontal cortex, primary auditory cortex, and corpus callosum obtained from schizophrenia patients and controls have pointed out the irregularity of proteins in oligodendrocytes, astrocytes, glial cells, and synapses. These were studies that particularly highlighted mitochondrial and synaptic proteins. Important proteins involved in cell signaling pathways include ATP synthase subunit alpha (ATP5A1), postsynaptic density protein 95 (PSD95), calcium/calmodulin-dependent protein kinase II, ephrin B, ciliary neurotrophic proteins, glutamate, and gamma aminobutyric acid (GABA) receptors [74–77].

Several recent reports have also examined patients diagnosed with schizophrenia and bipolar disorder. In these studies, using serum and plasma samples, irregularities in complement system proteins and lipid proteins were reported. Interesting findings include changing expressions of complement C9 (C9) and Interleukin 1 Receptor Accessory Protein (IL1RAP), Ankyrin Repeat Domain-Containing Protein 12 (ANKRD12), Cadherin 5 (CADH5) in serum and apolipoproteins in plasma [78–81]. Additionally, a meta-analysis also revealed downregulation of apolipoproteins [73].

Another focus of proteomic studies in schizophrenia patients has been to investigate post-treatment drug effects reflected in the serum and plasma proteome [82]. Proteomic analysis of plasma samples from patients with schizophrenia revealed that proteins that change in response to treatment are mostly associated with the immune and inflammatory systems [83]. Although antipsychotics are the primary treatment drugs for schizophrenia, these drugs may also have various side effects, especially on fat tissue metabolism. Proteomic examination of olanzapine, risperidone, and haloperidol drug treatments in rats prenatally exposed to MAM (methylazoxymethanol) provided important information about the adipose tissue proteome and demonstrated downregulation of proteins belonging to the TOR signaling pathway [84]. Additionally, studies conducted in post-mortem brain tissue samples and schizophrenia cell models have shown that antipsychotic drugs may have effects on two post-translational modifications: succinylation and malonylation [85].

An interesting proteomic study performed on dried blood spots of newborn babies investigated biomarkers that indicate disease susceptibility. Increased expression of Alpha-2-antiplasmin (A2AP), Complement C4-A (CO4A) and Antithrombin-III (ANT3) has been reported [86]. These results may constitute important data sources for proteomic studies with untreated schizophrenia patients.

10.7 Conclusion and Remarks

Recently, methodological, instrumental and software developments have been reflected in proteomics applications and have given researchers a deeper understanding of the molecular basis of diseases. In this chapter, we focused on studies using proteomic technology to investigate Alzheimer's disease, Parkinson's disease, and schizophrenia, three neurodegenerative diseases that seriously affect human life. Today's proteomics technology has the potential to reveal large-scale protein profiles of single types of cells or organelles from biological material. As of 2024, information on a total of 204229 human proteins is stored in the UniProt Knowledgebase, 20428 of which have been manually annotated and reviewed (Access date: 23.01.2024). Considering the enormous number and diversity of the cells that make up the human brain, the importance of data obtained from high-resolution mass spectrometers becomes increasingly important.

On the other hand, it should not be forgotten that the reflection of the neuropathological status on the proteome data depends on the process of combining and interpreting robust and reliable results. A meticulous study should be carried out in proteomic studies for sufficient sample size, good determination of sample inclusion and exclusion criteria, a good sample preparation workflow that requires minimal manipulation of the sample, and powerful statistical and bioinformatic analyses. Widely used and constantly updated applications such as STRING, Perseus and other informatics tools mentioned above, as well as new applications or modules such as STRINGApp and PerseusNet, continue to make significant contributions to the field of proteomics in general. However, the fact that proteomic data obtained on neurodegenerative diseases have not yet been strongly implicated into clinical routine suggests that more efforts are needed in wet laboratory studies and the development of more comprehensive informatics tools.

In summary, while MS-based proteomic studies provide rich findings that advance our general knowledge of neurodegenerative diseases, difficulties in presenting, interpreting, and integrating the large volumes of data collected slow the process of generating specific information about neurodegeneration that can be applied to the clinic. An overview of recent studies reveals the need for new proteomic analyses that will show protein-protein interactions, post-translational modifications, and alterations in the protein expression, especially for the determination of new diagnostic criteria and for better classification of disease subtypes in schizophrenia. Multidisciplinary collaborations involving researchers such as molecular biologists, chemists, and computer scientists are of great importance in overcoming the challenges in evaluating proteomic data analysis. In particular, the increased prevalence of user-friendly software and the easier applicability of these to proteomics will enable the data to be interpreted and presented rapidly.

Bibliography

[1] M. Downs, J. Zaia, and M. K. Sethi, "Mass spectrometry methods for analysis of extracellular matrix components in neurological diseases," *Mass Spectrometry Reviews*, vol. 42, no. 5, pp. 1848–1875, 2023.

[2] E. Fingleton, Y. Li, and K. W. Roche, "Advances in proteomics allow insights into neuronal proteomes," *Frontiers in Molecular Neuroscience*, vol. 14, p. 647451, 2021.

[3] B. C. Carlyle, B. A. Trombetta, and S. E. Arnold, "Proteomic approaches for the discovery of biofluid biomarkers of neurodegenerative dementias," *Proteomes*, vol. 6, no. 3, p. 32, 2018.

[4] M. D. Filiou, D. Martins-de Souza, P. C. Guest, *et al.*, "To label or not to label: applications of quantitative proteomics in neuroscience research," *Proteomics*, vol. 12, no. 4-5, pp. 736–747, 2012.

[5] M. G. Sürmen, S. Sürmen, A. Ali, *et al.*, "Phosphoproteomic strategies in cancer research: a minireview," *Analyst*, vol. 145, no. 22, pp. 7125–7149, 2020.

[6] F. Hosp and M. Mann, "A primer on concepts and applications of proteomics in neuroscience," *Neuron*, vol. 96, no. 3, pp. 558–571, 2017.

[7] A. Santos, A. R. Colaço, A. B. Nielsen, *et al.*, "A knowledge graph to interpret clinical proteomics data," *Nature biotechnology*, vol. 40, no. 5, pp. 692–702, 2022.

[8] C. Chen, J. Hou, J. J. Tanner, *et al.*, "Bioinformatics methods for mass spectrometry-based proteomics data analysis," *International journal of molecular sciences*, vol. 21, no. 8, p. 2873, 2020.

[9] P. Y. Lee, J. Osman, T. Y. Low, *et al.*, "Plasma/serum proteomics: depletion strategies for reducing high-abundance proteins for biomarker discovery," *Bioanalysis*, vol. 11, no. 19, pp. 1799–1812, 2019.

[10] P. Bastos, R. Ferreira, B. Manadas, *et al.*, "Insights into the human brain proteome: disclosing the biological meaning of protein networks in cerebrospinal fluid," *Critical Reviews in Clinical Laboratory Sciences*, vol. 54, no. 3, pp. 185–204, 2017.

[11] R. Raghunathan, K. Turajane, and L. C. Wong, "Biomarkers in neurodegenerative diseases: Proteomics spotlight on als and parkinson's disease," *International Journal of Molecular Sciences*, vol. 23, no. 16, p. 9299, 2022.

[12] A. P. Jain and G. Sathe, "Proteomics landscape of alzheimer's disease," *Proteomes*, vol. 9, no. 1, p. 13, 2021.

[13] E. M. Cilento, L. Jin, T. Stewart, *et al.*, "Mass spectrometry: A platform for biomarker discovery and validation for alzheimer's and parkinson's diseases," *Journal of neurochemistry*, vol. 151, no. 4, pp. 397–416, 2019.

[14] P. C. Guest, "Proteomic studies of psychiatric disorders," *Investigations of Early Nutrition Effects on Long-Term Health: Methods and Applications*, pp. 59–89, 2018.

[15] A. G. Woods, I. Sokolowska, A. G. Ngounou Wetie, *et al.*, "Mass spectrometry for proteomics-based investigation," *Advancements of Mass Spectrometry in Biomedical Research*, pp. 1–26, 2019.

[16] T. Sajic, Y. Liu, and R. Aebersold, "Using data-independent, high-resolution mass spectrometry in protein biomarker research: perspectives and clinical applications," *PROTEOMICS–Clinical Applications*, vol. 9, no. 3-4, pp. 307–321, 2015.

[17] A. Bilbao, E. Varesio, J. Luban, *et al.*, "Processing strategies and software solutions for data-independent acquisition in mass spectrometry," *Proteomics*, vol. 15, no. 5-6, pp. 964–980, 2015.

[18] O. Karayel, S. V. Winter, S. Padmanabhan, *et al.*, "Proteome profiling of cerebrospinal fluid reveals biomarker candidates for parkinson's disease," *Cell Reports Medicine*, vol. 3, no. 6, 2022.

[19] L. Ping, D. M. Duong, L. Yin, *et al.*, "Global quantitative analysis of the human brain proteome in alzheimer's and parkinson's disease," *Scientific data*, vol. 5, no. 1, pp. 1–12, 2018.

[20] T. Välikangas, T. Suomi, and L. L. Elo, "A comprehensive evaluation of popular proteomics software workflows for label-free proteome quantification and imputation," *Briefings in bioinformatics*, vol. 19, no. 6, pp. 1344–1355, 2018.

[21] C. Loureiro, M. A. R. Buzalaf, F. Moraes, *et al.*, "Quantitative proteomic analysis in symptomatic and asymptomatic apical periodontitis," *International Endodontic Journal*, vol. 54, no. 6, pp. 834–847, 2021.

[22] C. D. Wenger and J. J. Coon, "A proteomics search algorithm specifically designed for high-resolution tandem mass spectra," *Journal of proteome research*, vol. 12, no. 3, pp. 1377–1386, 2013.

[23] S. Tyanova, T. Temu, and J. Cox, "The maxquant computational platform for mass spectrometry-based shotgun proteomics," *Nature protocols*, vol. 11, no. 12, pp. 2301–2319, 2016.

[24] A. Palomba, M. Abbondio, G. Fiorito, *et al.*, "Comparative evaluation of maxquant and proteome discoverer ms1-based protein quantification tools," *Journal of proteome research*, vol. 20, no. 7, pp. 3497–3507, 2021.

[25] E. Oveland, T. Muth, E. Rapp, *et al.*, "Viewing the proteome: how to visualize proteomics data?," *Proteomics*, vol. 15, no. 8, pp. 1341–1355, 2015.

[26] H. Weisser and J. S. Choudhary, "Targeted feature detection for data-dependent shotgun proteomics," *Journal of proteome research*, vol. 16, no. 8, pp. 2964–2974, 2017.

[27] J. P. Schessner, E. Voytik, and I. Bludau, "A practical guide to interpreting and generating bottom-up proteomics data visualizations," *Proteomics*, vol. 22, no. 8, p. 2100103, 2022.

[28] P. Sinitcyn, J. D. Rudolph, and J. Cox, "Computational methods for understanding mass spectrometry–based shotgun proteomics data," *Annual Review of Biomedical Data Science*, vol. 1, pp. 207–234, 2018.

[29] N. T. Doncheva, J. H. Morris, J. Gorodkin, *et al.*, "Cytoscape stringapp: network analysis and visualization of proteomics data," *Journal of proteome research*, vol. 18, no. 2, pp. 623–632, 2018.

[30] J. D. Rudolph and J. Cox, "A network module for the perseus software for computational proteomics facilitates proteome interaction graph analysis," *Journal of proteome research*, vol. 18, no. 5, pp. 2052–2064, 2019.

[31] L. Gatto, L. M. Breckels, T. Naake, *et al.*, "Visualization of proteomics data using r and bioconductor," *Proteomics*, vol. 15, no. 8, pp. 1375–1389, 2015.

[32] H. Hampel, R. Nisticò, N. T. Seyfried, *et al.*, "Omics sciences for systems biology in alzheimer's disease: State-of-the-art of the evidence," *Ageing Research Reviews*, vol. 69, p. 101346, 2021.

[33] S. Rayaprolu, L. Higginbotham, P. Bagchi, *et al.*, "Systems-based proteomics to resolve the biology of alzheimer's disease beyond amyloid and tau," *Neuropsychopharmacology*, vol. 46, no. 1, pp. 98–115, 2021.

[34] A. M. Swomley and D. A. Butterfield, "Oxidative stress in alzheimer disease and mild cognitive impairment: evidence from human data provided by redox proteomics," *Archives of toxicology*, vol. 89, pp. 1669–1680, 2015.

[35] F. Di Domenico, E. Barone, M. Perluigi, *et al.*, "The triangle of death in alzheimer's disease brain: the aberrant cross-talk among energy metabolism, mammalian target of rapamycin signaling, and protein homeostasis revealed by redox proteomics," *Antioxidants & redox signaling*, vol. 26, no. 8, pp. 364–387, 2017.

[36] A. Tramutola, C. Lanzillotta, M. Perluigi, *et al.*, "Oxidative stress, protein modification and alzheimer disease," *Brain research bulletin*, vol. 133, pp. 88–96, 2017.

[37] M. Abyadeh, V. Gupta, N. Chitranshi, *et al.*, "Mitochondrial dysfunction in alzheimer's disease-a proteomics perspective," *Expert review of Proteomics*, vol. 18, no. 4, pp. 295–304, 2021.

[38] D. A. Butterfield and D. Boyd-Kimball, "Redox proteomics and amyloid β-peptide: insights into alzheimer disease," *Journal of neurochemistry*, vol. 151, no. 4, pp. 459–487, 2019.

[39] E. Drummond, S. Nayak, A. Faustin, *et al.*, "Proteomic differences in amyloid plaques in rapidly progressive and sporadic alzheimer's disease," *Acta neuropathologica*, vol. 133, pp. 933–954, 2017.

[40] C. F. Mendonça, M. Kuras, F. C. S. Nogueira, *et al.*, "Proteomic signatures of brain regions affected by tau pathology in early and late stages of alzheimer's disease," *Neurobiology of disease*, vol. 130, p. 104509, 2019.

[41] G. Sathe, M. Albert, J. Darrow, *et al.*, "Quantitative proteomic analysis of the frontal cortex in alzheimer's disease," *Journal of neurochemistry*, vol. 156, no. 6, pp. 988–1002, 2021.

[42] E. B. Dammer, D. M. Duong, I. Diner, *et al.*, "Neuron enriched nuclear proteome isolated from human brain," *Journal of proteome research*, vol. 12, no. 7, pp. 3193–3206, 2013.

[43] E. C. Johnson, E. B. Dammer, D. M. Duong, *et al.*, "Deep proteomic network analysis of alzheimer's disease brain reveals alterations in rna binding proteins and rna splicing associated with disease," *Molecular neurodegeneration*, vol. 13, pp. 1–22, 2018.

[44] E. S. Drummond, S. Nayak, B. Ueberheide, *et al.*, "Proteomic analysis of neurons microdissected from formalin-fixed, paraffin-embedded alzheimer's disease brain tissue," *Scientific reports*, vol. 5, no. 1, p. 15456, 2015.

[45] E. Drummond, S. Nayak, G. Pires, *et al.*, "Isolation of amyloid plaques and neurofibrillary tangles from archived alzheimer's disease tissue using laser-capture microdissection for downstream proteomics," *Laser Capture Microdissection: Methods and Protocols*, pp. 319–334, 2018.

[46] A. K. Carlisle, J. Götz, and L.-G. Bodea, "Three methods for examining the de novo proteome of microglia using boncat bioorthogonal labeling and funcat click chemistry," *STAR protocols*, vol. 4, no. 3, p. 102418, 2023.

[47] B. Olsson, R. Lautner, U. Andreasson, *et al.*, "Csf and blood biomarkers for the diagnosis of alzheimer's disease: a systematic review and meta-analysis," *The Lancet Neurology*, vol. 15, no. 7, pp. 673–684, 2016.

[48] L. Higginbotham, L. Ping, E. B. Dammer, *et al.*, "Integrated proteomics reveals brain-based cerebrospinal fluid biomarkers in asymptomatic and symptomatic alzheimer's disease," *Science advances*, vol. 6, no. 43, p. eaaz9360, 2020.

[49] G. Sathe, C. H. Na, S. Renuse, *et al.*, "Quantitative proteomic profiling of cerebrospinal fluid to identify candidate biomarkers for alzheimer's disease," *PROTEOMICS–Clinical Applications*, vol. 13, no. 4, p. 1800105, 2019.

[50] K. E. Wesenhagen, C. E. Teunissen, P. J. Visser, *et al.*, "Cerebrospinal fluid proteomics and biological heterogeneity in alzheimer's disease: a literature review," *Critical reviews in clinical laboratory sciences*, vol. 57, no. 2, pp. 86–98, 2020.

[51] K. K. Dey, H. Wang, M. Niu, *et al.*, "Deep undepleted human serum proteome profiling toward biomarker discovery for alzheimer's disease," *Clinical proteomics*, vol. 16, no. 1, pp. 1–12, 2019.

[52] H. Wang, K. K. Dey, P.-C. Chen, *et al.*, "Integrated analysis of ultra-deep proteomes in cortex, cerebrospinal fluid and serum reveals a mitochondrial signature in alzheimer's disease," *Molecular neurodegeneration*, vol. 15, no. 1, pp. 1–20, 2020.

[53] K. K. Dey, H. Sun, Z. Wang, *et al.*, "Proteomic profiling of cerebrospinal fluid by 16-plex tmt-based mass spectrometry," *Clinical proteomics: Methods and protocols*, pp. 21–37, 2022.

[54] E. Eldem, A. Barve, O. Sallin, *et al.*, "Salivary proteomics identifies transthyretin as a biomarker of early dementia conversion," *Journal of Alzheimer's Disease Reports*, vol. 6, no. 1, pp. 31–41, 2022.

[55] K. McNicholas, M. François, J.-W. Liu, *et al.*, "Salivary inflammatory biomarkers are predictive of mild cognitive impairment and alzheimer's disease in a feasibility study," *Frontiers in Aging Neuroscience*, vol. 14, p. 1019296, 2022.

[56] F. Yao, X. Hong, S. Li, *et al.*, "Urine-based biomarkers for alzheimer's disease identified through coupling computational and experimental methods," *Journal of Alzheimer's Disease*, vol. 65, no. 2, pp. 421–431, 2018.

[57] M. Inoue, H. Suzuki, K. Meno, *et al.*, "Identification of plasma proteins as biomarkers for mild cognitive impairment and alzheimer's disease using liquid chromatography–tandem mass spectrometry," *International Journal of Molecular Sciences*, vol. 24, no. 17, p. 13064, 2023.

[58] M. Aroso, R. Ferreira, A. Freitas, *et al.*, "New insights on the mitochondrial proteome plasticity in parkinson's disease," *PROTEOMICS–Clinical Applications*, vol. 10, no. 4, pp. 416–429, 2016.

[59] Y. Jang, O. Pletnikova, J. C. Troncoso, *et al.*, "Mass spectrometry–based proteomics analysis of human substantia nigra from parkinson's disease patients identifies multiple pathways potentially involved in the disease," *Molecular & Cellular Proteomics*, vol. 22, no. 1, 2023.

[60] V. A. Petyuk, L. Yu, H. M. Olson, and o. Yu, "Proteomic profiling of the substantia nigra to identify determinants of lewy body pathology and dopaminergic neuronal loss," *Journal of proteome research*, vol. 20, no. 5, pp. 2266–2282, 2021.

[61] S. Plum, B. Eggers, S. Helling, *et al.*, "Proteomic characterization of synaptosomes from human substantia nigra indicates altered mitochondrial translation in parkinson's disease," *Cells*, vol. 9, no. 12, p. 2580, 2020.

[62] M. G. Sürmen, S. Sürmen, D. Cansız, *et al.*, "Quantitative phosphoproteomics to resolve the cellular responses to octanoic acid in rotenone exposed zebrafish," *Journal of Food Biochemistry*, vol. 45, no. 10, p. e13923, 2021.

[63] M. G. Sürmen, S. Sürmen, D. Cansız, *et al.*, "Amelioration of rotenone-induced alterations in energy/redox system, stress response and cytoskeleton proteins by octanoic acid in zebrafish: A proteomic study," *Journal of Biochemical and Molecular Toxicology*, vol. 36, no. 5, p. e23024, 2022.

[64] İ. Ünal, D. Cansız, M. G. Sürmen, *et al.*, "Identification of molecular network of gut-brain axis associated with neuroprotective effects of pparδ-ligand erucic acid in rotenone-induced parkinson's disease model in zebrafish," *European Journal of Neuroscience*, vol. 57, no. 4, pp. 585–606, 2023.

[65] M. S. Rotunno, M. Lane, W. Zhang, *et al.*, "Cerebrospinal fluid proteomics implicates the granin family in parkinson's disease," *Scientific reports*, vol. 10, no. 1, p. 2479, 2020.

[66] Y. Zhao, Y. Zhang, J. Zhang, *et al.*, "Plasma proteome profiling using tandem mass tag labeling technology reveals potential biomarkers for parkinson's disease: a preliminary study," *PROTEOMICS–Clinical Applications*, vol. 16, no. 2, p. 2100010, 2022.

[67] R. Jiang, C. Rong, R. Ke, *et al.*, "Differential proteomic analysis of serum exosomes reveals alterations in progression of parkinson disease," *Medicine*, vol. 98, no. 41, 2019.

[68] S. Virreira Winter, O. Karayel, M. T. Strauss, *et al.*, "Urinary proteome profiling for stratifying patients with familial parkinson's disease," *EMBO molecular medicine*, vol. 13, no. 3, p. e13257, 2021.

[69] M. Figura, E. Sitkiewicz, B. Świderska, *et al.*, "Proteomic profile of saliva in parkinson's disease patients: A proof of concept study," *Brain Sciences*, vol. 11, no. 5, p. 661, 2021.

[70] M. Boerger, S. Funke, A. Leha, *et al.*, "Proteomic analysis of tear fluid reveals disease-specific patterns in patients with parkinson's disease–a pilot study," *Parkinsonism & related disorders*, vol. 63, pp. 3–9, 2019.

[71] M. Lualdi, M. Ronci, M. Zilocchi, *et al.*, "Exploring the mitochondrial degradome by the tails proteomics approach in a cellular model of parkinson's disease," *Frontiers in Aging Neuroscience*, vol. 11, p. 195, 2019.

[72] G. Costain and A. S. Bassett, "Clinical applications of schizophrenia genetics: genetic diagnosis, risk, and counseling in the molecular era," *The application of clinical genetics*, pp. 1–18, 2012.

[73] J. E. Rodrigues, A. Martinho, C. Santa, *et al.*, "Systematic review and meta-analysis of mass spectrometry proteomics applied to human peripheral fluids to assess potential biomarkers of schizophrenia," *International Journal of Molecular Sciences*, vol. 23, no. 9, p. 4917, 2022.

[74] G. Reis-de Oliveira, G. Zuccoli, M. Fioramonte, *et al.*, "Digging deeper in the proteome of different regions from schizophrenia brains," *Journal of proteomics*, vol. 223, p. 103814, 2020.

[75] E. Velasquez, F. C. Nogueira, I. Velasquez, *et al.*, "Synaptosomal proteome of the orbitofrontal cortex from schizophrenia patients using quantitative label-free and itraq-based shotgun proteomics," *Journal of proteome research*, vol. 16, no. 12, pp. 4481–4494, 2017.

[76] M. L. MacDonald, M. Garver, J. Newman, *et al.*, "Synaptic proteome alterations in the primary auditory cortex of individuals with schizophrenia," *JAMA psychiatry*, vol. 77, no. 1, pp. 86–95, 2020.

[77] V. M. Saia-Cereda, J. S. Cassoli, A. Schmitt, *et al.*, "Differential proteome and phosphoproteome may impact cell signaling in the corpus callosum of schizophrenia patients," *Schizophrenia Research*, vol. 177, no. 1-3, pp. 70–77, 2016.

[78] M. Oraki Kohshour, N. R. Kannaiyan, A. J. Falk, *et al.*, "Comparative serum proteomic analysis of a selected protein panel in individuals with schizophrenia and bipolar disorder and the impact of genetic risk burden on serum proteomic profiles," *Translational Psychiatry*, vol. 12, no. 1, p. 471, 2022.

[79] L. Smirnova, A. Seregin, I. Boksha, *et al.*, "The difference in serum proteomes in schizophrenia and bipolar disorder," *BMC genomics*, vol. 20, no. 7, pp. 1–14, 2019.

[80] E. C. Santa Cruz, F. da Silva Zandonadi, W. Fontes, *et al.*, "A pilot study indicating the dysregulation of the complement and coagulation cascades in treated schizophrenia and bipolar disorder patients," *Biochimica Et Biophysica Acta (BBA)-Proteins and Proteomics*, vol. 1869, no. 8, p. 140657, 2021.

[81] C. Knöchel, J. Kniep, J. D. Cooper, *et al.*, "Altered apolipoprotein c expression in association with cognition impairments and hippocampus volume in schizophrenia and bipolar disorder," *European archives of psychiatry and clinical neuroscience*, vol. 267, pp. 199–212, 2017.

[82] J. S. Cassoli, P. C. Guest, A. G. Santana, *et al.*, "Employing proteomics to unravel the molecular effects of antipsychotics and their role in schizophrenia," *PROTEOMICS–Clinical Applications*, vol. 10, no. 4, pp. 442–455, 2016.

[83] S. Garcia-Rosa, B. S. Carvalho, P. C. Guest, *et al.*, "Blood plasma proteomic modulation induced by olanzapine and risperidone in schizophrenia patients," *Journal of proteomics*, vol. 224, p. 103813, 2020.

[84] J. Kucera, K. Horska, P. Hruska, *et al.*, "Interacting effects of the mam model of schizophrenia and antipsychotic treatment: Untargeted proteomics approach in adipose tissue," *Progress in Neuro-Psychopharmacology and Biological Psychiatry*, vol. 108, p. 110165, 2021.

[85] B. J. Smith, C. Brandão-Teles, G. S. Zuccoli, *et al.*, "Protein succinylation and malonylation as potential biomarkers in schizophrenia," *Journal of Personalized Medicine*, vol. 12, no. 9, p. 1408, 2022.

[86] J. D. Cooper, S. Ozcan, R. M. Gardner, *et al.*, "Schizophrenia-risk and urban birth are associated with proteomic changes in neonatal dried blood spots," *Translational psychiatry*, vol. 7, no. 12, p. 1290, 2017.

[51] F. C. Sager [illegible] a pilot study [illegible] the [illegible] the [illegible] of [illegible] in treated [illegible] and [illegible] patients [illegible], *[illegible] and [illegible]*, vol. [illegible], no. [illegible], p. [illegible], [illegible].

[52] C. [illegible], J. [illegible], P. D. Cooper [illegible] Altered [illegible] in [illegible] associated with [illegible] and [illegible] volume in [illegible], *[illegible] of [illegible]*, vol. 247, pp. [illegible], 2017.

[53] [illegible] C. [illegible] A. [illegible] et al. [illegible] of the [illegible] and [illegible] patients [illegible], vol. 10, [illegible], p. [illegible], [illegible].

[54] S. [illegible] [illegible] modulation [illegible] in schizophrenia [illegible], vol. 224, p. [illegible], 2020.

[55] [illegible] effects of the [illegible] schizophrenia and [illegible] treatment [illegible] targeted [illegible], *[illegible] and [illegible]*, vol. [illegible], p. [illegible], 2021.

[56] [illegible] Tiles [illegible] and [illegible] of [illegible], *[illegible] Medicine*, vol. [illegible], 2022.

[57] [illegible] Cooper, S. [illegible], [illegible] et al., [illegible] risk and [illegible], *[illegible] Journal [illegible]*, vol. [illegible], no. 13, p. [illegible], 2012.

Index

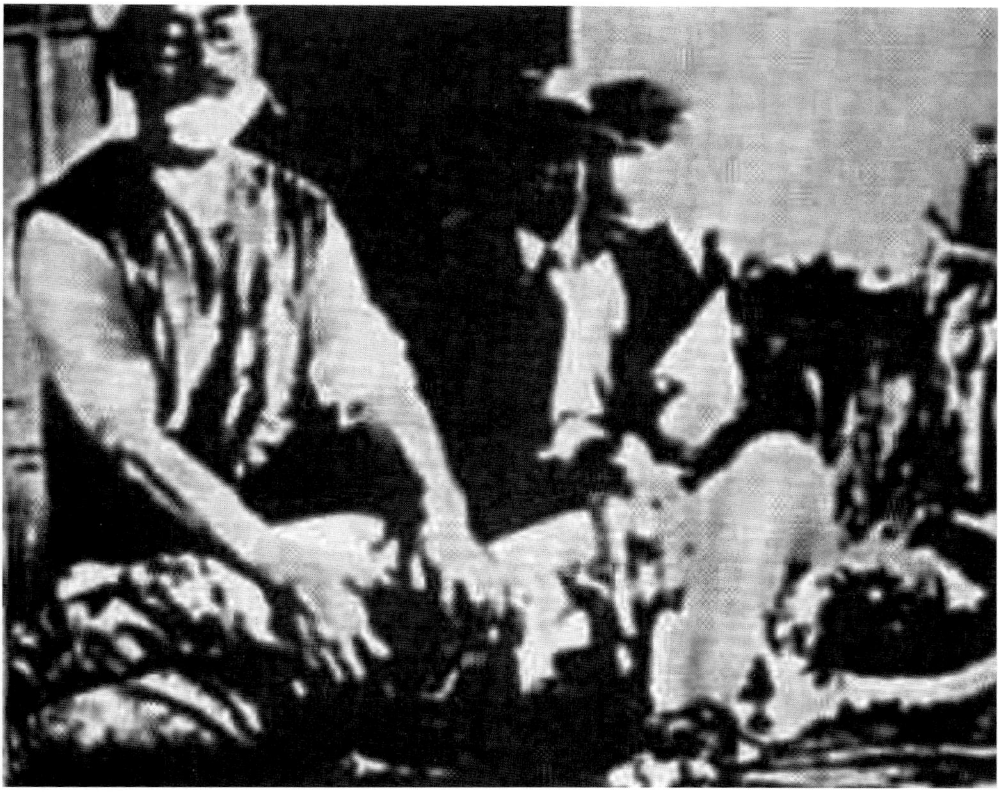

A poor-quality photo reportedly showing Japanese doctors carrying out a dissection on a live prisoner.

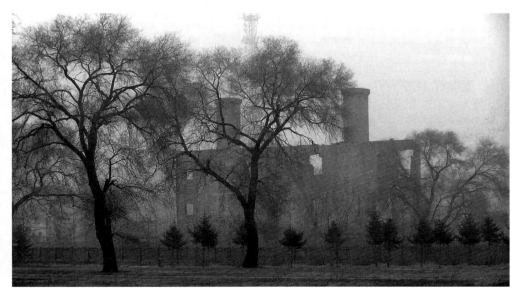

Ruins of a Unit 731 bioweapons facility building at Haben. (*Wikimedia*)

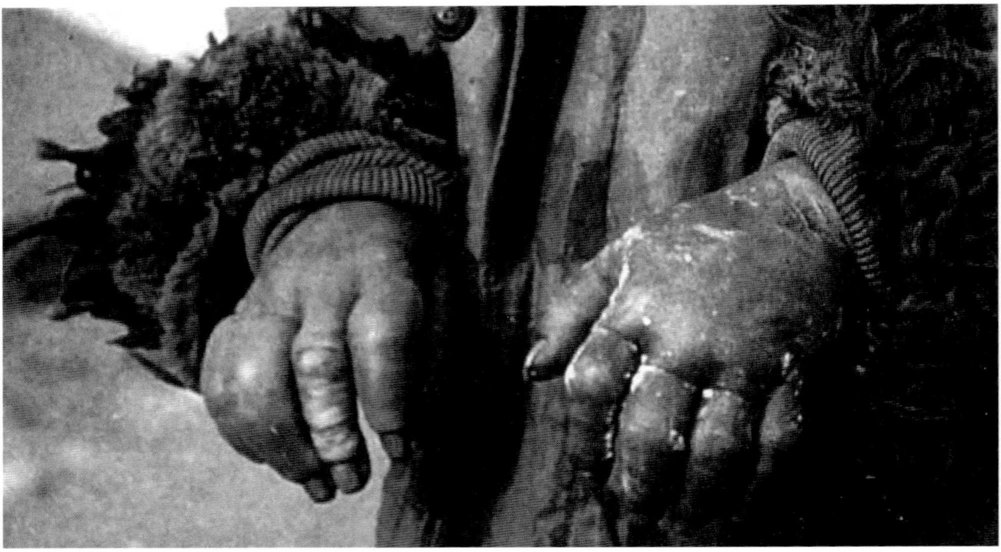
The frostbitten hands of a Chinese prisoner at Unit 731.

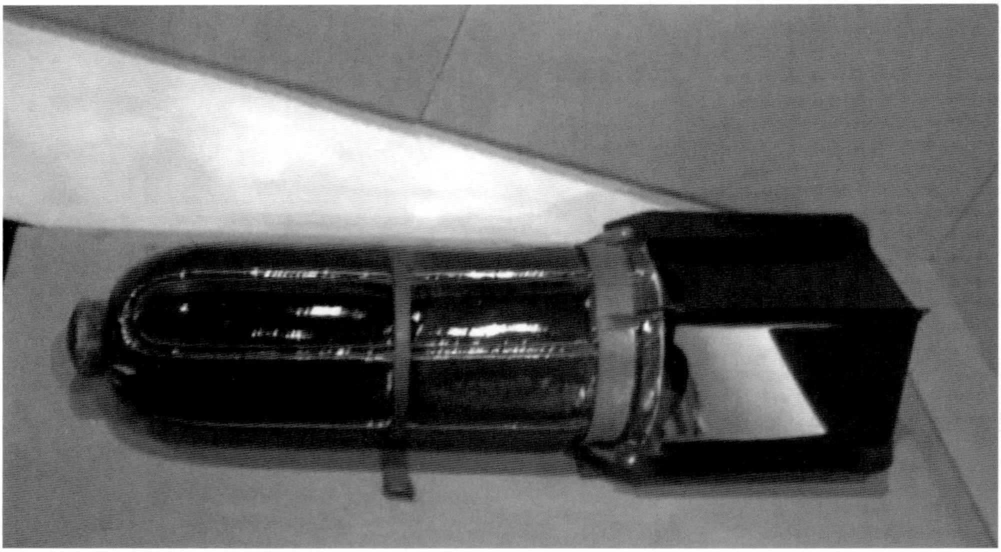
Example of a Japanese bomb designed to carry biological agents.

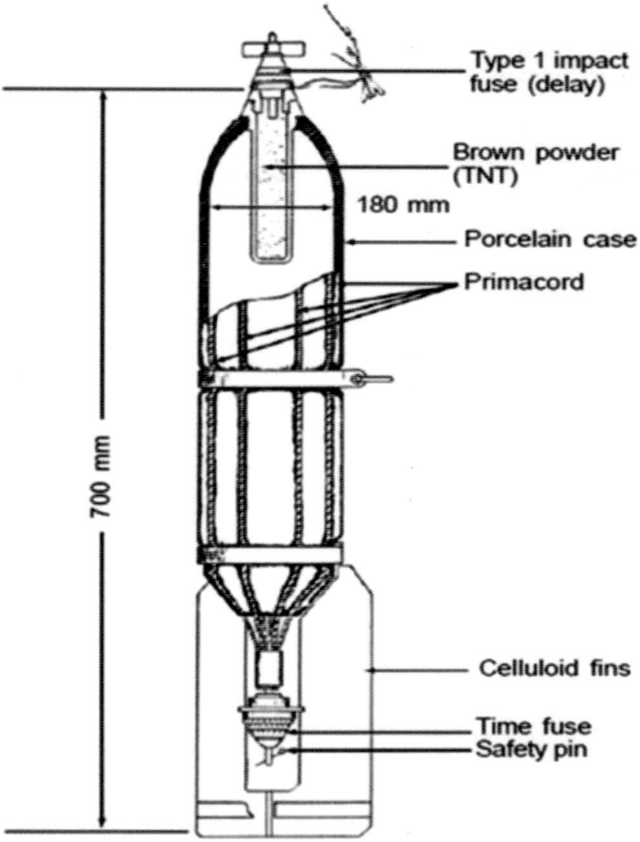

Japanese Type 50 Uji bomb used to deliver biological agents such as the plague and anthrax.

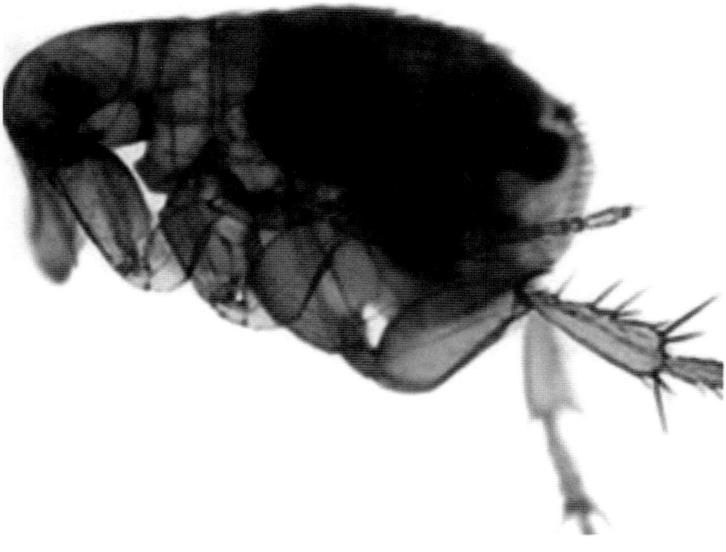

Oriental rat flea infected with *Y. pestis* bacterium, which appears as a dark mass in the gut.

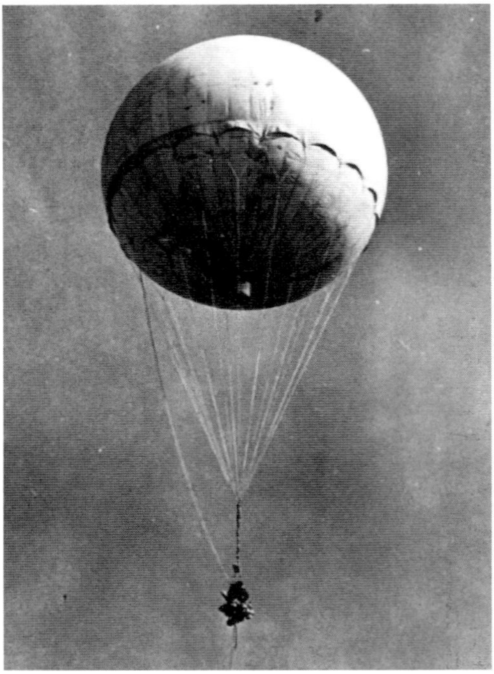

A Japanese Fu-Go balloon bomb pictured in flight. (*Wikimedia*)

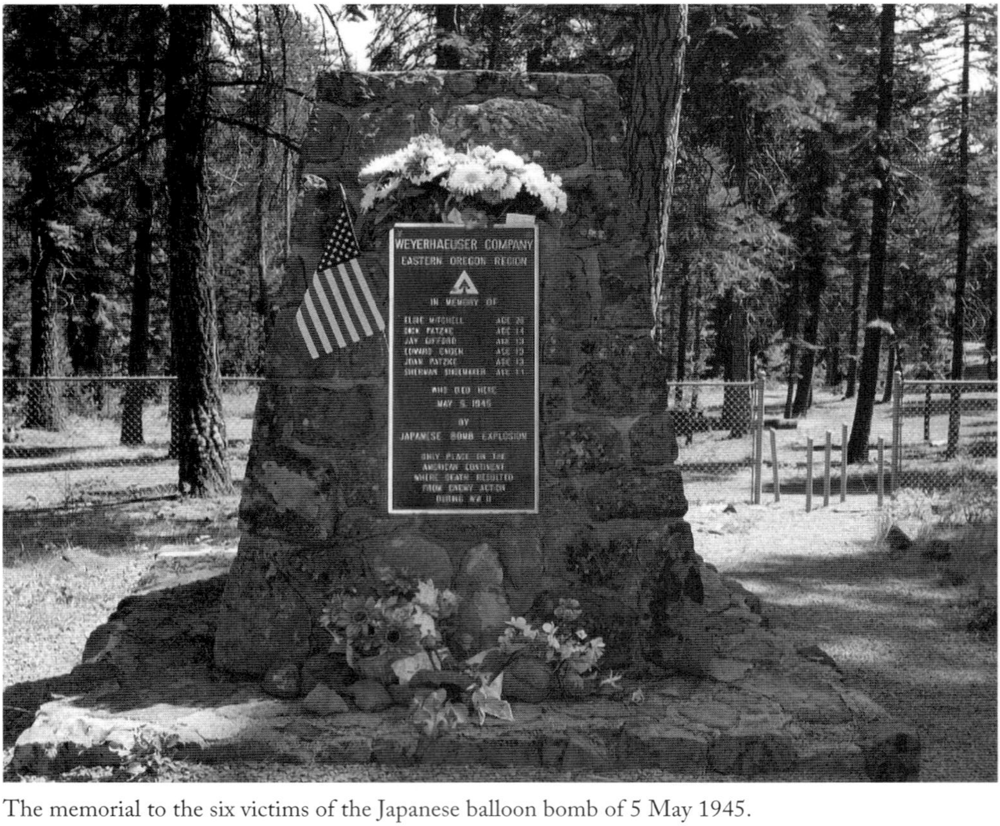
WEYERHAEUSER COMPANY
EASTERN OREGON REGION
IN MEMORY OF
MAY 5 1945
BY
JAPANESE BOMB EXPLOSION

The memorial to the six victims of the Japanese balloon bomb of 5 May 1945.

girls selected for these experiments were asked beforehand if they were virgins or not. They were told that they should answer the question honestly as the doctor would find out later anyway if he or she were not telling him the truth.

Mrs B, now aged 77, was at Stutthof in 1943 and recalled:

> 'It is extremely emotional, psychologically speaking to have to go into the details. Please understand I could never have any children. As I recall, they (the Nazi doctors) experimented with my vagina with different instruments and cuts. The pain was agonising. They gave me all sorts of medicines that made me nauseous. The pain was excruciating, and it made me so sick. My female parts no longer work. Because of this I could not have children. I had a husband, but I couldn't bear him any children and as a result he divorced me. They also put something in our food that made us ill and sterile. I was little more than a slave labourer in a munitions factory, a factory employee gave me a slice of bread that I wanted to give to my sister, who was dying from malnutrition. So, I hid the slice of bread in my sleeve. Well, the Nazi guard found it, and he began beating me across my face and my ears until blood began to pour from them. There was no medical attention in the camp, so my ears became badly infected. I was liberated in Kiel Germany Ostpreusen on May 4th, 1945. I was completely deaf when they took us to hospital. At the hospital they took good care of me, and they had to explain to me that I had no eardrums left in my ears. As of today, I am very hard of hearing. I had lots of surgery, but it has done me no good. In other words, I am now deaf. I am 100% deaf in my right ear, 80% in my left. Not only did I lose my hearing, which I so desperately needed in order to continue where I left off at the age of just 14 with my voice and singing education: my parents and my own dream was to become an opera singer. I had voice lessons as a child with promises and hope of an operatic career one day. My dreams never materialized.'

Mr E, now aged 69, was at Mogilev from August 1943 to October 1943 and recalled:

> 'I was subjected to medical experiments from the beginning of August 1943 until the end of October 1943 under the Nazi regime. In a camp where I was kept as a child, we did not receive any food for days. We cried out for food. Then the boss of the camp came up to us children. He distributed various desserts among us children. After a couple of hours, we realized that something was not in order with the food. I got very sick and suffered with cramps, I vomited, had diarrhoea, chills and fever. Many children died as a result of the poisoned food. Due to this heavily poisoned food my legs felt as if they would be paralyzed. I could not walk for several weeks and could only be carried. As soon as I recovered, I received numerous injections from a doctor into the right side of my mouth, close to my lower jaw. Why I was injected, for what and what substance was injected I don't know, since I was only 8 years old at that time. I still have a hole on my right cheek. The man who ordered all of this, his name was Knoblauch. After the war he was hunted down as a war criminal.'

Ms G, aged 81, was at Auschwitz from March 1944 to April 1944 and she recalled:

> 'Each day I was submerged in hot water. Whenever I tried to put my head out of the water in order to breathe, I was forced back into the water by Dr Mengele who used a stick to push me down into the water. This would last for ten minutes. I was immediately afterwards put into cold water and the same procedure was repeated. There were five people including myself undergoing the same process. After these daily sessions we were taken to barrack number 8 at Auschwitz, which was destined for those who were to die, to see how long we were going to survive. A

woman passing by saw me gesturing and crying for help through a hole in a plank of the wooden barracks. She loosened the plank and wrapped me. I was saved. I know nothing of the fate of the other four persons.'

Chapter 8

Human Taxidermy

An interview with Gustav Priebst, the son of a former member of the *Waffen* SS, in the summer of 1997, revealed the Nazi proposal for a form of racial biology museum. The Nazis were so convinced that they would emerge victorious from the Second World War that the proposal was subject to much discussion between the chief of the SS, Heinrich Himmler, Adolf Hitler and senior figures within the German medical profession, particularly from 1939 to 1943. Priebst's father told his son that there were two possible locations considered for the construction of the museum: Berlin, which was logical considering that Berlin was the capital of the Third Reich, and Munich, another location dear to Hitler as the birthplace of the Nazi Party. The construction was intended to go ahead after the Nazis had won the war, according to Priebst's father. If this sounds too farfetched to be true, then perhaps the exhibition entitled 'Physical and Emotional Appearance of the Jews', which opened at the Museum of Natural History in Vienna in 1939, should be seen as a precursor to an endeavour on a much grander scale. Actual design drawings for such an institution were never officially drafted, but the project remained the topic of frequent conversation between Himmler, Hitler and senior Nazi physicians who expressed great enthusiasm, seeing it as a celebration of the work they had conducted throughout the years of war.

After 1943 it became obvious that Hitler's plans to conquer and secure Europe were not proceeding as many had expected. Priebst's father explained to him that although the proposal for the museum was not completely scrapped, there was less discussion of the project due to greater concerns elsewhere. The fact that Himmler had raised the idea in the first place, along with the existence of a near-complete collection of human skulls and skeletons cataloguing almost all members of the human race, particularly the *Untermenschen* (sub-humans), gives credibility to an idea that had been thought to be hearsay or malicious rumour since the end of the Second World War in Europe in 1945. Naturally some will argue that what Priebst was told by his father in the years after the war was little more than fantasy, and that even the Nazis would not have gone as far as this. This overlooks the fact that the regime had murdered millions of people and conducted horrific medical experiments on thousands of others, in the process taking and preserving body parts and internal organs and embalming bodies and placing them into storage. Is it such a stretch to believe that they might have had plans to champion and display their work?

I asked Priebst whether his father had any ideas about what such a museum might look like. Priebst explained that the museum was a 'no expense spared' idea. The design was to be influenced by ancient Roman architecture, with steps leading up to a grand entrance hall with tall marble pillars on either side, possibly with either the Führer's personal seal or the SS *Totenkopf* carved in stone on the apex of the building. There would be a lavish reception area leading to vast marble-floored galleries featuring glass-case displays of skulls, complete skeletons and preserved organs with various explanatory plates and photographs. A separate anthropological section would house actual human taxidermy specimens set in life-like dioramas. Such an idea would have thrilled the likes of SS chief Heinrich Himmler and many other leading Nazis as a celebration of victory over the *Untermenschen* and the birth of a new Nazi Aryan race. At the close of my interview with Priebst he made the following remark:

> 'It would not have been anything like the museums you can see elsewhere in the world, there may well have been a coffee shop but no souvenir store selling lamps and wallets fashioned from the skin of the *Untermenschen* or human skull ashtrays from the

> concentration camps. Do you know that the Americans as moral as they attempted to appear in the conduct of their war made skull ashtrays from the boiled heads of dead Japanese soldiers? Yes, they cut off the heads, boiled them to remove the flesh and brains and they then sent these things home to their wives as trophies. What is the difference at the end of it all?'

Priebst is certainly correct to say that the American forces in the Pacific took home Japanese skulls which were then fashioned into ashtrays. I was offered one of these Japanese skull ashtrays privately for £500 back in the 1990s, with supporting photographs and documentation, which I declined.

Gustav Priebst's reference to the proposal for a human taxidermy gallery was not the only account I would hear on this subject during my years of research. While carrying out interviews with former members of the *Bund Deutscher Madel* (the Hitler Youth organisation for girls aged 14 to 18) I met the then elderly Hilde Hermann, who corroborated the account given by Gustav Priebst. In April 1942 Hilde had been a nineteen-year-old university student from Berlin. She recalled:

> 'I had been interested in human biology for many years and it was a subject which fascinated me, and I enjoyed it very much. I wanted to work within some context in human biology and the Reich at that time offered opportunities to bright young minds with a sound medical biology study background. When I graduated from university, I had hoped to maybe get work in one of our hospitals. At first, they tried to dissuade me from this career path, and they would say things like "surely marriage and children should be your first concern, you can play doctors and nurses later Frau". I was even offered work in an asylum, and I told them I did not want to work there. I had seen what it was like in the asylums, and they were not pleasant places to work. In fact, Hitler had instructed that those people in the asylums should be "cared for

in the correct manner that one should care for a lunatic". This was the cryptic way of communicating that these mental patients should be euthanised through whatever means. I did not wish to be a part in what I felt was a dreadful scheme, I did not wish to become a murderer. I almost gave up on any hope of gaining employment in the field I had studied for until I was offered a position within the laboratory of a pathology department in a local hospital. It was not quite what I had in mind, but I felt I could gain some useful experience. My friends would joke about it and they would say to me "Hilde, can't you see they are giving you shitty jobs in the hope you will just give up, go home and get married, make babies for the Führer and be bored ever after?". The reality was joking aside they were probably trying to find the nice way of telling me the truth. I remember vividly whilst still in the pathology department that one day a series of glass jars were brought in. The large glass jars contained a human brain in each. I was asked to take each brain out of its jar, examine it very closely looking for even the slightest of anomalies and make a report on each including an explanation on my conclusions. Some of the brains I examined were normal and I could find no oddities when compared to other donated specimens in the laboratory collection. Yet there were some brains with obvious damage, but not the kind of damage one would find normally. There would be the obvious signs of heavy trauma, of having been struck by a heavy blunt instrument which caused bleeding of the brain. The dark areas on some of these brains was where the bleeding had taken place. I knew that these people had been severely beaten about the head and that the injuries would have almost certainly caused death. Then there were brains with deformities that didn't match the brains of a normal healthy human being, they appeared diseased and abnormal to me. It was obvious to me that some of the brains had not developed fully from birth and therefore must have been taken from the corpse of a mental patient. More brains arrived the following day and I was told they were from eastern Europe. The paperwork that came with the jars stated Roma, Russian peasant, Polish Jews, criminals and partisans as the origin of source. We were to study each specimen carefully and write our reports accordingly. These were titled as special reports which were to be sent to and retained by the SS. We were told they were of special interest to Heinrich Himmler head of the SS. Himmler was very interested in this area of our racial science and had many other experts working in this field. I can remember how the one brain specimen looked very poor, it was very bloody and misshapen, and I asked whether this one had been damaged at the time of its removal from the corpse as it was barely useful for any analysis. One of the doctors there said to me "the damage to this specimen was not caused by the opening of the skull or indeed the scalpel and saw used to extricate it, this Frau Hermann is what happens when you are struck in the head by a 7.92-mm Gew 98 [Gewehr 98 – German bolt action army rifle] bullet. The bullet has struck the unprotected head at 760 metres a second (2,493 feet per second), impressive is it not?" The clear fluid the brain was sitting in was dark like the colour of red wine, it was disgusting to look at. As the bullet impacted the victim's head it forced fragments of skull bone inwards like lots of little splinters. As the bullet continued through the brain itself the path of the bullet had caused expansion outwards, it looked like a piece of offal from an animal. Perhaps the most sinister side of things was when we were invited to special meetings with leading physicians involved in racial science. As a junior I was asked to attend as it was said I might learn something more useful than just the study of organs removed from dead bodies of those who it was said were the enemies of the German race. I was apprehensive about these meetings as I had no idea as to the nature of the discussions which would be held. I remember the first meeting very well as beforehand a physician within the

> SS came to give me a short interview. He explained I was a very lucky girl to have been selected and I was selected on my clinical merits and not my pretty face. This unnerved me somewhat, but I remained composed and just smiled at the man and thanked him for such a compliment. I was told the meetings were more a series of conferences and that they would be held behind closed doors, and they would be secret. I was warned quite strictly that none of the content of the discussions held within these secret meetings should be repeated to anyone including my parents, boyfriend or friends. I was told that the consequences of talking about anything would be extremely serious and I would be well advised to heed the warning he was giving me. I told him I would not repeat anything, in fact I gave him my word as it frightened me a little as the tone of his voice and the look on his face made me very aware of how serious he was. At the end of this interview, he asked me to send in the next junior, he shook my hand and thanked me for my time then just said "that is all Fraulein, heil Hitler."

I opened the door and left the room and told the next junior a young man named Herbert that he was next. The next day while working nothing was even mentioned between us about the interview of the previous day, we were too scared to even talk about it between ourselves. The actual conference as it was called was held two weeks later in a building in the suburbs of the city (of Berlin). This was not Wannsee nor was it connected with the Wannsee conference and was held in what looked like an ordinary grand house in the suburbs. We had been given a hotel stay for the night and everything we ate and drank was paid for by those organising the conference or meeting whatever you wish to call it. It was quite nice as I had never received this kind of treatment before. Several cars were laid on to collect us the following morning and take us to our destination. When we arrived at 11am in the morning we had to wait outside the gates of this grand building until three guards came out and checked our identity papers and checked that we were not carrying any weapons. I thought it was ridiculous as why would we be carrying any weapons, if any of us had been assassins who were we going to assassinate as we had no idea who would be chairing the discussions. We were counted into the courtyard by the guards and more of them appeared. There was fifteen of them all together escorting us, and these were not ordinary soldiers, they wore the black SS uniforms. They didn't say anything to us other than "come this way in an orderly line". We were told to wait outside the front door until two men in smarts suits introduced themselves as Doctor Theobald and Doctor Rifke. They asked us inside and shook us each by the hand thanking us for giving our time and how delighted they were to see us. Inside the building there was this grand concourse, paintings adorned the walls along with huge swastika drapes. It was quite some house and I guessed it belonged to one of these doctors. We went through several doors and along a network of corridors until being asked to come inside and take a seat in what looked like a very ornate company boardroom. As we took our seats there was the rattle of a trolley which sounded as if it was crammed with crockery. A woman in a dark jacket and skirt came into the room with this trolley of cups and saucers and a coffee urn. She placed several sugar bowls on the large table in front of us and the cups and saucers were distributed to each of us. The two doctors stood at another doorway which obviously was another entrance into the room, and they were quietly talking, and I noticed one looking at his pocket watch. One of the SS guards came in with several folders which I assumed contained paperwork. These folders were on the table where at the moment there were empty chairs, so we were waiting for others to arrive, at least that's what we assumed. The coffee was poured into our cups, and we helped ourselves to sugar and cream. The young man named Herbert was seated next to me and he went to light himself a cigarette was quickly informed "young sir, there is no smoking here would you kindly wait until later". Herbert sat there rather awkwardly with this lighted cigarette in his hand and no way of extinguishing it. One of the SS guards noticed his predicament and came over and took the cigarette from him and dispensed it out of the window before closing it. The two doctors told us to relax enjoy our coffee that we will begin the discussion very soon and apologised for keeping us waiting. It must have been an hour later as I began to feel like I needed to go to the toilet, and I knew I could hang on no longer. I felt embarrassed to have to get up from my seat and ask Doctor Rifke "could I please use a toilet". He just said to me "yes, of course you can Fraulein" before calling the woman who had brought the cups, saucers and coffee in for us. I heard Doctor Rifke say "Diana, please escort her to the ladies' room". This rather stern-faced woman who I guessed to be in her fifties told me to "come this way, follow me but we must be quick as the Reichsführer will be arriving very shortly." I was just about to say to "who the Reichsführer of the SS Herr Himmler"? but I stopped myself as I just thought to myself "hell, Himmler himself is attending". The lady's washroom was bigger than the entire ground floor of my parents' home, it was huge. It was a relief to have used the washroom and then be escorted back to the meeting room. I took my seat and refused a third cup of coffee for fear of needing the toilet yet again. The combination of nerves and anxiety gnawed away at me as I sat waiting for this discussion to begin and what I knew to be our special guest arriving. Two guards entered the room took their places either side of the door and after a slight pause in walked that instantly recognisable figure that was the Reichsführer of the SS Heinrich Himmler. We all stood bolt upright and gave our "heil Hitler" salute. Himmler came in removed his cap placing it to his side on the table. Himmler looked around the room, smiled and wished us a good morning and apologised for being so late and that other matters had ran into his time. He ran into a lengthy speech regarding the virtues of the research work being conducted by the excellent physicians both senior and junior across the whole of the Reich regarding racial sciences. That "it was extremely important that each one of us understood the value of experimental medical research work and its various related disciplines including that of genetics." He mentioned that "much work had already been carried out involving many thousands of German citizens who gave their time voluntarily." These Germans he explained "were of course pure blood line." He then went on to refer to what he termed as "the other races and the importance of understanding their medical and genetic make-up which could only be fully explored through medical and surgical research by approved physicians all across the Reich." These other races were 'contaminates' as he referred to them which must under no circumstances be permitted to affect the blood lines of pure Germans even if they possessed many of the same physical attributes of the pure Germans. These fine specimens of the *Untermensche* (sub-humans) were he said the proverbial "wolf in sheep's clothing that only further in-depth research through medical and genetical means could fully expose." He went on to add that "in this sense experimentation, and the gathering of specimens for study etc was entirely legitimate." Then came one of the main segments for the discussion. Himmler announced that he had held several consultations with some of Germany's leading animal taxidermists with the regard to the preservations of complete human specimens which could best illustrate to the future German race the physiological differences between the German Aryans and the *Untermensche*. He explained that "it was entirely feasible to carry out taxidermy on human specimens as it was with animals and that these could then be displayed at purpose-built institutions celebrating the German race." The Doctors present including many of the senior medical people all agreed what a good idea it would be and when could work begin in this area. Of course, we all had to look as if we were enthused by the proposal but inside, I was thinking to myself that this was something out of a horror story, it was not normal behaviour to even suggest something like this. I certainly did not feel comfortable with the idea of having to assist in the creation of some form of human taxidermal display. There had been many whispered rumours about this idea, and it was nothing new at all, it really wasn't but it wasn't talked about openly. Then there was the question of what might happen if the Allied powers learned of the plans for these institutions. Himmler addressed the question by saying that "all preliminary research and technical work on this proposal will be secret and that a small number of bodies would be subject to taxidermy in order to ascertain the conditions by which the bodies should be displayed, most notably the conditions such as heat and humidity as animal skin was different to that of human skin and reacts differently to the process of taxidermy. The heads were the most important part and research would have to be very thorough into the discovery of the best methods of preservation as in some native head-hunting cultures human heads were known to shrink and distort and this would be of no use to us." One of the juniors questioned the subject of decay which might take place within a human taxidermy specimen and how might this be addressed. Himmler looked across to Doctor Rifke and just gave him a nod at which Doctor Rifke said "thank you Reichsführer. There will of course be no internal organs present within the displays. Each individual display will be much like an artificial human skeleton where the skin is then stretched over this artificial skeleton. We may use plasterwork for this purpose. The actual heads we hope to use, and removal of the brain organs is a straightforward process, as are internal parts of the mouth such as tongue and skin. We simply recreate these, yet we have to experiment and consult on the best means of preserving the vital heads. We will be experimenting with several techniques and chemicals and will be consulting with the taxidermists who are among the finest at their craft in the Reich. It was at this point that a Doctor Walter Bauer stood up and addressed us with an example of how human taxidermy was perfectly feasible. This Doctor Bauer explained:

> "There is one successful specimen of human taxidermy in existence. This specimen is known as 'El Negro' or in broader terms 'The Negro'. The specimen is of course a colonial acquisition dating back to the 1800s. The specimen was an illegally exhumed African native warrior which had been subject to mounting using wire,

> wood and newspaper. The specimen was then shipped to Paris in a container of animal taxidermy specimens. The body was exhibited at Number 3, Rue Saint France. This negro specimen ended up being transported to Spain and it was and still should be regarded as a European colonial artefact. Arrangements are being made for our representatives to see this 'El Negro' specimen and to learn possible techniques which may be employed towards our own endeavours. The Führer himself is aware of these points and may request the loan of the actual 'El Negro' specimen for study here in Germany."

A junior again then raised the question of the difficulties of mounting human skin as it dries out it is extremely difficult to stretch over anatomical replicas and does not look natural due to discolouration and distortion. Doctor Bauer continued:

> "Yes, that is a very valid point, but I can assure you we will discover the best method of preserving as much of the actual anatomy as is possible. We shall experiment and it will be a process of elimination until the best method is procured."

Another junior asked Doctor Bauer if the Spanish would be prepared to loan the actual "El Negro" specimen and how best could such a fragile artefact be shipped to Germany for study.

Doctor Bauer replied:

> "The SS would be totally in charge of the acquisition of the specimen should permission be granted by the Spanish authorities at the museum where it is held. We cannot personally guarantee cooperation, but I am sure the Führer could persuade them to be compliant in this matter should we desire to obtain subject to loan the actual specimen itself. Fees of course would have to

be discussed with the Spanish, but I cannot see this being an issue at all."

Bauer then asked "Reichsführer do you wish to add anything to this part of our discussion?"

Himmler just reiterated with the following remarks:

"We have access to any of the materials we require, should the Führer make a personal request for any particular artefact which may have essential value to our work then I can assure you it will be retrieved as and when required through either peaceful or forceful means."

At that the meeting was drawn to a close as Diana entered the room to collect the cups and saucers from the table. The Reichsführer of the SS stood up and thanked us all for our participation and he shook our hands before leaving. We had to wait for a further thirty or so minutes before we could leave the room which had become stuffy with perspiration due to the closed windows and the weather being pleasantly warm outside. I was glad it was over, and I felt quite uneasy, and I felt slightly dejected over it all. The thought of going back to the hospital and having to sit at a desk poking human brains and other organs and dissecting them looking for abnormalities I couldn't intelligently detect filled me with dread. It was putting me off medicine completely, I hadn't envisaged being a butcher of humans, I had wanted to help the living not dissect the dead. I understood fully at this point the evil that I had somehow inadvertently become a part of. Shortly after I returned home, I sat down in my room, and I wrote everything down despite being warned against it. I had a sharp memory as I had worked as a secretary, there were parts I could not fully recall but what I have said above is virtually all of it. At the time my parents were very curious but as much as my parents pestered to know where I had been and what had been said I didn't tell them. I explained it was secret and if anything got out accidentally, we might all be arrested and worse even executed. I sat them down two years after the war and told them everything. It took two long years for me to be able to talk to my own parents about it all. They were very shocked but not surprised as in their hearts they knew exactly what had been going on with thousands of people vanishing from the city. We all saw how Jews had their homes and businesses confiscated, how they were beaten in the streets, made to wear those stars on their clothing and then taken away. They were not going to holiday camps were they, it should have been obvious to most especially by 1943, even the most ignorant of German citizens could not have been that stupid. Besides there was many a drunken soldier on leave from the front who bragged about how many Jewish pigs he had slaughtered. People ask me today how I cope knowing what I had been involved with as a young woman. The answer is a simple one I turned to God after the war and every day I have asked his forgiveness despite the fact I never hurt anyone, and I had no choice but to do what I was told at that hospital where I worked as a young girl. Yes, I could have quit but then they would have wanted to know why? I had a friend who feigned depression saying the work had started to destroy his health, they took him away and I later discovered he had died. They told me he had died due to a blood infection, but I know that wasn't true, they took him away thinking he was a mental case and they murdered him as depression was a mental state which couldn't be tolerated, you couldn't be an Aryan if you were suffering from such a condition. This was the problem you were faced with every day back in those times, there was no escape, no escape at all.'

The nephew of one of the prominent German animal taxidermists who was approached by associates of the SS agreed to reveal some information provided I respect his request for anonymity. Having agreed to this he was more than happy to talk about how his uncle was approached for information on ways that corpses might be preserved and mounted for display. He recalled:

'My uncle was an expert of his particular craft. He had produced some excellent taxidermy specimens of large animals which included boar, bears and wolves. This was a specialist discipline back then and it required knowledge and skill that few people had. It was associates of the SS who approached him for information, and he had to explain to them that to successfully preserve the skin of a human being would be very difficult for many reasons. Animal hides were of course different to human skin as animals had fur for one thing whereas human skin does not. Animal hides do not shrink badly if treated correctly. You could not use animal skin preservation formulas on human skin as the two were completely different. Only the skin of pigs had a similar genetic makeup to that of humans, yet it was still challenging. It seemed that the SS were looking to acquaint the finest taxidermists and have them put their minds together to solve all the issues that would inevitably arise. My uncle told them that while the problems could be solved, and a satisfactory method found to perform taxidermy on corpses he could not guarantee that deterioration of some form would not occur either soon after or at some timescale after the procedure. Specimens would have to be placed within a temperature-controlled environment where heat and humidity were strictly controlled and subject to close monitoring. My uncle was curious to know the ideas behind all the questions he was being asked on various preservation methods and methods employed in other parts of the world including those used by some native tribes. My uncle had studied all these things as a young man and had seen shrunken heads which originated from head hunting tribes. These heads had the brains removed and were deliberately shrunken as they were often worn by the natives in ceremonies. I know these men visited my uncle's home and his workshop where he carried out his work on several occasions. Then the visits suddenly stopped and this he told me was around December of 1943. He made enquiries to find out if he should continue his own research work. The same week these men returned and asked for all of his written notes that he had prepared and any test materials he had been supplied with. The test materials he had been given were small sections of skin with which he could conduct tests with various formulas that might help skin retain elasticity, texture and colour. One of the major problems was that the natural colour of human skin tends to change, it often becomes an unnatural hue of white as if it had been bleached. There was little that could be done about this, and he suggested the use of alternative methods of colouring where discolouration occurred. Having to re-colour cases of entire large specimens would be a very time-consuming process requiring someone with a specialist knowledge to carry out the work. In the end the whole sordid idea was cancelled due to the reasons of the time required, the sheer expense involved and the fact that suddenly the war was not going Hitler's way. A project such as that the Reichsführer of the SS Heinrich Himmler was proposing and eager to push ahead on could only become a reality if it was certain that Germany would win the war. 1943 was a catastrophic year for Germany and many of these proposals were consigned the to the rubbish bin. The materials and texts written by my uncle were taken away and they were destroyed by incineration. He was politely asked to talk no more about the idea and if there was a change of mind the authorities would be in touch, but they left him alone after this.'

I asked what his uncle's feelings about the whole idea had been? Was he supportive of it or not? The nephew replied:

'I don't think he was comfortable with it all, more that he was put under pressure to be involved. He couldn't have refused as these were powerful people connected with the Reichsführer of the SS. To have refused on the grounds of morality would have suggested he disagreed with the regime, and he may have been given an ultimatum either do as we ask, or you will get trouble. That is how the Third Reich operated, they utilized the fear of retribution from above to get what they wanted'.

Another source revealed that mental patients from Germany's lunatic asylums had been euthanized and a selection of the corpses placed in storage in freezers. The bodies had been gutted just like pigs. The brains and internal organs were sent out for medical research purposes to various universities in the Reich. Many of these gruesome specimens would remain locked in cupboards at institutions around Germany, only to be accidentally rediscovered decades after the end of the Second World War.

Sadly, there is no concrete evidence in existence to prove that the Germans were looking to create a hideous museum as discussed above. There were groups and individuals who made sure any documents which did exist on this subject were destroyed so that they could not be found by the Allies. We can be excused for thinking that it all sounds very farfetched, but we must also remember that the death camps were once just a rumour that people thought was too horrific to be true, but turned out to be real. There is still so much about the Third Reich that we have yet to discover.

Conclusion

Whether the forced medical experiments conducted on concentration camp prisoners by Nazi German physicians throughout the Second World War served any useful medical or anthropological purpose has been the subject of continued debate since the end of the Second World War. Some have argued that certain aspects of the research proved of some value in the advancement of modern medical and surgical disciplines, including the development of effective medicines for combating diseases and infections resulting from all manner of wounds and day to day injuries. However, prisoners incarcerated in the death and forced labour camps of Nazi Germany were in a state of such dire physical and mental poor health, and were receiving totally inadequate nutrition and/or medical care, as to call any results of experimentation into question. Generally, a healthy, fit individual with a sufficient intake of adequate nutrition and access to professional medical aftercare would respond to medical experiments in a completely different way to a malnourished, traumatised prisoner.

It is also possible that some of the Nazi doctors were offered a more lenient prison sentence in exchange for their cooperation and information about their medical research, which may have proved beneficial to the Allies after the war. For example, the Nazi scientists identified the dangers to human health posed by organochlorine pesticides such as DDT before anyone else. They also sought to discourage alcoholism and the smoking of tobacco among the German population, understanding the risks that over-consumption of alcohol and tobacco posed to a person's general health and wellbeing, and indeed, certain organs in their body. It was also German scientists who confirmed the link between asbestos and lung cancer, and who developed the first high-powered electron microscope for medical research. They also promoted the idea of females self-examining their breasts for lumps, the early signs of the possible onset of breast cancer. The Nazi leadership fully endorsed such campaigns to benefit the health of their citizens. So we can see how advanced many areas of Nazi German medicine were.

To give another example, nerve surgeon Dr Susan Mackinnon required assistance to help her complete an operation. The manual she reached for to provide the essential reference material was Pernkopf's *Topographic Anatomy of Man*, written by Austrian professor of anatomy Eduard Pernkopf, a volume widely regarded as the finest example of anatomical diagrams in the world. However, this manual was formulated from the findings gained from examining the bodies of hundreds of people murdered by the Nazis during the Second World War. The precisely drawn, incredibly detailed diagrams were made by observing the dissected victims' bodies.

There is also the question of whether the big post-Second World War drug companies profited and benefitted from the Nazi human medical experimentation programmes. It is very likely that some of them did, even covertly, but whether any of them would ever admit to this is another question entirely.

Whatever value (if any) there may have been in terms of scientific knowledge, the Nazi German medical experimentation programme was never anything more than '*une science diabolique*' the awful effects of which many victims are still suffering today.

The fact that the Reichsführer of the SS Heinrich Himmler, backed by many of the Nazi physicians, expressed so much enthusiasm for the creation of a post-war house of horrors in the form of a race and biology museum seems incredible, but the Nazis came frighteningly close to the creation of just such an institution. That they did not succeed in winning the war is something for which we must be eternally grateful.

Chapter 9

Imperial Japanese Human Medical Experimentation

DRAFT WARNING TO ALL JAPANESE

The Governments of Australia, Canada, France, the Netherlands, New Zealand, the United Kingdom and the United States of America, on behalf of all Governments at war with Japan, hereby issue a solemn warning to the Japanese Government and people. These Governments declare that it is the inescapable duty of the Japanese Government and its people to protect Allied prisoners of war and civilian internees from acts of violence and harm and to safeguard them from starvation and death. These Governments declare that they will hold the Japanese Government, as well members of the Japanese military, naval, and air forces, no less than the commandants and guards at all prisoner of war and civilian internee camps, the Japanese gendarmerie and all other persons who have contact with Allied prisoners of war and civilian internees, individually and collectively responsible for the safety and welfare of all Allied nationals, prisoners of war and civilian internees in Japanese custody.

The Japanese Government on many occasions has publicly and solemnly declared to the nations and people of the world that it accords prisoners of war and civilian internees good and humane treatment. If at the end of hostilities it is found that the Japanese authorities have not safeguarded from harm or have wilfully exposed to danger the Allied personnel in their keeping and the solemn declaration of the Japanese Government are thereby proved

> to have been without foundation, the Allied Governments declare that any individual, regardless of position or status, guilty of having permitted starvation and death or guilty of having maltreated or having permitted the maltreatment of any Allied prisoners of war, internees or citizens, whether in a battle zone, or lines of communication, in a camp, hospital, prison or elsewhere, will be ruthlessly pursued and brought to punishment. This is the firm and fixed intention of the Allied Governments.

The above statement, delivered to the Japanese government with the declaration of war with Japan in the Second World War, is impressive and sends a very blunt and clear message. Yet despite the Japanese openly defying every condition, there was relatively little follow up after the war and only a handful of Japanese were ever punished for war crimes. This was despite the fact that many thousands of Japanese committed unspeakable acts of violence, sadism, torture, rape, mutilation and murder. It is worth noting that Germans accused of either direct or indirect involvement in war crimes are still actively pursued around the world, while Japanese war criminals have been consistently overlooked or even rehabilitated.

It is interesting that in some situations those accused of war crimes have been welcomed for the knowledge they possess. German rocket scientists were taken to the USA after the end of the Second World War and exempted from prosecution in exchange for their input into American space programmes. A similar approach was taken with Japanese scientists involved in human medical experimentation, raising difficult questions about whether the value of their knowledge is more important than the lives of those affected by their wartime activities, the survivors of which have lived with the consequences ever since.

Imperial Japan's role in the Second World War from 1941 is notorious among historians as having been conducted with the utmost violence, cruelty, brutality and savagery. As early as the Russo-Japanese War of 1904–05 the Japanese had been responsible for many sickening acts that were clearly war crimes. After battles Russian soldiers were found dead having been mutilated by the Japanese. Some of the dead Russian soldiers had hammers and sickles carved into their backs and chests, rifle cartridges hammered into their eye sockets, fingers, toes, ears, tongues and genitals sliced off and one body had an anti-tank shell inserted into the rectum and pushed in so far it exited into the stomach. It was also noted that fingernails had been torn out and feet had been burned. The examination of the Russian corpses revealed that they had very likely been alive when the torture had been carried out. Many of the acts perpetrated by the Imperial Japanese military against Allied prisoners of war and civilian internees during the Second World War were similar.

Japanese medical authorities, like their Nazi counterparts, carried out vivisections and mutilated live human subjects. The Japanese had their own supply of human guinea pigs for medical experiments, having conquered most of Asia and the Pacific. Captured Allied prisoners of war and civilians of the conquered territories were herded into jungle camps, either in the areas of Japanese military occupation, or in Japan itself. Initially brutal and often fatal medical experiments, if they can be labelled as such, were conducted within the jungle camps and there are many eyewitness accounts of atrocities carried out under the warped guise of obtaining some form of medical knowledge. A prisoner of war at Khandok described how another perfectly healthy and able-bodied prisoner was selected. He recalled of this event:

> 'The prisoner was tied to a tree outside the Hiari Kikan office a Japanese doctor and four Japanese medical students stood round him. They (the Japanese) then began pulling out the tied prisoner's fingernails one by one. Once they had done this, they then sliced open his chest and removed his heart. The doctor then proceeded to give a practical demonstration.'

The diary of a captured Japanese officer was found to contain a similar incident to that described above:

> 'The two prisoners who had escaped from the camp last night were soon recaptured in the jungle. To prevent them from escaping a second time pistol shots were fired at the feet of both prisoners, but it was difficult to hit them. The two prisoners were later dissected while still alive and conscious by Medical Officer Yamaji. The livers of the two prisoners were taken out, and for the first time I saw the internal organs of a human being. It was very informative.'

Women were not spared by the Japanese. An eyewitness recalled that the Japanese found a young woman hiding in some grass. They proceeded to beat and strip her of her clothing before taking her to a hut with no side walls on. As two of the Japanese held the girl down on the ground another took out his sabre from its scabbard and cut off the woman's breasts. The same Japanese soldier then slit open the woman's abdomen to reveal her womb. The witness recalled that the girl screamed for some seconds before lying still and quiet. The Japanese, having killed the girl, then set the hut with her body inside on fire.

Private Jack Mates, who had been serving with the British 14th Army when captured in the jungle fighting against the Japanese, recalled:

> 'They seemed to enjoy the fact that they could do what they wanted with us and that included the infliction of pain merely for the sake of it. For example, they carried out these parades where one of the bastards wearing these silly round glasses and a white doctor's coat would tell us all to line up, we would be naked, and we would have to bend down and touch our toes. This bastard would then walk along the row of men, and he would stick this thing inside each man's anus. It resembled a thermometer only it wasn't one of those as it was much thicker but made of glass. This glass thing was put up each man's backside and it was not cleaned

or sanitized for each man. There were men suffering from piles who would protest to the doctor telling him that this would cause them terrible pain and discomfort but any man who did protest was immediately beaten up by the Jap guards who were always at his side. He would also kick the men as they were beaten to the ground. The men who protested were then taken to the nearest tree stump or other object the Jap doctor thought was adequate, they were then bent over it and had this glass thing forcibly shoved up their backsides. It left us in pain and discomfort but for these men it was particularly agonising. There were combat medics within our ranks, and they could not understand what this practice was all about or what the Japs hoped to gain from it. In their opinion it was done as just another form of humiliation, to degrade and dehumanize us even further than what they already had at that time.'

Sergeant Martin Cother, another member of the British 14th Army unlucky enough to have been captured by the Japanese during the fighting in the Burmese jungle recalled:

'Due to the extreme conditions and lack of decent food and vitamins your body would sometimes be covered in sores, ulcers and insect bites. I had a particularly nasty ulcer on my right leg which kept filling with pus. The Japs noticed things like this and while you were standing on parade, they would stab ulcers and boils on your body with a stick. We had our own medics amongst us but they were given no bandages or medicines with which to treat us, so often wounds would become horribly infected. One of the Japs came to me one morning after this ulcer I had burst. He poured some petrol onto a dirty piece of rag and insisted it was tied around my wound. It was as much as I could do to stand on that leg, but he shouted and gestured that if I didn't get up and go to work with the other prisoners, he would set light to the rag. So, you just had to force yourself to get up and carry on. The wound became badly infected to the point where this Jap doctor who came to the camp once a month began to take an interest in efforts by our own medical staff to combat the problems we had in our camp. Our medic was a good chap, but he had nothing with which to help us with and he tried to argue his case with the Jap commander of the camp and this doctor who visited every month. There was a lot of shouting as the Japs lost their tempers which they always did if you tried to reason with them. I was taken to a hut across the parade area and placed on a table so as the Jap doctor could have a look at my leg. He examined my leg and then left returning several minutes later with a leather case. The leather case had all these surgical instruments inside and some of these were taken out. He muttered something to the guards who quickly seized me and held me down. The Jap then started cutting around the area of the ulcer. I was given no pain killing drugs or anything and the pain was excruciating, yes, I screamed out in agony but was soon punched unconscious by the Jap guards who both took it in turns to rain blows on my head. I came to back in our prisoner barracks hospital. It was not by any means a hospital, just a bamboo and foliage hut where the sick were placed either to recover or to die. My leg was in a bad way and the man we called Doc was convinced that the leg would have to be amputated. I don't know where he got it from, but he managed to get this clear alcohol solution and managed to steal some salt from the Japs. The salt was agony when placed on the wound, but it dried it up and helped it to actually heal. I remember Doc saying to me when I was in terrible pain with a fever on top of it over the next week or so "now, now don't fret Cother, I will be making a report about this incident, they will pay for it one day." Sadly, we lost Doc to disease just two months prior to our liberation.'

In many of the jungle camps prisoners were subjected to medical torture which served little purpose than to perhaps gain some understanding of how much suffering a human being could tolerate before reaching the point of death. The Japanese doctors who visited these remote, disease-riddled camps understood fully as physicians how to inflict maximum pain upon an individual. It appears the Japanese doctors gained sadistic pleasure from tearing out the finger and toenails of prisoners. If a prisoner passed out during the procedure he would be dragged outside where water would be poured over his head to bring him round, then the procedure would then be continued. One can only imagine the excruciating pain experienced. One witness recalled:

> 'They took this one fellow into a hut and this short fat little Japanese wearing a white doctor's coat began pulling out the prisoner's fingernails. This was done with a pair of ordinary tool pliers. After each nail was wrenched from the finger the doctor would examine the prisoner's heart rate with a stethoscope. He would then write down notes on a clipboard he had with him. Once they had pulled out all his fingernails they started on his toenails. Each time the poor sod passed out through the pain they dragged him out in full view of the other prisoners and poured water over his head. He came round a couple of times but after that they could not bring him round, so they began kicking and beating him. The prisoner never regained consciousness and died, a small mercy as his wounds would have become horribly infected and he would have probably ended up having to endure amputations which in turn would have proved fatal as they did in many cases. Those camps were filthy places, rife with all kinds of disease, infection and flies. Most of the flies had been feeding off the human excrement in the latrines and these alone led to the deaths of many prisoners as they brought disease into the camp. The camps were no place to carry out any form of surgery as the smallest of cuts often turned into suppurating wounds.'

Prisoners were routinely brought into huts where Japanese doctors performed vivisections, removing livers, kidneys and hearts while the victim was still alive. This material was not harvested for the purposes of medical research, but for consumption by the Japanese officers and doctors carrying out the procedures. There are countless eyewitness testimonies from Allied prisoners of war and captured Japanese soldiers regarding the Japanese practice of cannibalism. The Japanese regularly augmented their food supplies by cannibalising the bodies of prisoners of war and civilian internees, yet they were forbidden to cannibalise their own dead. Human flesh and/or organs were consumed with rice when fish, pork or other meats were unobtainable. There are accounts of Japanese doctors having removed organs from live human beings before cooking the organs with rice and vegetables and distributing this among the soldiers, who remarked that the flavour was somewhat dull. The officers and soldiers themselves were never permitted to take part in these procedures, which clearly were not medical in nature but were undertaken as such. One Japanese officer wrote that he had even consumed the testicles of one murdered prisoner. These were fried in oil with vegetables, boiled rice was added, and they were served to him in his quarters. After sampling the testicles, he recorded that they did not taste good at all and that they had a sponge-like consistency. Cannibalism became more frequent in the closing stages of the Second World War when the Japanese became cut off from their regular supplies.

Under the organisation of what was known as Unit 731 the Imperial Japanese Military of the Second World War conducted some of the most barbarous acts perpetrated against human beings in the name of medical and military science. Two years after the beginning of a parallel programme in Nazi Germany, the Japanese began using captured Allied servicemen along with the civilian populations of conquered territories, in their own human medical experiments. The types of human medical experimentation carried out by the Japanese bore many similarities to those of Nazi Germany, and it is likely that the regimes shared the data from their respective work, which included injecting various diseases and toxins, controlled dehydration, hypobaric chamber experiments, biological weapons testing, vivisection, amputation and standard weapons testing. Away from the notorious Unit 731 were the Japanese Allied prisoner of war camps, often situated in remote areas of the jungles of Asia, where doctors were given a free hand to do as they pleased with their prisoner subjects, many of whom were already suffering the effects of their brutal treatment, severe malnutrition, dysentery and tropical disease. In these squalid jungle POW camps Japanese doctors effectively subjected their captives to a catalogue of medical tortures which served no purpose whatsoever other than that of the infliction of unnecessary suffering which often led to death. The experiments carried out on POWs in the camps differ slightly from those conducted by Unit 731, as it appears there were no particular medical or surgical objectives. Thousands of Allied POWs and civilians were effectively murdered in this manner. The names listed below were Japanese veterinary surgeons who carried out vivisections on live Allied prisoners of war at the outdoor dissecting ground of No.100 Army Corps based at Hainking (Changchum), Manchuria. It is illustrative of the contempt the Japanese had for their prisoners of war that veterinary surgeons were permitted to conduct dissections: the prisoners were viewed as animals. The names of these individuals were given by witness Takeshi Nishimura in a report on Japanese war criminals in August 1946. It was reported that these individuals carried out dissections on Allied, Chinese, Indian, Burmese and what were termed 'local' prisoners of war, and that the individuals were dissected while fully conscious, with no anaesthetic being administered beforehand, and while crawling with pests. The prisoners were opened up from throat to navel by means of a scalpel, and their organs were carefully inspected for signs of disease or other infection before being removed for closer analysis. Once the procedures had been conducted the prisoners were dragged away and cast into a pit dug into the ground. Some were still alive at this point and no attempts were made to end their suffering by mercy killing. Unsurprisingly, there were no survivors of these dissections, carried out by those Japanese individuals named below:

Motoji Yamaguchi – former veterinary surgeon major
Yujiro Wakamatsu – former veterinary surgeon major-general.
(Forename unknown) Hozaka – former veterinary surgeon lieutenant-colonel.

I could find no record indicating that the above-named individuals were ever arrested and/or interviewed by the Allied authorities tasked with investigating Japanese war crimes at the end of the Second World War. In all likelihood these men were never questioned about their involvement in the above-mentioned crimes at the No.100 Army Corps barracks, despite eyewitness accounts confirming their guilt.

Unit 731

As early as the mid-1930s, with aggressive Japanese incursions into China, the Japanese Imperial Army carried out biological warfare and medical testing largely on the civilian population under the authority of General Shiro Ishii, the lead physician at what became known as Unit 731. Originally the conception of the much-dreaded Japanese Kenpeitai (military police), the unit was commanded solely by General Shiro Ishii, who had served as a combat medical officer in the Kwantung Army, thus developing a special interest in medical disciplines, particularly those associated with the military. Funding for Unit 731 was very generous, coming directly from the Japanese government, and this funding continued right up until the end of the Second World War. The Japanese Emperor Hirohito was well aware of Unit 731 and its activities and the fact that his government was responsible for not only funding its day-to-day operations, but also the murders that were taking place there. The death toll as a result of these vile so-called experiments is not known, but sources quote in excess of 400,000 victims. Unit 731 was short for Manshu Detachment 731, but was also often known as the Kamo Detachment, the Ishii unit after its infamous lead physician, and more officially as the Epidemic Prevention and Water Purification Department of the Kwantung Army, a ridiculously tame moniker for one of the most murderous organizations of the pre-war and Second World War period.

Unit 731 was established by the Japanese Imperial military as a covert biological and chemical warfare research branch. From its establishment in 1936 Unit 731 became primarily engaged in the use of human beings for lethal human experimentation and biological weapons research. Unit 731 was based in the Japanese-occupied Pingfang district of Harbin which was the largest city in the Japanese puppet state of Manchukuo (now north-east China). The unit had active branch offices throughout China and south-east Asia. Unit 731 began its work during the Second Sino-Japanese War, which began in 1937, and continued until the Japanese surrender in 1945. Such was the lethal efficiency of Unit 731 that there were no survivors among those used in the various medical programmes; only witnesses survived, among them some of the Japanese medical and military staff involved in the programmes.

Chinese citizens were routinely taken by Japanese soldiers operating with Unit 731. They would be taken to the compound, beaten senseless, deprived of food, water and rest in what amounted to a slow dehumanization process, at the end of which each subject was referred to simply as a 'log' by the Japanese. A variety of tests were carried out on those taken to the Unit 731 compound, including experiments in which various diseases were injected into individuals, controlled dehydration, hypobaric pressure chamber testing, vivisection and organ procurement, amputation and standard weapons testing. Such tests were considered of high value from a medical perspective to the Japanese military who were operating largely in tropical/jungle conditions, where infection, particularly from wounds received in battle, was a major concern. The best methods of amputating limbs which were either severely damaged or had become infected, and indeed any post-operative care, could only be discovered from research gained through practical experience. Like Nazi Germany in Europe, the Japanese conquest of the Far Eastern and Pacific territories meant they soon accumulated huge numbers of not only Allied military prisoners of war, who included Indians, Chinese, Russians, Burmese, British, Australians and Americans, but also thousands of civilian men, women and children. The indigenous people of Japanese-conquered territory were not spared the horrors of human experimentation, and nor were the babies born to women raped by Japanese soldiers in every Japanese theatre of operation. Where biological weapons testing was concerned the Japanese military were careful never to use such weapons in areas of Japanese occupation. Most of the biological weapons were tested in China in areas populated by Chinese citizens. This ensured no food or water sources used by the Japanese would become contaminated.

Waging war against an enemy through biological means is certainly nothing new in the history of warfare. In the ancient world, if an enemy had barricaded himself into a secure and seemingly impenetrable fortress, rotting or diseased human or animal carcasses and human excrement were flung over the walls using crude catapult weapons. The intent was to cause an outbreak of disease among the defenders within and force their surrender. Local water sources were also poisoned with rotting carcasses, urine and faeces. These were found to be effective methods against an enemy behind walls who could otherwise not be dislodged or forced to the negotiating table. These age-old methods of waging war under primitive conditions were used by the Japanese in China, Asia and the Pacific.

What types of human medical experiments were carried out by the infamous Japanese Unit 731? Firstly, the medical staff, particularly the young Japanese medical students employed in Unit 731 operations, were very different from the lowly soldiers often selected to guard the prisoner of war camps in the jungles of Asia and the Pacific. These students were among the most intelligent Japan had to offer. They would have enrolled in this barbarism with a full understanding of what it involved. The main focus of Unit 731 was germ/biological warfare involving the use of particularly virulent strains of diseases such as anthrax, bubonic plague and cholera. The Japanese regime had no moral aversion to the use of bacteria and diseases as a means of waging war against an enemy, and had conducted in-depth research into biological warfare well in advance of the country's entry into the Second World War on 22 September 1940. The view was that the fact that such weapons and research had been banned by the Geneva Convention of 1925 was in fact a verification of their effectiveness – this warped philosophy reflected Japanese imperial thinking of the time.

The Unit 731 installation was built in Manchuria, which meant that the unit was separate from the Japanese mainland, a useful precaution when dealing with some of the world's deadliest diseases and bacteria. Initially the main victims gathered and taken to the Unit 731 facility were Chinese, but later huge numbers of Allied prisoners of war became available. The Japanese were hoping to become world-leaders in the use of biological weapons. It was Shiro Ishii who organized a secret research group, known as the 'Togo Unit', to commence work in Manchuria. Shiro Ishii, far from being an unknown, was very famous among professors in Japan. Many of Ishii's peers had heard rumours that he was using human subjects for experiments related to the military. Almost every form of disease was subject to experimentation under Ishii's expert guidance. Ishii's team had conducted experiments on animals including pigs, goats, cows, horses, cats and dogs, but it was decided that in order to ascertain the effectiveness of any vaccine developed that human test subjects would be necessary. Ishii established his main research operation at Harbin. Harbin was chosen as it would enable Ishii to access a steady stream of POWs for his research work, and also allow him the luxury of working without interference from the authorities in Tokyo. Ishii carried out this work in the full knowledge that he could have conducted the same experiments in Tokyo without the use of POWs and obtained far more accurate results due to the more modern equipment available there. Harbin gave Ishii the secrecy he insisted on, along with an endless supply of human guinea pigs. Ishii operated under the alias of Hajime Togo during the course of his work at Harbin. Ishii's older brother, who acted as his private secretary, used the alias of Hosoya. It was discovered that all of Ishii's officers used aliases while working at the secret Harbin facility. The idea of bacterial warfare was solely Ishii's. He had returned from a trip to Europe in 1930 and immediately initiated steps for funding bacterial warfare, both offensive and defensive. Most microbiologists in Japan were connected in some way or another with Ishii's work. He mobilised most of the universities in Japan to assist in research for his unit. In addition to the Tokyo Army Medical College, these included the Kyoto Imperial University, Tokyo Imperial University, Infectious Disease Research Laboratory, Tokyo and others. The following is a list of all the staff who served under Ishii at Harbin:

General Shiro Ishii (director) – Commanding Officer
Major General Hitoshi Kikuchi – Chief, 1st Section
Colonel Kiyoshi Ota – Chief, 3rd Section
Colonel Hatushige Ikari – Chief 2nd Section
Colonel (forename unknown) Nagayama – Chief, Clinical Section
Colonel Tomasada Masuda – Chief, Administration
Major (Forename unknown) Hirasawa – Test Pilot (Aeronavigation)
Colonel Takashi Muraka – Chief, Education
Colonel Saburo Sonada – Chief, Education
Colonel Kokan Imazu – Chief, Administration
Colonel Masataka Kitagawa – Chief, Administration 2nd Section
Colonel (forename unknown) Eguchi – Chief, Administration 4th Section.
Major Yashiyasu Masuda – Pharmacy
Major (forename unknown) Tanabe – Chief, General Affairs
Major (forename unknown) Takahashi – Chief ,General Affairs

The Togo Unit had been proposed in 1930 in response to Japanese observations that the Western powers were conducting their own research into the development of biological weapons. One of Ishii's main supporters within the Japanese Imperial Army was Colonel Chikahiko Koizumi, who would rather ironically later be appointed as Japan's Minister for Health from the period 1941 to 1945. Koizumi himself had joined a secret poison gas research committee as early as 1915, during the First World War, and he, along with other members of the Imperial Army, was said to have been impressed by the successful German use of poison gas such as chlorine during the Second Battle of Ypres, in which the Allies suffered 5,000 deaths and 15,000 wounded as a result of chemical weapons attacks.

Unit Togo was located and commenced its work in the Zhongma Fortress, a prison and experimentation camp in the village of Beiyinhe, some 62 miles south of Harbin on the South Manchuria railway. The individuals transported to Zhongma included common criminals, bandits, anti-Japanese partisans and those labelled as political opponents to the regime. Most of those labelled as being political opponents of the Japanese Empire had been forced to incriminate themselves through confessions wrung from them by the dreaded Kempeitei. It was noted that the prisoners were generally well fed on a diet of rice, wheat, meat and fish, and were even occasionally given alcohol in order for the subjects to be in the best of physical health at the beginning of the experiments. Then, over a period of several days, the prisoners were drained of blood and deprived of even the most basic nutrition and water. Their state of deterioration was recorded at every stage and during this period some were vivisected without any anaesthetic. It was also at this time that some of the prisoners were deliberately infected with plague bacteria. These bacteria were often administered through using infected fleas. Other bacteria were experimented with, and once injected the victims were then observed to see how rapidly the bacteria took hold in the body and the effects on the individual. Some subjects, despite being critically ill, were forced to perform certain tasks such as answering questions, completing puzzles and lifting heavy objects from one side of a room to another. These tests were carried out to determine how well the victim could function and for how long before total incapacitation and death occurred. Prisoners were also injected with animal blood and urine to see whether or not this had any value within the biological weapons programme. Bacteriological bombs were also developed. For example, prisoners would be tied to trees and the bombs, which were little more than cannisters containing various contagious diseases, were then dropped by aircraft near to the test subjects, but not so close as to kill them instantly. The Japanese were interested to observe the effect of disease-infected shrapnel on the subjects.

Japanese plans to infect San Diego with the bubonic plague were also hatched at Unit 731. The planned operation, rather colourfully known as Cherry Blossoms by Night, was proposed for September 1945. The means chosen to deliver the bubonic plague bacteria was using aircraft flown by Kamikaze (Divine Wind) suicide pilots. The plan was in its advanced stages when it was cancelled by Hideki Tojo, who would later be hanged for other war crimes. At the time of the cancellation Japan's primary focus was on the defence of its country as opposed to any offensive operations. The Japanese surrender in August 1945 was another factor. China was not so fortunate and plague bombs developed from tests carried out by Unit 731 were actually used against its cities by the Japanese. These plague bombs carried bacteria such as bubonic plague, anthrax and cholera. Some of these plague bombs resembled conventional aerial bombs, but the internal mechanism was redesigned to accommodate containers to hold infected insects. Another means of deployment of biological weapons was through aerosols to be carried by aircraft.

The results of these attacks are evident in the statistics. For example, outbreaks of the plague were reported in Changde in north-central China and Ningbo in eastern China. It is known that some 3–400,000 Chinese people were killed by this method of biological warfare from the Japanese military. The post-Second World War US government attempted rather unsuccessfully to cover up the scale of these Japanese atrocities, which outlines the military importance of the work carried out by Unit 731. The legacy of Japan's biological warfare programme is that many of these deadly disease-containing bombs lie buried and undiscovered in the Chinese countryside today. Furthermore, hundreds of Chinese are still suffering from the effects of Japanese biological weapons. A 71-year-old Chinese woman named Wang Juhua was interviewed in 2005. Reporter Geoffrey York travelled to Zhongzhu in China to speak with her. What the American reporter saw shocked him, and he recalled:

> 'The elderly woman shuffled across the yard of her village home. Swarms of flies were buzzing around her legs as she removed a simple tissue dressing to reveal one of the festering wounds on her leg. When the tissue was removed it exposed what looked like a chunk of raw, decaying flesh. The old lady cleaned the wound with a crude tea water solution and some disinfectant powder before covering the wound with a fresh piece of tissue paper. Twice a day she would carry out this ritual which gave some short relief from the constant pain of her swollen and blackened legs. For six decades she has had to endure the agony of these wounds which will blight her life sadly until death.

The elderly woman explained:

> "I was just eight years old when the Japanese attacked us. I was out feeding our cattle and walking through the grassland. I did not see anything but once I returned home, I felt my legs itching and I scratched them. Small red dots began to appear on my legs and these then became blisters. As I grew older the wounds became worse and for three years I was confined to bed as I could not walk. The wound is always itchy and painful, as if some insects

or small animals are biting me. It is always worse when I am out working in the fields, but I have to work if I want to survive."

Wang's wounds have never been properly diagnosed yet local experts believe the wounds are due to exposure to anthrax or glanders or possibly a combination of the two. The nature of her wounds has meant that she has suffered social isolation. Even some of her relatives were unwilling to live with and assist her. Wang explained that "due to the sight of my wounds and the flies people became sickened by me. In the past there were people in the village who had similar wounds, and we would visit each other, but now there are hardly any of us still alive."

In a neighbouring village another survivor 72-year-old Wu Chahua lives. Her face is twisted and distorted by scars that began as small holes and blisters around the time when the Japanese began deploying their germ weapons. Wu recalled:

> "It was one day in 1943, I saw pieces of paper falling from a Japanese aircraft. It was not long after that I became ill, and my skin began to rot. I have been unable to find the name of my illness, but doctors believe it to be a typhoid fungus. Many other people caught the same disease, and my head also feels dizzy, I can't walk properly, and I fall over. Those Japanese devils have brought me lifelong misery and pain, I hate them very much."

Liu Chen Huang was ten years old when he witnessed what later transpired to have been a carefully coordinated germ warfare attack on his village by Japanese aircraft.

He recalled:

> "I remember it as if it were only yesterday. Even as a youngster I had to go out to work in the fields gathering rice with my family. It was summertime in mid-1943 we began noticing many Japanese

twin-engine aircraft flying in the vicinity of our village. It was our opinion that they were on reconnaissance flights and maybe their interest was in the nearby town. We would always run and take cover when we saw them as often, they would shoot at you if they saw you. We had heard many stories of Japanese planes machine-gunning people out working in the countryside so we did not take any chances, we would always run and hide in the ditches until the planes flew on. The type of planes that came over were the bomber aircraft with two engines. I would be fascinated by them by also very afraid of them too. I recall one occasion when two of these Japanese bombers came over. The army must have noticed them visiting us regularly, so they had decided to set up some guns hidden in the trees and give them a greeting the next time. As we took cover, we could see the Japanese planes fly over then there was the sound of machine gun fire. We could not see from our hiding place whether it was the Japanese planes firing or the guns of our army. The sound of firing went on for some seconds then there was the sound of something crashing down into trees and then the ground. We could not hear any planes, so we came out of the ditch and looked around. Around a quarter of a mile away there was smoke rising up into the sky. Of course, word soon got to us that one of the Japanese planes had been brought down. The Japanese aboard the plane had been killed. There was rumour that members of our local defence force had captured the pilot alive but executed him soon after. I never discovered if this was true or not. The Japanese plane became a focal point for us youngsters and despite being warned to leave it alone by our parents we young people went and climbed upon it and tried to tear parts from it. It remained where it was for around a month before it was taken away presumably for scrap. We had no Japanese planes come over for some time after this incident which we felt was odd, but we carried on with our working in the fields. The one morning we were all up early, we had a simple breakfast before heading out into the fields to work. It was a pleasant sort of day warm with hazy sunshine. We had been out for around two hours when there was the sound of engines approaching very fast from an easterly direction. We stood there saying to ourselves "what is it?" and "where is it?" as we could not see an aircraft anywhere. The reason we couldn't see it was because he was flying so low that he was below the horizon. By the time we saw the aircraft it was too late to do anything, there was this roar of the two engines, followed by a very loud whoosh sound and the aircraft was trailing what looked like a spray, some form of fine mist. My father shouted, "he has been shot in his radiators as he is trailing steam". So, we were not concerned at all by this as we thought it's another Japanese plane that has been shot and will probably crash nearby. We heard no other sounds this time and we began to continue with our work again. As the morning progressed, we all began to feel unwell. I felt like something had bitten me and I began to scratch my arms and my face which soon became very reddened and inflamed. My mother, father and sister all felt the same discomfort and we decided to head home. I recall the next morning feeling very unwell, in fact all of us felt very unwell and we were unable to go out and work that day as a result. A doctor was summoned to the village as other villagers were falling ill at the same time and some of the older villagers died. The doctor could not understand what was wrong with us. We felt generally very unwell, and our bodies began to develop sore areas which then became like blisters which would swell up and burst. Unlike a normal blister these would not heal. The skin would remain raw and weeping and extremely sore and itchy. Other symptoms included watery stools, constant thirst, poor vision and severe fatigue. The reality was our local doctor's knowledge did not stretch as far as the symptoms we were all experiencing. It was only after the passing of some weeks it was suggested that the Japanese planes, we had seen including the one we saw being shot down had been carrying some sort of biological weapon. We required more specialist treatment which meant we would need to see doctors in the city hospital. This was totally denied as there was the concern that whatever we had could be spread among the population if we went there. Instead, we were treated like farm animals, we had to be treated at a distance with drugs we didn't even know the names of. We were instructed to take them in the prescribed manner, and this is what we had to do. We made some slight improvement, yet we were never really well after that attack and the sores continued to be a recurring problem on our bodies. These sores seemed to appear particularly in the moist areas of the body, the armpits, feet and groin. They would always appear as blisters to start with soon becoming suppurating wounds overnight. To still be suffering from the effects of something which happened now so long ago is deplorable. Both my mother and father have gone now but up until the day they died they suffered. My sister and myself have received no compensation for our suffering for all these years. The reason for this is quite simple. The Allied powers mainly America and Britain attempted to create a cover up and pretend the Japanese biological weapons attacks didn't happen. They desperately wanted the research material for themselves, so no Japanese were prosecuted and instead they were recruited by their former enemies. The Western Allies were afraid that the Russians might learn more about the Japanese biological weapons and their effects upon humans and were prepared to tell lies in order to get their hands on the materials they needed. Today people are waking up to these dirty deeds and it brings the question of what else have they lied to the world about? They could have helped us the victims, but they chose to ignore us instead to protect their own evil interests. I can forget to a degree but forgive I can never do. Apart from our suffering we as with others were ostracized within our own communities. People who were unaffected treated us like a leper colony. In some instances, we were herded into our own allocated villages where we could not leave, we couldn't travel anywhere, and no one could visit us. It was little more than a prison camp. The Japanese who did this to us should have been living like that not us. But no, the Americans took them away, gave them nice houses, highly paid jobs in their biological warfare labs and in some instances new identities so as they could never be prosecuted.'

Liu Chen Huang at this point leans forward places his head in his hands and weeps. His son who has sat quietly beside his elderly father suddenly holds up his hands gesturing that "this is enough he can talk no more on this occasion".

A 72-year-old former Japanese army medical assistant who had worked at the Nanking facility for a short period while in China recalled during an interview with the *New York Times* newspaper in March 1996 how he had been involved in a project to develop plague bombs which could be used against the Allied forces during the Second World War. The elderly man insisted on anonymity before agreeing to speak of his work. He recalled:

'It was exciting, and it left an impression on me because it was my first time. A Chinese prisoner had been deliberately infected with the plague as part of the research project I was involved with. After the prisoner had been administered the plague bacteria a period of time was allowed to elapse so as the bacteria could do its job within the prisoner's body. He was kept separate from all of the other prisoners for obvious reasons. It was decided after a period of time that the prisoner would be cut open so as we could ascertain what the disease actually did to the internal organs. No anaesthetic was given to the prisoner as there was concern that an anaesthetic drug may have an effect on the results of the procedure. The prisoner was a Chinese male of thirty years of age, he was tied down naked to a table fully aware of what we were about to do to him. The fellow knew it was all over for him, so he did not resist as he was led into the room and tied down. Only when I picked up the scalpel did he begin to scream. I proceeded to cut him open from the chest to the stomach, he screamed terribly, his face contorted in agony. He made this unimaginable sound; he was screaming so horribly. But then finally he stopped screaming. This was all in a day's work for the surgeons, yet it left a very deep impression on me.'

Like so many Japanese doctors and surgeons involved in the biological weapons research programmes the elderly Japanese man was not prosecuted after the war despite having been captured, questioned and admitting to war crimes. The post-Second World War US administration agreed to offer immunity from prosecution in exchange for any records, details, or results of the experiments they carried out.

Another anonymous source claimed to have carried out work on the actual design of plague bombs for the Japanese Imperial Airforce. The anonymous source explained via an email:

'The bombs weren't really bombs in the conventional sense. In most cases a bomb is a simple steel container with fins, explosive filling and a fuze to accomplish detonation. These bombs kill people or destroy buildings through blast and/or fragmentation. There were bombs designed for use against armoured targets and bombs for use against enemy soldiers. These conventional bombs had steel casings which ranged in size, weight and the thickness of the metal. When it was proposed by our military that a plague or germ bomb was a good method of attacking an enemy especially the enemy civilian population, we had to come up with a method by which the bacterium could be deployed. Experimentation was conducted on the possible use of artillery shells as a means of releasing biological or germ agents against an enemy or his territory. Artillery shells were found to be ineffective for the purpose of biological warfare primarily due to the fact they required thick metal casings in order to not break up upon the stresses of firing. Therefore, powerful explosive fillings were required which in turn destroyed the cargo within. There was no practical means of successfully configuring artillery shells at that time to carry biological or germ agents. Artillery shells were best suited to chemical applications where gases were formed upon combustion of the explosives. It was found the incendiary effects of the explosive fillings might destroy the bacteria. We did not wish to waste time trying to perfect something which was not feasible at that time, so we concentrated on what you call plague bombs. These plague bombs could easily be constructed from a relatively lightweight material such as porcelain or aluminium and they only needed a small charge with which to break open the casing and release the contents. It was discovered that porcelain was the best material for the construction of these bombs. The use of high explosive such as that carried in a conventional aircraft bomb as with artillery shells would have destroyed the contents. With a plague bomb the payload was infected fleas such as those taken from rats. Fleas are an incredibly hardy insect and could be placed within a thin glass or porcelain container within the aluminium casing. Corn and other grain were also placed within the plague bomb cannisters to attract rats once the bomb had dispersed its contents to the ground. The idea being that rats would be attracted to the corn and in turn would become infected by the payload of plague infected fleas. A small initiating charge was all that was needed to burst both the container wall and the fragile porcelain flask containing the infected insects. Once this container had burst the fleas would fall and settle on the ground where they would also be picked up by dogs and cats. These plague bombs would have to be delivered at low level. The problem with plague bombs is that it was a painstaking task harvesting the numbers of insects required for the bombs. A technician suggested placing the corpses of rats or other animals infected with plague insects, yet fleas will only remain on a living host and will jump off a dead one. So, there were problems with these ideas, but they were effective once created as tests proved this. The bombs designed to carry such diseases as anthrax were far simpler devices. The disease could be contained within the same porcelain, glass or metal container as the plague bombs. The bombs were cylindrical in shape with stabilising fins at the rear and fitted with a short bursting charge and fuze. There were many other forms of disease and bacteria considered for use in bombs. Corn and grain were also used as a means of carrying bacteria and diseases as a payload within our bioweapons. Weapons containing infected grain was used against the Chinese who were unaware that this bounty from the sky we were dropping on them was potentially deadly. There were instances where the grain was dispersed over a village or town, and this was eagerly collected up by the citizens without any of it being analysed beforehand. When samples of grain dropped by our aircraft was analysed under proper laboratory conditions, they then discovered the pathogens. Any disease which would have debilitating effects upon the enemy, or his people was worth pursuing as it only takes a few successful bombs to infect a large city, again this was proven to be true by their deployment against the Chinese. In my view it was not a criminal act, you fight wars to win them by any means, don't you? It is like the two atomic bombs dropped on my country, if we had had them first and a means to deploy them, we would have most certainly used them. Biological weaponry is no more barbaric than a weapon which kills through extreme heat, blast and radiation in my opinion.'

From US Army Intelligence reports it appears the main plague bomb, as it was referred to, was known as the Type 50 Uji Bomb. The Type 50 Uji bomb had a length of 700mm and diameter of 180mm. The bomb weighed 25 kilograms and was fitted with a Type 1 impact fuse with delay. Stabilisation of the bomb was achieved through celluloid fins fitted to the rear of the bomb along with a time fuse safety pin also fitted into the central rear section of the bomb. The bomb did indeed have a case made from porcelain and not glass or aluminium, yet as stated above various case materials were trialled to find the most effective method. The bomb was capable of carrying a 10-litre payload. The nose cone was fitted with a brass metal impact fuse fitted with a delay. Fitted to the fuse was a load of 500 grams of TNT. In cases where the tail fuse and internal prima cord failed to function, the explosive train contained within the nose section of the bomb would detonate when the bomb impacted the ground, the bomb thus dispersing its payload. It is reported that some 500 bombs of this model were manufactured in 1940–41, and extensive field trials were carried out during the period 1940 to 1942 at Unit 731's proving ground near Anta, Manchuria. For safety reasons during the proving tests the bombs were detonated on the ground in static tests before being dropped from aircraft. In the initial test phases bombs with no biological payloads were carried and the bombs were filled with containers of dye solution and suspensions of non-pathogenic organisms. The later test programmes were conducted with the use of a suspension of *B. anthracis* spores as the payload. In the aircraft drop tests with a wind velocity of 5 metres per second (11.5mph) and bombs being detonated at an altitude of 200–300 metres it was observed that the payload would be dispersed over an area of 40–60 metres by 600–800 metres. A proportion of the Type 50 Uji bombs were adapted to carry a payload of up to 30,000 fleas which had been infected with the *Y. pestis* bacteria. *Yersinia pestis* is a gram-negative, non-motile coccobacillus bacterium without spores that is related to both *Yersinia pseudotuberculosis* and *Yersinia enterocolitica*. It is a facultative anaerobic organism that can infect human beings via the oriental rat flea. The dispersal method for the explosive opening of the bomb had to be redesigned so that it did not kill the fleas. The redesigned bomb was wrapped with a 4-metre length of prima cord.

Prima cord was nothing more elaborate than hollow cord filled with an explosive material. It required initiation via a detonator and was capable of initiating the detonation of other explosive materials. A fuse would explode the prima cord at an altitude of 200–300 metres, thus liberating the bomb's payload. After some considerable research and much trial and error at Anta, the dispersal method for the bombs was perfected to the point at which 80% of the fleas contained inside survived. These redesigned Uji bombs were undoubtedly the most effective of the biological weapons created by the Japanese in terms of being able to inflict sickness and death on the largest number of Chinese who were targeted with the bombs.

The devices which became known as the Fu-Go Balloon bombs (A-Type used by Imperial Japanese Army and B-Type by the Imperial Japanese Navy) first made their appearance in the skies over the US between November 1944 and April 1945. These Japanese balloon bombs were the first ever weapon system with intercontinental range, pre-dating the intercontinental ballistic missile. They were originally conceived to carry incendiary or high-explosive payloads to the enemy heartland, yet they did not prove very successful. Of the 9,300 balloons launched from sites on coastal Honshu only 300 were found or observed in the US, Canada and Mexico. The original intention of these crude weapons was to deliver incendiary devices to the US in the hope they might land in forests and crops with the obvious outcome of causing destructive fires. Other balloons carried high explosive, which posed a threat to anyone tinkering with one of the devices when discovered on the ground. A US media censorship campaign prevented Japanese intelligence from learning any useful results from the balloon launches, yet on 5 May 1945, six civilians were killed by one of the Japanese balloon bombs near Bly, Oregon. The six victims were the only fatalities in the continental US resulting from these balloons. The victims were Elsie Mitchell (26), wife of minister Archie E. Mitchell; Edward Engen (13), Richard Patzke (14), Jay Gifford (13), Sherman Shoemaker (11), and Joan Patzke (13), who were out in the woods picnicking when they noticed the strange balloon object. The group then attempted to pull it out of the woods. Reverend Mitchell heard the explosion and quickly ran to the scene where he discovered the bodies. The families of the victims were awarded compensation by the US government and a memorial was erected at what today is called the Mitchell Recreation Area. The US government, while not overtly concerned by the appearance of the balloon bombs carrying incendiary or high explosives, nevertheless had real concern that the Japanese might deploy balloons carrying biological or germ payloads. In a letter to Lieutenant Colonel M. Moses, a Lieutenant Colonel Gaylord W. Anderson, US Army Medical Corps, addressed several points of concern relating to this issue, writing:

(1) In accordance with verbal request of Captain Baker, the undersigned on 27 December 1944 proceeded in company with others to the Naval Research Laboratory to examine two Japanese balloons that had landed on the Pacific Coast. The presence of the undersigned was requested because of the possibility that such balloons might have been intended as biological weapon devices.

(2) It is the opinion of the undersigned that these balloons are probably not designed for biological warfare for the following reasons: (a) The loading of these balloons with a bacterial charge would accomplish nothing unless a device were available for spreading bacterial organisms in flight. There was no evidence to suggest that such spraying or spreading devices had been present. Release of bacterial organism's incidental to the landing of the balloon would accomplish nothing in view of the fact that balloons have an incendiary device to destroy the bag, the fire resulting being sufficient to destroy any bacterial organisms that would contaminate the soil around the point of landing. (b) Another conceivable method of spreading infection would be to have balloons carry infected animals.

This is extremely unlikely in view of the fact that the balloons are designed to travel at an altitude at which animals would die due to the lack of oxygen and extremes of cold unless the balloons were equipped with elaborate heating and oxygen supply apparatus. There was nothing about the balloons to suggest the presence of such apparatus. (c) The chief bacterial organism which could be disseminated by rodents in particular would be plague. Inasmuch as the ground squirrels throughout the west coast and even as far as east as the Dakotas are already infected with the plague, nothing would be accomplished by the introduction of an occasional plague-infected rodent such as a rat.

(3) The possibility of their use to introduce infected insects cannot be dismissed. On the other hand, if such had been their intent, it seems unlikely that they would have been sent over at the present season of year even on a trial basis.

For The Surgeon General: Gaylord W. Anderson, Lieutenant Colonel, Medical Corps Assistant.

The letter stresses the importance of the two main factors of temperature and oxygen in the successful deployment of live and therefore effective bacterial/germ weapons to the US mainland via the balloons. The balloons did not have the capability to fulfil the role of bacteriological weapons for use against the US as they could not carry the necessary apparatus. Even had more elaborate methods of delivering germ/bacterial payloads to US soil been available, such as via an aircraft or unmanned missile type weapon such as the German V1, it is doubtful whether a successful delivery could have been achieved and whether the results would have been worth the considerable efforts required of Japan at a time late in the Second World War when the country was focussed more on defence than attack.

The possibility of the Japanese use (and US counter use) of botulinum, the active toxin of *C. botulinum*, as a biological weapon was also discussed by the US military authorities. The substance *C. botulinum* is so toxic that, mixed with an inert material in the proportion one to twenty, it could be employed to kill or incapacitate all persons within a given area, effectively clearing the way for an invasion.

Techniques:

> *C. botulinum* can be cultured in a broth of meat and bean meal under a two-inch covering of mineral oil in brewery vats. The hot broth is run directly from the cookers, through the filters, and into the vats under the covering of oil while still hot, and seeded with spores of *C. botulinum* while still hot enough to destroy vegetative organisms, which will establish conditions under which this organism will be able to overgrow all others and produce a toxin of high potency.
>
> Daily tests to monitor the development of toxicity are carried out during the fermentation process. For this purpose, mice have been the preferred test animal and 1/10cc of dilutions of 1:10,000; 1:100,000; 1:000,000 should be employed.
>
> As soon as the maximum toxicity has been reached, the media is filtered by suction, and salted out with ammonium sulphate. The toxin comes to the surface as scum; the bulk of the media can be drawn off from below, and the sludge run into centrifugal extractors. The extracted toxin should be mixed with four to five times its weight of the inert powder with which it is to be later diluted (preferably silica of a maximum diameter of eight microns), frozen with dry ice, and dried in high vacuum. The addition of the inert material before drying is for the purpose of preventing clumping, as it is desirable to have the dry toxin in as finely divided a state as possible.
>
> The dry toxin is mixed with a fine, inert powder in such proportions as to make a final dilution of about one to twenty to

> one to forty; loaded into large steel drums of one-ton capacity, so constructed that they can be transported in aircraft and so that the toxic powder may be discharged into the air by the use of compressed air in a small cylinder.
>
> The night before (twenty to thirty hours would be best) an invasion, during the hours of darkness, aircraft dump a few tons of this powder into the air to the windward of the target area. The dust is carried over the target area by the wind and is not easily breathed but settles on everything. Anyone getting any of it on the mucous membranes, the cornea of the eye, or into the lungs, or stomach will be poisoned with the toxin. The illness does not strike until six to twenty-four hours have elapsed after absorption; so that there would be little chance of the enemy against whom it was used discovering the nature of the attack until too late. Used as a means of defending Japanese held islands in this manner it would be possible to keep any hint of the nature of the attack from reaching other enemy bases.
>
> The toxin could also be used against shipping or enemy warships by laying down a haze of the dust on their course, so they would steam directly through the contaminated haze.
>
> The advantages of using silica as the inert dust is simple; silicon creates deposits with the sufficient fineness; coarse material, such as glass sand, is easily reduced down to the required fineness; silica grains of a diameter of eight microns or less will remain suspended in the air for hours and will penetrate the smallest cracks and crevices and cannot be kept out of dwellings. In the dry state it does not pack or clump, and it has no tendency to draw moisture which may be present in the air.

At point in the discussion there was an address as to the morals of the possible US military usage of such weapons which were viewed by many to be inhumane. The US declared non-agreement with this notion and in actual practice it would probably such weapons should be considered to be more humane than any weapon(s) now employed (possible reference to future deployment of the atomic bombs). Those persons receiving large doses of the toxins will almost certainly die, but the chances are most of the victims would get sub-lethal doses of the toxin. They would be made ill, but most of them would only suffer temporary incapacity and recover without need of any treatment. The illness itself takes the form of placid paralysis and there is no pain or injury to tissues. Recovery from infection takes place within forty-eight hours to one week, and there are few after affects. The only real objection to any proposed counter-usage by the US military forces would be that of sportsmanship, but such considerations can have little weight in a situation of total war where phosphorus bombs are standard equipment.

The victim simply falls to the ground, blind and helpless, and depending on the dose, will either die or recover, but for the time being, he will be of no use whatsoever to his unit.

The big advantage is that it will make possible the taking of strongly held positions without the complete destruction of valuable resources and installations, thus preventing an enormous waste of materials. It has been advised that such a weapon should not be used against civilian populations unless it is done in order to bring the war to an end at one stroke. Otherwise, there is the chance the enemy might discover the nature of the attack and by their awareness be able to guard against it in future.

Tests of the air distribution of the dust may be made by mixing the same grade of silica that is used with the toxin with methylene blue, discharging it into the air from different altitudes and observing the distribution by exposing pieces of white cloth throughout the test area and noting the number of grains picked up on each piece.

Things were not all plain sailing for the Japanese, as back in the autumn of 1934, a prison break occurred at the Nanking facility which put the facilities' secrecy in severe jeopardy. This prison break was followed by an explosion the following year in 1935, an act considered to have been one of sabotage which led Shiro Ishii to cease his operations at the Zhongma Fortress. After discussions with the Imperial Japanese military hierarchy, it was decided that Ishii should relocate to Pingfang, 15 miles south of Harbin, where he could set up a new operation at what would be a much larger facility with which to continue his work. Again, those who believe that the Japanese Emperor Hirohito was somehow detached from the actions of the Japanese military government will be surprised to learn that it was Hirohito who issued a decree authorizing the expansion of Ishii's unit and its integration into the Kwantung Army as the Epidemic Prevention Department. In fact, Hirohito's brother, Prince Mikasa, toured the Unit 731 headquarters in China. Prince Mikasa even wrote in his memoirs that he had watched films showing how Chinese prisoners were made to march on the plains of Manchuria where poison gas was then released upon them.

In addition to Unit 731 there was also the establishment of a biological warfare development facility which was known as the Kwantung Army Military Horse Epidemic Prevention Workshop which was later referred to simply as Unit 100. A chemical warfare facility known as the Kwantung Army Technical Testing Department, later referred to as Manchuria 516, was also created. Following the Japanese invasion of China in 1937, sub-units of the biological and chemical warfare programmes were situated in many Chinese major cities and these included Unit 1855 in Beijing, Unit Ei 1644 in Nanking, Unit 8604 in Guangzhou and later Unit 9420 in Singapore. These units were all part of Ishii's network, which at the height of the various operations comprised some 10,000 personnel. Medical doctors and professors from all across the Japanese Empire were encouraged to joint Unit 731 as there were rare opportunities within the organisation to conduct experimentation on human beings. Evidence that the subjects had been dehumanised in the eyes of the staff working in these units is provided by the fact that the units were referred to as 'lumber mills' and the victims of experimentation as 'logs'. On a day when the death toll was high, staff might joke among themselves that 'many logs were felled today'. However, according to one junior uniformed civilian employee of the Japanese Imperial Army who worked at Unit 731, the project was internally known as '*Holzklotz*' which is German for log. Another irony perhaps was the fact that the corpses of the expired victims were then disposed of via incineration. Staff also referred to the victims of Unit 731 as 'Manchurian monkeys' or "Long-tailed monkeys', writing their reports as if the experiments had been conducted on monkeys rather than human beings.

American historian Sheldon H. Harris claimed that the Togo Unit employed brutal methods to secure human organs for study. The guards would be ordered to find a fit and healthy man, woman or child. The prisoner would be taken from his or her cell and forced to sit in a chair where they would be restrained before one of the guards split the prisoner's skull with the blow of an axe. The head would then be prised apart, and the brain extracted. It would then be taken away for research and once that particular piece of research had been completed the brain was disposed of by being tossed into an incinerator. Nakagawa Yonezo, a professor emeritus at Osaka University, had studied at the Kyoto University during the Second World War and while he was there, he had seen footage of human experiments and executions at Unit 731. Yonezo later testified as to the 'playfulness' (if it can be referred to as such) of the experiments when he recalled:

> 'Some of the experiments had nothing to do with advancing the capability of germ warfare, or indeed that of medicine. There is such a thing as professional curiosity: what would happen if we did such and such? What medical purpose was served by performing and studying beheadings? None at all. That in my personal view was just playing around, the actions of the bored. Professional people too like to play around.'

Perhaps one example of this 'playing around' is this account from a member of the Japanese army who served as a guard throughout the existence of the Nanking facility. The soldier's name was Ishiwaru Ikeda, and at the time of writing he was 88 years of age but had vivid memories of the things which he had seen at the Nanking facility. I had made contact with the elderly Ishiwaru during my research for a previous book focussing on the jungle war against the Japanese. Ishiwaru had connections with other former Japanese who had an association with Unit 731 during the Second World War, but none of them were prepared to talk. Therefore, the rarity and historical value of Ishiwaru's recollections cannot be stressed enough. Ishiwaru recalled the following:

> 'The soldiers would get bored at times and here we were surrounded by all these people who were not really viewed as worthy human beings. They were often viewed with disdain, like an animal simply waiting for you to take its life in order to eat it. There were no emotions of care towards these people, they were enemies of our nation mostly, so the taking of the lives of one or two of these people was not seen as something worth punishing us for. It was something that was often overlooked if you like. Beheading with swords was popular. I remember one late afternoon, there had been storms and it had been raining for most of the day, we were bored and restless. One of the guards suggested killing a prisoner with his sword to experience what it was like as he had never had the chance to kill with his sword up until that point. Other guards argued that we couldn't do it to any of the healthy logs as the physicians may get angry about losing a good log for their research. It was decided to take one of the old Chinese who may not have long to live as it was. That was it, they went and brought an elderly Chinese man from one of the cells. He knew what was going to happen as Sergeant Kuchii was standing with his sword unsheathed as the man was led into a room used for washing. There was a drain where the blood could flow without us having to clean up too much mess afterwards, so they ordered him to kneel down over the drain. Sergeant Kuchii placed the

blade edge of his sword on the centre of the back of the man's neck. As he raised his sword, I could see that it was so sharp that just from resting the blade on the man's neck it had drawn blood. All it took was a single blow which did not appear that forceful and the man's head fell severed from the shoulders of the torso. There was a lot of blood, Sergeant Kuchii quickly retrieved the severed head holding it by a small tuft of greying hair. We were all curious to see if the eyes or mouth might move, but the eyes were fixed, and the mouth was quite still. Sergeant Kuchii held up the head and began to ask it questions. He argued that the brain could still function for some minutes after being severed from the body. He explained he had been told this by one of the doctors at the facility and he was curious as to whether or not there was any truth in the matter. After questioning the severed head and receiving no reaction from it he simply threw it down and kicked it before ordering some guards to remove it. They asked what they should do with the head and the body of the dead man, and they were instructed that they could do what they wished with it as it was their property now. They were told to "get it out of here, get rid of it by any means". I heard rumours later that the head had been cast into a river while the body had parts cut from it and were cooked before being fed to the unsuspecting prisoners some of whom were relatives of the dead man. In reality we learned nothing from this execution other than how effective Sergeant Kuchii's blade was.'

Following the above disclosure, I asked the elderly former Japanese soldier if he had witnessed any of the actual human medical experiments carried out at the Nanking facility. Drawing a deep breath, the old man looked down at the floor momentarily before lighting himself a cigarette. He then recalled of the human medical experimentation:

'There were many experiments carried out with various poisons and diseases. The types of poisons and diseases varied from those found in nature within plants, fish and animals or that of a synthetical nature, manmade as you say. Some of the prisoners selected did not always come quietly, some fought the guards as they were brought out of the cells and the guards were forced to beat them, sometimes they were beaten unconscious which the physicians then got very angry about shouting at the guards "you idiots, how are we supposed to make accurate observations if the subject is asleep"? On the one occasion the doctors waiting to carry out an experiment with a natural toxin ordered the two guards to return a beaten and unconscious prisoner or log back to his cell and bring another one out. He told the two guards if the subject was not conscious on this second occasion, he would carry out the experiment on "you two", referring to the two guards. A second male prisoner was brought out and placed in a chair where he was restrained with leather straps to prevent him from moving. The experiment involved the injecting of tetrodotoxin which is found in the Fugu or Pufferfish. The physician drew out the poison from a glass phial into a glass syringe with a long needle attached to it. The prisoner didn't fight as he knew it was useless, yet the doctor told him that he was giving him a vaccination for disease. As he reassured the prisoner with his lies, he slid the needle into the vein in the prisoner's forearm and injected the poison. It was then a case of observing what would happen. From what I could see nothing really happened, the prisoner remained very still and did not cry out or say anything. I learned later that this poison paralyzes a human being breathing, they are acutely aware of everything going on around them, they remain fully conscious but unless resuscitated they literally suffocate. I witnessed doctors injecting solutions containing mercury and even acid. These prisoners screamed out in agony and convulsed often foaming at the mouth like a rabid animal. The one prisoner

> I recall fought so violently due to his agony he bit half of his own tongue off; he had even swallowed it as the doctors checked for it in his mouth after he died. There was blood coming from the nostrils too, it was not the most pleasant of things too see but the young doctors were extremely fascinated and excited about these experiments on the prisoners. Usually, reports were made on the amount of poison administered, how long it took to take effect, what those effects were and how long it took for the subject to expire. The corpses were then sent for vivisection where various organs were removed to observe the effect of the poisons on those organs. Tests were carried out to ascertain the levels of toxicity found in organs such as the liver, kidneys, brain and heart. All these things were written down and placed into files for future reference. There was a lot of work conducted on poisons and from those few poison experiments I witnessed the prisoners did not necessarily die quickly, sometimes they took hours even days to die from the effects. If a prisoner survived the first injection of poison a higher dose would be administered.'

Like the Nazi German human medical experiments, the Japanese conducted many experiments into the effects of hypothermia. Such experiments were carried out as a means of understanding and treating the various forms of hypothermia experienced by army personnel on the ground in winter conditions, air crews operating at high altitudes and naval personnel who faced the risk of exposure to extreme temperatures as an occupational hazard. At Unit 731 former physiologist Yoshimura Hisato was the main authority on hypothermia experiments on human beings. Before his career with the infamous Unit 731 Hisato was a lecturer at the Kyoto Imperial University Faculty of Medicine. He was employed by the Imperial Japanese Army as an army engineer – a researcher who in effect was treated like an officer but not a professional military serviceperson. At the Unit 731 facility Hisato pursued his keen interest into hypothermia and its effects upon the human body, conducting all manner of hypothermia-related experiments on prisoners. In one such experiment a prisoner was forced to have his legs submerged in a vat of freezing water to which ice was added. The prisoner was forced to remain with his legs submerged in this vat until they had frozen solid, and a coating of ice had formed within the skin itself. This would have taken a few hours to occur, and the agony experienced by the individual would have been incomprehensible. When Hisato was satisfied that the prisoner's legs were frozen solid, he was pulled from the vat. An eyewitness to this experiment recalled how the limbs were then struck a blow with a cane and the sound of the cane hitting the limbs was like that of striking a tree trunk. The same experiments were carried out with the prisoner's arms immersed in the same freezing cold vat of water and ice. In addition to the freezing of limbs Hisato experimented with various methods of rapidly rewarming the frozen limbs of a prisoner. These rewarming methods included pouring boiling water on to the frozen limbs, holding them in close proximity to an open fire or leaving the prisoner in a cell overnight to ascertain how long it might take for the prisoner's blood to thaw. Often the result was gangrene, leading to death or the loss of the affected limbs. Many of the victims of Hisato's experiments who required amputations were treated like meat in a butcher's shop. They were dragged on to a table, held down and the limb sawn off with no anaesthetic. Hisato surmised in a few such cases that anaesthetic would not be necessary as the prisoner's limb was suitably anaesthetised through the freezing process. This was ridiculous but typical of the attitude of the Japanese towards their prisoners. It is a sad irony that the medical world today understands that the most effective way to treat frostbite is to warm the affected limbs in water at 100–122-degrees Fahrenheit. This was discovered as a result of work carried out at Unit 731.

Experiments were also carried out with sexual diseases such as syphilis and gonorrhoea. These were two particularly unpleasant sexual diseases and as many prisoners were left deliberately untreated purely for observational purposes the diseases caused widespread complications within the bodies of the subjects. As the effects of the diseases increased all manner of treatments were administered to the infected prisoners to ascertain the best methods of treatment and/or cure. Some of the supposed treatments, however, were quack practices which served no real purpose and often condemned the test subjects to a slow and agonising death. Ishiwaru recalled seeing male prisoners who had been deliberately infected with the herpes virus, and how long fine metal rods would be inserted into the penis. Ishiwaru told me that these fine metal rods had a coating of either barbs or a sandpaper-like substance. They were drawn back and forth, and he recalled that blood and sometimes even pus would discharge from the male subject's penis. These same rods once used were then used on prisoners who had no infection to see how rapidly the disease took hold in the genitals. He also recalled that some of these rods were inserted into the anus of both male and female prisoners. This was really torture, as it was already known that both syphilis and gonorrhoea could be treated with drugs, though the treatment period could be as long as five days to six months. Many Allied servicemen who had contracted these sexual diseases were treated while being able to carry out their normal duties. Ishiwaru recalled:

> 'There was a particular fascination with the sexual diseases. One of the senior medical staff at Nanking referred to sexual diseases as a western plague and that the British and American societies in particular were guilty of the propagation of sexual diseases throughout Asia. Yes, he blamed the white colonialists saying that before the arrival of these people with their immoral promiscuous lifestyles sexual diseases were not a prominent factor within Asian societies. So, there was a lot of interest in how sexual diseases occurred in the genitals and body as a whole and prisoners were infected with these diseases to ascertain how debilitating the effects were once the disease had developed. Prisoners were forced to carry out everyday tasks and they were carefully observed for the effects of pain, fever and fatigue brought on by the disease.

> A number of treatments were developed but these were never intended to have been beneficial to the prisoners. Once a treatment was proved successful the prisoner who had served as the guinea pig for the particular experiment was killed often by sword or bayonet and the other prisoners who were still suffering with the disease were left to suffer. Only the Japanese military were given treatment where it was required for sexual diseases. I recall one prisoner with a severe and advanced herpes infection. He had been stripped naked so as his afflictions could be seen at all times. His genitals were a mass of weeping sores, and these had spread around his body from what I can remember. Because he was unable to wash and stay clean these sores had spread around his mouth too, it was hideous. Due to the conditions men like these would not survive for very long and this man died after a few weeks. After death the man's genitals were vivisected, it looked like they were pulling strands of spaghetti out from the testicles. Everything was examined as the doctors wished to discover if the disease had any influence on fertility.'

It is worthy of note that the insanitary conditions Japanese soldiers operated under were exacerbated further by poor personal hygiene among the Japanese military. Many Allied veterans of the war in the Far East recalled how one could actually smell how close the Japanese were in the jungle. Private Paul Hopper recalled:

> 'They had this peculiar dirty smell about them. How can I describe it? It was like dirty socks and onions mixed together. We knew they didn't wash that much as neither did we, but we washed ourselves at any opportunity we could yet the Japs it seems didn't bother. So, you knew they were nearby just by that certain odour they all seemed to possess.'

The Japanese soldiers' basic lack of hygiene put them at far greater risk of disease than their western counterparts. The fact that Japanese soldiers also raped any women they happened to chance upon also contributed to the spread of sexual diseases through the ranks of the Imperial Japanese Army. A British Army doctor recalled that almost every Japanese soldier captured alive by his unit had some form of sexual disease and that it was shockingly prevalent within their ranks. Rather than issuing orders to prevent the rapes and the subsequent spread of unpleasant sexual diseases, the Japanese high command appeared content to ignore this problem, as the threat of women being raped was considered a useful psychological weapon against those considering resistance, and a fitting punishment for the females of enemy nations, particularly those of the west. According to one Second World War British Army source, within the Japanese army medical field kit treatments for sexual diseases were more commonly found than those for the treatment of snake bites.

The Japanese fascination with the reproductive aspects of human biology mirrored that of their Axis partner Nazi Germany, albeit on a much cruder and more violent scale. Many pregnant women were retained at the Nanking facility and most of those subjected to often fatal human experimentation were young Chinese females. As familiarity developed through regular correspondence with Ishiwaru, he began to open up more and more about what he had seen in Nanking. Some of the most horrific were carried out on pregnant women brought into the facility. Ishiwaru recalled:

> 'The Japanese at the time hated the Chinese who were viewed as little more than dogs. It was like the Nazi's hatred towards Jews in Germany. Yes, it was particularly virulent and only today we look back in considerable shame at what we did to a people who by all intents bore little cultural difference to our own. Pregnant Chinese women were brought into the facility, many of them were frightened and concerned for the unborn children they were

carrying. The fear and anxiety clear to see on their faces as they were brought in and placed in cells. Those women in the early stages of pregnancy were nurtured as if the seed of flowers. They were fed well and kept under constant medical observation as their pregnancy evolved. I am sorry to reveal that horrible things were done to some of these women, things I could never condone even as a Japanese soldier, we were not all beasts and I have to reiterate I by no means agreed with the things that happened at Unit 731. As difficult as it is to talk about, I witnessed how one pregnant Chinese woman who had reached the terminal phase of pregnancy was brought into the surgeon's room. This was little more than a concrete room with an operating table in its centre. The woman was calm until they (the doctors present) made her remove her clothing then lie down on the surgeon's table. As they began to restrain her by the use of straps with buckles on to her head, wrists and ankles she attempted to struggle and began shouting and screaming "what are you going to do with me, please don't hurt me, have mercy, have mercy". It was difficult to see what was happening as one of the doctors had his back to us preventing us from seeing what the other one was doing, there were also bars obstructing my view inside the room. The woman continued to scream out for a few minutes when she went quiet, yet the doctors were still standing over her and you could see their arms moving as if they were cutting something. The one passed something to the other and this object was placed in a large metal bowl that looked like a wok used for cooking. The cell door opened and as the doctor walked past us, we all saw that in the bowl he was carrying away was the body of the woman's unborn infant. I recall the body being covered in blood and showing no signs of life. I know some of these infant bodies and smaller foetuses were placed into preservative fluid in glass containers ready for medical study. I do know that before the end of the war the doctor who carried out the surgery on this woman was killed by Chinese partisans as he attempted to flee. Other than that, I do not know what became of the other doctor as I did not know anything about him. Many doctors and surgeons young and old came and went during the existence of the unit and many young medical students were brought to the facility to observe the work going on there and some were actively encouraged to participate in some of the activities.'

At the Nanking facility many of the female prisoners were subjected to sickening abuses including repeated rape at the hands of their Japanese guards. The Japanese guards singled out the youngest Chinese females. The women were often taken from the cells where they were kept and subjected to all manner of humiliation at the hands of the off-duty soldiers who had an unlimited supply of sakei (rice wine). There appeared to be little discipline among the soldiers on days where they were excused military duty and those soldiers who were on duty and responsible for guarding the female prisoners often took part in the selection of suitable young girls. One witness who wished to remain anonymous recalled Japanese sexual brutality at the Nanking facility:

'As an ordinary low-ranking soldier, I followed every order to the book, as we were taught in our training. Any hesitation would mean severe punishment a beating or even death depending upon the circumstances. Many of us had time away from our military duties as did other soldiers including our enemies. I recall a Sunday evening in the spring of 1942 there was a big celebration and food and Sakei was brought in for us all. After consuming the food and drinking the Sakei of which there was lots some of the soldiers wanted women. The military had brothels of course which the soldiers were permitted to use but here there were some very beautiful female prisoners. Most of these girls were Chinese and as we viewed them as little more than dogs, we were permitted to take a small number of these women out of the cells for our amusement. There were some females who had been subjected to infection. They had been deliberately injected with diseases and they were kept separate from the others. We could not for obvious reasons use these infected women but there were many others to choose from. It was a simple case of going into the cell blocks picking who we wanted, and the guards would order that woman to come out. They would then be taken to the soldier's barracks rooms. I recall there was one young soldier he had not been with us very long and he took too much time choosing a woman as I think from his reactions he had never been with any woman before. The corporal in charge shouted for him to "hurry, hurry pick one now you fool, why are you waiting?" This young soldier reminded me of someone at a restaurant unsure of what meal to order. After a couple of minutes, the soldier received a hard slap across the face from the corporal who grabbed a random woman by her arm and dragged her out of the cell and shouted at him "here, this is your woman take her boy". The women were herded across to the soldiers' barracks and I admit to being shocked by what I witnessed. I did not want a woman as I was married with a young wife, but I saw what happened with the Chinese women. They were treated like meat they were slapped and stripped and raped. The soldiers would rape one woman then swap the woman he had picked for another his friend had just raped. The Sakei did not seem to stem their virility and the raping went on until well into the early hours. When the women's ordeal was finally over many of them had blackened eyes from beatings and had cuts and bruises about their bodies. I even saw teeth marks on the breasts of more than one of the women as we escorted them back to the cell blocks. Many of them were sobbing and limping as we walked them back. I felt a sense of sadness for these women, yet I could not express this for fear of being punished myself. There was nothing I could have done for them for these women the situation was hopeless and few of them would survive for very long. I know that one of the young women taken that night had died. The reasons could not be ascertained as to why so her body was taken for dissection by one of the student doctors. The doctor opened the lower abdomen and the area around the sexual organs where he found much damage and his conclusion was the woman had expired due to internal bleeding. Reports such as these were all documented meticulously for various research purposes. I heard many years after the war that some of this material was read by doctors of the western nations when examining criminal accounts of rape and the varying degrees of internal or external damage which can occur from non-consensual sexual activity. What many do not understand is that there were very brutish Japanese soldiers who raped women in what to me were peculiar ways. They would insert their penis into the anus for example. This is something which happened frequently, but I never understood why as to me such an activity was something I thought of as dirty, something that only homosexuals did. They raped women orally too and some of these women received injuries to their throats due to the use of excessive thrusting. These women dared not complain of these injuries for fear of being subjected to vivisections. They often had to endure the pain of what would be permanent injuries for them. I was questioned after the war many times by British and American personnel who wanted information on the activities of Japanese physicians at the facility. What they then did with this information and documents recovered I don't know. I do know that the information was given covertly as the governments collecting this data did not wish for word of it to get out for mostly political reasons at the time. This was back in the 1950s and 1960s you see. The medical research carried out on human beings by both our military and that of Germany our ally was seen as highly valuable material even if it had to be kept away from public knowledge for as many years as possible, it was considered highly secret and quality information could lead to better treatment for us at the

> hands of the Allies after the war, so information was traded quite freely by those involved who had been captured. I knew of some of the doctors who preferred to take their own lives rather than be subject to interrogation by the enemy. They took their lives in the traditional manner of Hara Kiri, ritual disembowelment by the use of a sword.'

The treatment of women prisoners at the hands of the Japanese was confirmed by many British and American medical staff attached to the Allied armed forces in the Far East theatre of operations. Many of the victims had suffered permanent disfigurement at facilities and the various jungle camps spread throughout the captured territories. For example, one American nurse named Hannah Colwyn, who had been attached to US forces in the Philippines, recalled after the liberation encountering many young Filipino women with genital mutilation, disfigured limbs and deep scarring about their bodies, all as result of what the Japanese termed 'medical experiments'. Hannah described a typical case she was witness to:

> 'Even today it is something which fills me with revulsion. That human beings could do such terrible things to fellow human beings. I was brought up in Wisconsin, USA in a very family orientated god-fearing environment. I knew I would witness horrific things in the course of my duties as a junior within a mobile medical surgical unit. I had braced myself for the gunshot, bayonet, blast and fire injuries which were the normal afflictions of the battlefield, I didn't kid myself it would all be a bed of roses, I knew the score and what I had signed up for. Yet, I was sickened by the cases of the young Filipino girls who had been raped and sodomized, had their leg muscles and sections of their bones cut away in so called medical procedures. Such procedures had damaged these poor girls for life, some I knew from their injuries would never be able to have children. Yes, they had been opened

up like laboratory rats and had crude hysterectomies performed on them many of which required corrective surgery later. I recall the one girl had bamboo splinters in her vagina and these had become infected. What evil son of a bitch could do such a thing was one of the things which went through my mind at that time. It was incredibly difficult for me to control my emotions, I felt extreme anger and sadness. It's difficult to contain these emotions when you see these things. We had heard so many stories of Japanese brutality but to see it for myself was another thing. The girl explained that a Japanese soldier had assaulted her with a piece of bamboo, he inserted it into her vagina with such force that fragments broke off inside of her, he was drunk and thought it was an amusing thing to do. Other Japanese soldiers laughed and took photographs. She had witnessed other young women who had tried to resist being beheaded with swords and their bodies then cut up into pieces. One girl I saw had also been injected with an unknown fluid directly into her left eye with a needle. She told me how a Japanese in a white doctor's coat injected her. She had been tied down before the procedure and a clamp was placed over her eye to prevent her from closing her eyelid. There was no anaesthetic, and she explained there was a severe burning sensation as the needle was inserted into her eye, the pain became so intense that they had to shove cloth into her mouth to stifle her screams. She could no longer see out of that eye, and she explained her vision in that eye was like a milky white. We could not ascertain as to what had been injected into the girl's eye, but we suspected it may have been some form of caustic chemical such as sodium hypochlorite as there was evidence of retinal burning of the kind caused by a bleach-like chemical. It was sickening and afterwards when I had time to myself, I sat quietly trying to think why these horrific things had been done to these unfortunate young souls. They had undergone painful and humiliating abuses and it was evident many were suffering from what we would term today as being severe Post Traumatic Stress Disorder. Many of the girls could not stop shaking, they jumped at every sudden movement and were alarmed by many ordinary everyday sounds. Many were withdrawn and tearful and some later took their own lives by jumping off cliffs onto rocks, they couldn't live with what had been done to them. I am 90 years of age now, the Second World War ended so long ago yet even today I remember and cry for those poor girls. Their chances of leading normal lives, marrying and having children after what had happened to them was very slim. I also heard stories mostly from the women I treated of men being forced into having sex with one another by the Japanese. The males in question were of all nationalities and the Japanese guards would select two male prisoners and tell them if they did not do what they were told then they would be cut open while still alive. So, the two men despite their extreme fear and loathing of what they were being ordered to do would have to perform oral sex and penetrate one another as the Japanese guards watched, laughed and shouted obscenities at them. The men were also forced to insert sticks in one another's anus and the guards would be in hysterics of laughter. Such stories disgusted me as this was not the behaviour of civilized human beings. The problem was I was not one to keep quiet. I reported these things up the chain of command to my superiors as they should be just for the record, and I was basically told to "shut up and do your job and say nothing". I found this even more offensive that someone was ordering me to "shut up and say nothing". I kept my peace so long as I was in the service but once I left, I told everyone I talked to about it. The problem was after the war nobody wanted to know about these things, it was a case of "well, the war is over now let's just get on with life". Today, all these decades on there are good people such as yourself who want to hear and record these stories no matter how horrific they may be. These stories should be heard not to persecute the young Japanese of today but remind them of what their grandfathers did and what Emperor Hirohito represented as it is nothing to be proud of at all.'

Whether or not all of the independent medical experimentation carried out on human beings by the Japanese was reported to the central Unit 731 authorities is not entirely clear. Today it is extremely difficult to gain access to original translated Japanese files on the activities of Unit 731 and its ancillary operators. This in some ways is perfectly understandable as Japanese society of today is reluctant to revisit a past it would rather forget.

At the war's end in 1945 any Japanese citizens either military or civilian who were found to have had any connections with the operations of Unit 731 and had been captured by the Russians were sent for trial at the Khabarovsk War Crimes Trials, which took place in the far easterly Russian industrial city of Khabarovsk from 25–31 December 1949. Of the twelve defendants tried by the Russians, all pleaded guilty to their crimes, receiving prison terms ranging from two to twenty-five years, to be served in the Siberian labour camps. Being sent to hard labour in Siberia was a death sentence in itself as few Japanese could tolerate the deadly Siberian climate or the harsh labour they would have to endure throughout their incarceration. In 1956 those still alive were repatriated back to Japan. There was some speculation that even with the Soviets deals were made, and Japanese prisoners could earn early release, or a more lenient sentence, provided they were prepared to give the Soviets information on their work carried out while with Unit 731.

The American treatment of the former Japanese war criminals of Unit 731 was a total contradiction in view of their horrific crimes. Secretly the Americans employed Japanese Unit 731 staff, as their research was viewed as valuable in the creation of the US's own biological weapons programmes. As the early post-Second World War peace was interrupted by the onset of the soon-to-be Cold War between Soviet Russia and the Western powers, the Western military powers understood the value of Japanese research into the application of biological (and chemical) weaponry as a means of waging war. More importantly, the militaries of the West were keen to understand whether the Japanese had indeed developed drugs or treatments as a means of countering the effects of these abhorrent and inhumane weapons of war. If so, none of the research could have been conducted without the use of human guinea pigs. This understandably did not sit well with either the Russian or Chinese governments following the end of the Second World War and the whole affair is still an affront to all those who perished at the hands of the Japanese in some of the most agonising and degrading ways imaginable. Russia and China have both since invested in their own independent research programmes into the application of both biological and chemical weaponry.

As relations between Russia and the West continued to sour, both sides allocated huge amounts of resources in the field of biological and chemical weaponry, despite the questions of the moral ethics associated with such weapons.

Retired US Army Major B.W Horrowitz, who had been involved in the gathering of intelligence on Japanese biological and chemical weapons, recalled:

> 'There was a reluctance by all of the nations who had been involved in the war against Japan to execute Japanese civilian or military personnel who had admitted involvement in both the human medical experiments and those conducted into biological and chemical weaponry. There was a tremendous amount of value in these areas of research. As abhorrent and disgusting as the medical experiments were there were the big American, British and German pharmaceutical giants who stood to profit from what the Japanese had discovered of a medical and/or disease control context. The research, it was said, was valuable in order to counter the threats of diseases in the world population of the future, in that sense what occurred is forgivable, that is how I understood it all. As for biological and chemical weapons they were seen as the

next option down from using atomic weapons. Both biological and chemical weapons have that fear factor, nobody wants to be on the receiving end of them, do they? The problem with acquiring all of the research material and any of the actual stockpiles of the weapons themselves after the Japanese surrender was that you can't keep all of these things to yourself for long no matter how good your security is. Exclusivity where these weapons were concerned was short lived. Nations such as Russia once they had perfected biological and chemical weapons, they then exported them to sympathetic allies and once the Cold War began and the Warsaw Pact was formed all of those individual countries were allocated both biological and chemical weapons often in return for other materials or money. It would seem any nation that hated the western powers were supplied with the same kinds of biological and chemical weapons the Japanese had used against the Chinese people. Even China itself understood the value of these weapons purely from a victim perspective and developed their own through information gained from their former enemy. It just illustrates how dumb us humans are, we are not happy unless we can find a better way to kill or maim one another. Nothing will ever change in that respect, and it can only ever get worse in my opinion.'

In a formerly secret military report dated November 1956 and entitled 'Summary of New Information About Japanese Biological Activities' the following was recorded:

(a) It was found that an organisation completely separate from Pingfan had carried on a considerable amount of research in the veterinary biological warfare field. At the present time ten members of this group are engaged in preparing a report that will be available sometime next August.

(b) General Ishii, the dominant figure in the biological warfare program is writing a treatise on the whole subject. This work will include his ideas about the strategical and tactical use of biological weapons, how these weapons should be used in various geographical areas, (particularly in cold climates), and a full description of his theory of biological warfare. This treatise will represent a broad outline of General Ishii's twenty years of experience in the biological warfare field and will be available in due course.

(c) It was disclosed that were available approximately 8,000 slides representing pathological sections derived from more than 200 human cases of disease caused by various biological weapons agents. These had been concealed in temples and buried in the mountains of southern Japan. The pathologist who performed or directed all of this work is engaged at the present time in recovering this material and the photomicrography of all of the slides. He will be preparing a comprehensive report in English, with descriptions of the slides, laboratory protocols, and case histories. This report will be available in due course.

(d) A collection of printed articles totalling about 600 pages covering the entire field of natural and artificial plague has been received; there is also on hand a printed bulletin of approximately 100 pages dealing with some phase of biological weapon or chemical warfare. These documents are both in Japanese and have not been translated.

(e) The human subjects used at the laboratory and field experiments were said to have been Manchurian coolies who had been condemned to death for various crimes. It was stated positively that no American or Russian prisoners of war had been used at any time (except that the blood of some American POW's had been checked for antibody content), and there is no evidence to indicate that this statement is untrue. The human subjects were used in exactly the same manner as other experimental animals, i.e., the minimum infectious and lethal dosage of various organisms was determined on them, they were immunised with various vaccines and then challenged with living organisms, and they were used as subjects during field trials of bacteria disseminated by bombs and sprays. These subjects also were used almost exclusively in the extensive work that was carried out with plague. The results obtained with human beings were somewhat (last word in report was not legible).

Afterword

This book, while not an exhaustive study, I hope will provide some useful knowledge of the various human medical experiments performed on human beings by the Axis partners of Nazi Germany and Imperial Japan during the Second World War. Of course, the Japanese military were active in this area of research well in advance of their entry into the Second World War as an ally with Nazi Germany, and as such had perfected methods of delivering biological weapons to enemy soil, which is evident from their rampages through China from the start of the Second Sino-Japanese War (7 July 1937–2 September 1945). Japan's ally Nazi Germany, and indeed even the Western combatants, were somewhat slow in recognising the offensive values of biological weapons, if only from a terror weapon perspective. Hitler, at least initially, expressed little serious interest in this area of weaponry, although he was more aware than most of the effectiveness of chemical munitions on the battlefield, having fallen victim to a British mustard gas shell attack in the Ypres Salient on 14 October 1918 during the First World War. The Nazis' use of Zyklon B, the highly poisonous insecticide used in the gas chambers of the murder factories such as Auschwitz in Poland, was never experimental in quite the same way as those weapons containing the plague bacteria as deployed by the Japanese. As the Second World War progressed Nazi Germany had produced stockpiles of the nerve agents tabun, sarin and soman, yet oddly had never opted to deploy these on the battlefield, despite the means of deployment via aircraft, artillery shells and the *Nebelwerfer* mortars being available. Nazi German medical experimentation was mostly directed towards racial genetics and physiology.

The accounts given by those who suffered as a result of falling victim to either Nazi German or Imperial Japanese medical experimentation make for very difficult reading. These people were human beings much like you and I and it is extremely difficult to comprehend that any group of human beings could do such terrible things to another in the name of science, geography, race, and/or political or cultural differences. What is perhaps the proverbial rubbing of salt into the wound for many of the survivors is the fact that their tormentors were given anonymity from justice for their crimes. They would never face a war crimes tribunal or feel the hangman's rope around their necks, purely due to the fact that they possessed knowledge considered of value to the victorious Allies, who were already falling out of bed with one another before the ink had even dried on the German and Japanese surrender documents. The human race, as it stands today, appears to have learned little from the violence and destruction of the relatively recent past. War persists in blighting the human race and there are of course powerful faceless entities within the shadowy realms of the world elite who stand to prosper from the cultivation, exploitation and destruction of human life wrought from these wars, just as the politicians, governments and drug manufacturing giants prospered by way of knowledge from the human medical experimentation conducted by Nazi Germany and Japan in the wake of the Second World War. Where there are billions of pounds or dollars to be made, or critical information to be acquired, human suffering is deemed an acceptable trade-off, thus the human conscience can soon be found discarded in the gutter alongside the false moralities being perpetrated via social media outlets, the news and the world press today.

Of all my work over the course of a great many years of research into the social and military histories of conflict I have found the interviews compiled for this particular volume arguably the most troubling. The fact that many victims are still suffering from the terrible things done to them by fellow human beings, the post-traumatic stress disorder, the nightmares which still disturb their sleep to this day, the inability to live their lives as fully as many of the unpunished perpetrators were able to... it all seems very wrong. When you sit and talk with these people their pain and suffering is visible and reaches out to you through their eyes and their emotions, and it stays with you and reminds you of the importance of both recording their stories and presenting them to the wider world. These stories and accounts should never be locked away in some personal archive where there is a danger that they may be overlooked. This is already happening in some parts of the world where 'real history' is considered 'just too distressing'.

I would like to thank all those who have assisted with the creation of this book, which has been one of the more demanding projects I have embarked upon. I hope that in some small way it serves as a lasting tribute to those brave souls who have come forward to tell their stories: they are now the history and without them there would be no history books from which we future generations can learn.

Acknowledgements

I would like to offer heartfelt thanks to all those who either agreed to be interviewed for the formulation of this work or contributed otherwise privately owned material. Special thanks to Anna Dann and her family for acting as liaison for the German side of this project and for valued assistance with translation of various archival documents and letters, and Haruto Sasaki for acting as liaison for the Japanese contributions and translation of archival documents and the Japanese Embassy, Piccadilly, London.

Bibliography

The following articles and published works were consulted for the production of this book:

Nazi Medicine and Research on Human Beings, Professor Volker Roelcke, 2004.
Conference on Jewish Material Claims Against Germany – personal statements from victims of Nazi medical experiments, online resource.
Select documents on Japanese Biological Warfare 1934–2006, compiled by William H. Cunliffe.
The Knights of Bushido – A Short History of Japanese War Crimes, Lord Russel of Liverpool.
Banzai You Bastards – Jack Edwards.
Howstuffworks.com (online resource)
Pacificatrocities.org (online resource)

Archival resources consulted

The National Archives, Kew, Richmond, Surrey.
The Imperial War Museum Department of Documents, London.
The Yad Vashem Archives, Jerusalem, Israel.
Arolsen Archives – International Centre on Nazi Persecution, Bad Arolsen, Germany.
The German Federal Archives, Koblenz, Berlin, Germany.
The National WW2 Museum, New Orleans, USA.